Medical Theory and Therapeutic Practice in the Eighteenth Century

Edited by Jürgen Helm / Renate Wilson

Medical Theory and Therapeutic Practice in the Eighteenth Century

A Transatlantic Perspective

Edited by Jürgen Helm / Renate Wilson

Franz Steiner Verlag Stuttgart 2008

Die Drucklegung des Buches erfolgte mit Mitteln aus dem TransCoop-Programm der Alexander von Humboldt-Stiftung.

Bibliografische Information der Deutschen Nationalbibliothek
Die Deutsche Nationalbibliothek verzeichnet diese Publikation in der Deutschen Nationalbibliografie; detaillierte bibliografische Daten sind im Internet über <http://dnb.d-nb.de> abrufbar.

ISBN 978-3-515-08889-3

Gedruckt auf säurefreiem, alterungsbeständigem Papier
Druck: Laupp & Göbel GmbH, Nehren
Printed in Germany

CONTENTS

INTRODUCTION AND ACKNOWLEDGEMENTS

Jürgen Helm and Renate Wilson

Medical thinking went through far-reaching conceptual changes during the eighteenth century, which led to departures from theoretical assumptions of long standing and to a range of often contradictory developments. The waning tradition of medieval and early modern Galenism, its humoral pathology and their attributes and qualities of matter competed with new insights provided by anatomical investigations. Analogous developments in iatrochemistry and iatromechanical theory and the nascent discipline of physiology battled the remnants of the Aristotelian intellectual edifice and its postulate of the organic integrity of body and soul. The collection of essays presented in this volume proceeds on the assumption that on the ground – and at the bedside – there may have been less discord in eighteenth-century medical practice in Europe. The iatromechanical followers of Friedrich Hoffmann held therapeutic views that differed relatively little from those of their colleagues subscribing to the psychodynamic school of Georg Ernst Stahl.

In most settings theoretical considerations were only one of the factors determining medical treatments and procedures. Specific therapeutic choices were guided by transmitted, local and individual stores of practical knowledge, by the expectations of patients, and by economic considerations. Also of interest are implicit or explicit preferences for particular therapies in defined social and religious settings and networks.

The opportunity to examine the apparent disjunction between theory and therapy in several geographic and linguistic medical contexts was provided by a cooperative grant of the German Alexander von Humboldt Foundation, which complemented a research grant of the US National Library of Medicine. This conjunction of support from both sides of the Atlantic enabled the editors of this volume to convene a conference examining aspects of medical theory and practice in eighteenth century Europe and North America. Our transnational approach, although limited to the German and Anglo-American sphere, is reflected in the background of the authors. Taking into account today's multilingual audiences, the publisher and the editors agreed to present over half of the contributions in English. To facilitate access, summaries are provided in both English and German at the end of this volume.

The resulting collection of essays is divided into four sections. The first attempts to provide insight into the complex relationship between medical theory and medical practice. Jole Shackelford traces Paracelsian uroscopy in George de Benneville's Medicina Pensylvania; Marion Maria Ruisinger examines the conflict between the venerable tradition of bloodletting and the pressure of new anatomical knowledge; Andreas-Holger Maehle illustrates the nascent experimental pharmacology of the eighteenth century; and Karin Stukenbrock examines the possible influences of modified medical theories on dietetic practice.

The second section focuses on the physician-patient relationship and therapeutic uncertainty. While Michael Stolberg demonstrates the patient perspective by examining their choices of physicians, Jürgen Helm examines the medical reasoning medical practitioners used to buttress the effectiveness of preferred therapies.

A third section deals with different forms and problems of the *Materia medica* in the eighteenth century. Robert Jütte lays out the context of the still widespread practice of using human tissue and fluids in eighteenth century therapy; Almut Lanz and John K. Crellin, respectively, present the pharmaceutical therapies of Friedrich Hoffmann in Germany and of a Silesian emigrant, Abraham Wagner, in colonial North America; Renate Wilson examines the tradition of German medical *Fachprosa* and its use in the transmission of therapeutic knowledge to the growing and multilingual North American medical markets.

In a final section, medical theory and practice are contextualized within eighteenth century religious and social settings on both sides of the Atlantic. Fritz Krafft shows the origin and the development of the image of "Christ as Apothecary" and of "postmortal remedies" in Lutheran theology. Allen Viehmeyer lays out the religious background of two spiritualist sectarians, Abraham Wagner and George de Benneville; and Elisabeth Quast investigates a Pietist network of noblewomen in Berlin and their role in the distribution of the so-called Orphanage pharmaceuticals.

In analyzing a complex field of medical practice, some of the papers concentrate on two colonial dispensatories and receptures that illuminate the therapeutic practices and medical orientation of two dispensing physicians in British North America. Others fit more closely into familiar topics in the European history of medicine. In her concluding remarks, Mary Lindemann uses the category of "context" to build a bridge between these settings and examine current historiographical trends in the history of medicine and therapeutics.

Finally, a few words on some of the conventions established in producing this bilingual volume may be in order: In order to accommodate not only two different languages but their different lexigraphic and print conventions, we have adopted German rules of punctuation and spelling for the German-language contributions but follow US practice for the English-language texts. For ease of access, the bibliographic references at the end of each contribution follow a uniform German research format. We ask readers for their indulgence where these conventions are not always fully observed. Finally, we note that in order to ensure appropriate access to original texts, the footnotes for the English-language contributions provide the original German wording for citations translated in the text and for supporting citations from German-language authors. The editors thank the contributors to this volume for the additional labor involved in these often complex and lengthy bilingual notes.

As noted, the contributions to this volume are based on the papers read at a two-day conference held in the Franckesche Stiftungen at Halle/Saale (Germany) in October 2005. We thank the Francke Foundations for their generous hospitality and the College of Physicians of Philadelphia and in particular Ed Morman for hosting an earlier working conference on the Wagner and de Benneville manuscripts in 2004. Both meetings were part of a cooperative research project supported by the Alexander von Humboldt Foundation (III-TCFO-DEU/1113677; Principal Investigators: Jürgen Helm, Renate Wilson), matching some of the funds provided by the National Library of Medicine of the Institutes of Health (1 G 13 LM07664-01; Principal Investigator: Renate Wilson). We also thank the Schwenkfelder Library for access to unpublished correspondence of Abraham Wagner and George de Benneville.

Our appreciation for their careful work goes to Bill Templer and Antje Matthäus, who translated the articles by Michael Stolberg and Marion Maria Ruisinger and by Almut Lanz, respectively. In particular, the editors are indebted to Elisabeth Quast for her substantive and technical contributions. She not only processed and formatted both the English and the German text and collated the index, but forced the wide range of bibliographic citations into one consistent and, we hope, accessible format.

Halle and Baltimore, Summer 2008

Part I:
Theory and Therapy

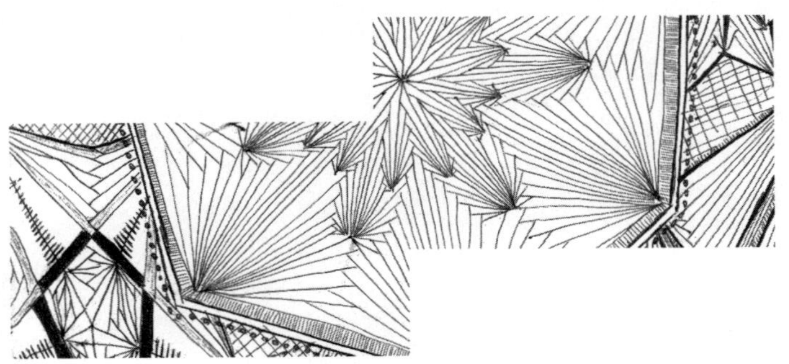

PARACELSIAN UROSCOPY AND GERMAN CHEMIATRIC MEDICINE IN THE MEDICINA PENSYLVANIA OF GEORGE DE BENNEVILLE

Jole Shackelford

Recent study of a German-English, dual-language medical manuscript compiled in colonial North America by the immigrant physician and religious leader George de Benneville (1703–1793) has revealed a wide-ranging and sometimes perplexing pharmaceutical therapeutics for the German community in Eastern Pennsylvania in the middle of the eighteenth century.[1] The manuscript is bilingual English and German with Latin technical terms and bears the title "Medicina Pensylvania or the Pensylvania Physician" in English and "Medicina Pensylvania Oder der Pennsylvanische Land Artz" in German and may date to the 1770s. It is introduced by a German language *Ad lectorem benevolum* and a 3-language *materia medica* and comprises a large, facing page German-English formulary and therapeutic manual occupying roughly 150 folia (physical pages), depending on how this is reckoned.[2]

The kinds of drugs listed and recommended throughout the entire *Medicina Pensylvania* indicate that de Benneville's medicine was an eclectic blend of Galenic herbal and chemiatric therapy, standard for the eighteenth century, with occasional intrusions of folk medicine.[3] Indeed, the bulk of this compilation comprises lists of *materia medica* and drugs, instructions for their manufacture,

1 For the digitized version of the bilingual de Benneville manuscript, see "Eighteenth-century Colonial Formularies: The Manuscripts of George de Benneville and Abraham Wagner," College of Physicians of Philadelphia Digital Library. Website address: http://www.accesspadr.org/cpp/.

2 The manuscript also includes various later additions, which are not proper to the originally-compiled *Medicina Pensylvania* and are not addressed in this paper. The manuscript resides at the Library of the College of Physicians of Philadelphia. Page references to this manuscript are complicated by its history. As a physical document, it is about 170 pages, beginning with a cover sheet with inscription and including all sections. The pages are paginated beginning with page 1. Thereafter, the manuscript is paginated such that facing English and German pages have the same number. With this in mind, references to this text will be made using the native pagination to enable the user of the physical document to find pages easily, but supplemented with a bracketed physical side number that was used to index the page images of the digitized manuscript (see note 1 above), which can be readily consulted online. Thus, [002] is the English title page, the *Ad lectorem benevolum* begins on [005], and the paginated portion begins on fol.1 [040] and runs to fol.149 [337] (the facing page system breaks down in the final pages to fol.150), with a few intervening blank pages that were not imaged. In general, on the website the German pages have odd and the English pages have even image numbers. All English-language quotes are from the digitized English version.

3 I use the term chemiatric here to refer to drugs that were prepared by chemical procedures and incorporated into sixteenth and seventeenth-century chemical pharmacy, regardless of how they might have been used therapeutically. The importance of this distinction is considered in SCHNEIDER (1972).

and descriptions of diseases and practical treatments without an underlying theoretical development or identifiable theoretical basis. However, several sections, totaling roughly 46 pages, reveal a practical chemiatric approach to diagnosis and healing that is unambiguously grounded in the medicine of the eccentric and radical German physician Theophrastus Paracelsus (1493–1541). These are a first section under the heading "astralis and astrabolismus diseases" (fol. 66–69 [170–177]), a second under "tartarous diseases" (fol. 69–76 [176–191]), and finally a very jumbled, in some places incoherently translated uroscopic manual (fol. 137–149 [312–337]). Moreover, textual connections between these portions and the German *Ad lectorem benevolum* that serves as an introduction, all of which are demonstrated below to derive from a seventeenth-century edition of a book by a German physician named Johann Hayne (fl. 1570s), suggest that this Paracelsian medicine was an integral part of the compiler's medical conception.

At first sight, these portions seem oddly out of place in an eighteenth-century medical manual, since they reflect astrological medicine and a reliance on uroscopy that are more in keeping with medieval and early modern methods than with the new medical approaches of the Enlightenment period. However, the table of contents for this compilation clearly shows that these sections were to be integral parts of a completed but never printed book, implying a coherent underlying vision of medicine. Although the extant form of the compilation is somewhat at variance with the proposed contents, the table of contents nevertheless reveals what must have been the intended structure of the final product.[4]

I am not speaking here merely of chemical recipes that harken back to Paracelsian chemical medicine but were later adapted to Galenic theory, or even to the ownership of Paracelsian books.[5] I mean rather what appears to be a Paracelsian clinical medicine, a therapeutic theory and pharmaceutical practice that were intimately tied to the Paracelsian conception of human physiology and

4 The title page with table of contents (in facing page English and German) divides the treatise into four parts: I. The theory and practice of chemical pharmacy; II. Medical simples, their characteristics, and dosages; III. Directions and descriptions for preparing various compound drugs, along with a list of diseases they are to be used for, "including in particular astral afflictions and painful humoral diseases" ("Nebst die astralischen zufällen und flüssige schmertzhafftige kranckheiten ins besonder" [003]); and IV. Instructions on diagnosing diseases by inspection of the urine and assessment of the pulse.

5 Such remnants of Paracelsus' medicine were not uncommon and have been identified for seventeenth-century colonial chemists and physicians associated with George Starkey and John Winthrop, Jr. For example, Cotton Mather's library contained books by Paracelsus and other chemiatric authors. See BEALL & SHRYOCK (1954), 62. My thanks to Lisa Boult for bringing this to my attention. GEVITZ & SULLIVAN-FOWLER (1995) point out that seventeenth-century New England medicine exhibited both Galenic and Paracelsian components. However, like many other historians, they identify "Paracelsian" with "uses chemically-prepared drugs," with no attempt to discern whether such drugs were employed within a Paracelsian or Galenic paradigm (see esp. 91, 94). For a discussion of what constitutes Paracelsianism, see PUMFREY (1998), esp. 26–27, and SHACKELFORD (2002a), 35–36. NEWMAN (1994), 39–53, briefly discusses the place of alchemy and chemical medicine in New England.

pathology and not reduced to a neoGalenism or twisted into another seventeenth-century theoretical system. Core components of this medicine are Paracelsus' tartar theory and an organically integrated diagnostics and chemiatric treatment traceable to Paracelsus' lectures and writings. The presence of this Paracelsian material in an American colonial medical manuscript suggests that a living tradition of chemiatric practice that derived from Paracelsian pathology and therapeutic method, as it is presented in Paracelsus' lectures on uroscopy and his treatises on tartar diseases, may have thus far escaped the notice of scholars of seventeenth and eighteenth century European medicine, who have tended to view the Paracelsian tradition in terms of medical and religious theory rather than a sustained practice. I aim here to establish that these sections reveal in de Benneville's medicine vestiges of such a Paracelsian therapeutics.

Tartar Diseases: Paracelsian Pathology in the *Medicina Pensylvania*

The concept of "tartarous diseases," namely diseases that arise from a buildup in the body of material residues called tartar, immediately suggests Paracelsian pathology, since this concept occupies a central place in Paracelsus' writings.[6] The origin of de Benneville's term "*astrabolismus*," which appears in the *Medicina Pensylvania* in connection with tartar diseases, is obscure, but the term "astralis" itself is clearly the English translation offered for the adjective "*astralisch,*" which appears on the German facing page, and simply means astral. The text reveals the long-held belief that human physiology is affected by astral and planetary influences and that pathological conditions can be linked to them causally, which is the theoretical basis for Renaissance astrological medicine. De Benneville offers specific remedies to combat astral diseases of the head and chest, for astral fevers, delirium, lethargy, mania, palsy and epilepsy, fits and falling sickness, fainting and palpitations of the heart, vomiting and dysentery, and to counter the bite of a venomous animal that has become mad through astral causes.[7] Clearly, he was drawing on an established astro-therapeutics.

The connection between astrological medicine and tartar theory within the Paracelsian medical tradition becomes clear if we consult an early seventeenth-century medical work by Heinrich Nolle (fl. 1606–1619), *Systema medicinae hermeticae generale* (*Hermetic Physick* in English translation). This book is a product of the Paracelsian medical tradition and is roughly contemporary with the ideas and methods described by Johann Hayne (de Benneville's source for this portion of the *Medicina Pensylvania)* and thus serves both as a convenient review of Paracelsian medical theory and as background to understanding de

6 Book 3 of his *Opus Paramirum, "De origine morborum ex tartaro"* (1531), his more mature *Das Buch von den tartarischen Krankheiten* (1537/1538), and one of the books of his *Carinthian trilogy*, composed in 1538.

7 De Benneville (2005), fol. 66–68 [170–175].

Benneville's medicine.[8] A brief survey of Nolle's explanation of astrological causes and tartar diseases will make de Benneville's use of these concepts more intelligible.

Nolle divides the causes of diseases into categories, and the one that pertains to our discussion is what he terms the substantial cause of "extrarious" etiological agents, namely those arising external to the body and entering it to produce disease. He refers to this cause as "either an impure tincture, or a Meteor," in order to draw attention to the macrocosmic-microcosmic correspondence that governs Paracelsian medicine. The "causes" of real atmospheric phenomena (*meteora*) are the same as those that govern the generation of some kinds of diseases in the human body, specifically those that de Benneville called tartarous diseases.[9]

According to Nolle, "meteors" can be either volatile or coagulated. Volatile ones are commonly called exhalations and are either dry, sulphurous and fiery (hot and dry by nature), or else they are moist, of a "mercurial and aqueous nature" (cold and wet).[10] Obviously these are direct descendants of the two kinds of exhalations that Aristotle identified in order to explain the origin of brittle minerals and ductile metals, which subsequently provided the foundation for the sulphur-mercury theory of composition that is common to medieval Arabic and Latin alchemy.[11] Such exhalations are aroused by their own heat or through the influence of the stars and planets, causing atmospheric and subterranean macrocosmic phenomena.[12] They are inhaled, imbibed, and eaten by humans and result in various diseases, "some of them being Mercurial, cold and moist; others sulphureous, hot and dry."[13] Following the principles of Paracelsus' correspondence idea, atmospheric meteors generate diseases in the body's corresponding superior region, namely the head and brain, and the subterranean ones generate diseases of the inferior chest and abdominal regions.

8 Heinrich Nolle, *Systema medicinae hermeticae generale in quo I. medicinae verae fundamentum, II sanitatis conservatio, III morborum cognitio, & curatio methodo explicantur* (Frankfurt, 1613). Owing to the difficulty of obtaining the Latin edition, I have made use of Henry Vaughn's English translation (NOLLE 1655), which is ample for the level of detail and accuracy needed for the present study. Nolle taught in Giessen from 1606 until he was found to be too sympathetic to Weigelian (i.e. Paracelsian) religious heterodoxy and forced to leave. He later received his M.D. in 1618 at Marburg, then a hotbed of Paracelsian and Rosicrucian thought. Therefore, he is as good a measure as any of the state of Paracelsian medicine in late sixteenth and early seventeenth-century Germany, when it was being elaborated as a systematic approach to healing. For an introduction to Nolle and the medical milieu at Marburg, see MORAN (1991), 122–129; and GILLY (1998).

9 NOLLE (1655), 34, 37.

10 NOLLE (1655), 38.

11 On Aristotelian matter theory and its relationship to medieval alchemy, see NEWMAN (2001).

12 NOLLE (1655), 39.

13 NOLLE (1655), 40. These parts of the body "do exactly quadrate and correspond with the airy Region, and the subterraneous Concavities of the earth."

Nolle devotes Chapter Five of his book to coagulated meteors, which he also calls tartars. Tartar in the human body is a mucilage with particular chemical characteristics: acrimonious, corrosive, aluminous, acid, and styptic. This mucilage is a mixture of solid (earthy) and liquid parts and eventually putrefies in the body, "from whence come worms and other innumerable symptoms." However, if a "supervenient spirit of Salt," separates the juice from the earthy part, the tartar coagulates and collects "in those places which are most apt to receive it."[14] Thus, the chemistry of salts in the body is implicated in the genesis of tartar diseases.

Tartar gets its name by analogy to the chemical tartar that forms on the insides of wine barrels. But this is not merely analogy, for the two kinds of tartar are but forms of a general substance that is normally dissolved in the fluid portions of animals and plants. All fruit juices have tartar, but it is most abundant in the juice of the grape. One can readily identify it through evaporation or distillation as the reddish solid that remains on the bottom of a laboratory vessel. What you see on surfaces where wine has sat for a time is the portion of the tartar that coagulated and adheres to the wood of the barrel. Previously this tartar was dissolved in the wine and is responsible for giving both red and white wine its color.[15]

According to Nolle, tartar also is found in human juices. Just as the chemist can separate tartar from wine by distillation, and nature separates it through long storage in the barrel, nature also can separate it from human blood and chyle, which is the milky nutriment matter that is passed from the stomach to the liver for further refinement into blood. When this tartar is separated and coagulated, it obstructs the passages and leads to diseases. All this is congruent with traditional Galenic theory.[16] The Galenists or "dogmatical physicians," as Nolle calls them, attribute the formation of tartarous obstructions to excessive coldness of the stomach and hotness of the liver; a too cold stomach will leave tartarous mucus in the chyle, which will then be further concocted in the blood, owing to the too hot liver, and then stick to the inner parts of the body, forming obstructions and lodging in the joints. The joints are especially liable to this process, since all parts of the body sustain themselves by drawing to them that part of the nutriment that most resembles them, and the "naturally glutinous and mucilaginous" joints readily attract "this Salsuginous and Tartareous matter." When the body is unable to expel this matter, stiffness and the "acute intolerable paines" of gout and arthritis follow.[17]

Thus far Nolle's account is phrased in terms that an orthodox Renaissance or early modern Galenist would find agreeable and conforming to the received university medical tradition. Tartar theory becomes distinctly Paracelsian when diverse kinds of tartar are identified with various kinds of chemical salts. But even

14 NOLLE (1655), 41.
15 NOLLE (1655), 42–43.
16 NOLLE (1655), 44.
17 NOLLE (1655), 45–46.

these can be thought of in terms of the traditional humors, and it is a matter of historical interest that the two explanatory frames seem to blend at key points. This suggests that the actual development of Paracelsian theory may have been far less a radical deviation from traditional medicine than it was made out to be by those of its practitioners who sought to distinguish themselves from ordinary physicians, like Nolle, or those traditional physicians who came later and had their own reasons for drawing a sharp dichotomy between chemical and humoral pathology. In the case at hand, Nolle attributes the nature of the disease and severity of its symptoms to "the nature and condition of the Tartar." He notes that one kind of tartar is identified by the Galenists as a salty phlegm, but there are also other species: a nitrous and bitter salt that causes bitter choler (yellow bile), "a vitriolated acid salt which predominates in acid phlegme and melancholy," aluminous tartars, and so on.[18] Nolle does not therefore reject humors, but rather finds the chemical salts to be the real agents that give them their properties and are thus more useful designations, especially since these can be used to characterize the diseases.[19]

Nolle divides the class of tartars into two groups, innate tartar, which is formed during fetal development, and "adventitious" tartar, which comes into the body from the environment. Adventitious tartar is further subdivided into four types corresponding to the elemental regions that produce them: (1) what comes from the earth (minerals, roots, plants, etc.), (2) what comes from the water (mainly fish), (3) what comes from the air (the flesh of birds and beasts), and (4) what "comes from the Firmament, which the spirit of Wine, in respect of its subtilty, doth most resemble." This last kind acts through the air we breathe, along with vapors arising from the earth and the water, and produces "those acute and pernitious Astral Diseases, the Pleurisie, the Plague, the Prunella, &c."[20]

Here we begin to see the intimate connection in Paracelsian medicine between the subjects of the three parts of the *Medicina Pensylvania* that concern us here, namely astral diseases, tartar diseases, and uroscopy. Astral diseases are really a subset of what Nolle called meteoric diseases, which include those arising from tartar. Uroscopy is not itself discussed by Nolle, but the theoretical basis for it in tartar theory is implicit. We see this clearly in his account of the body's digestions as separations of pure nutriment from impure wastes to be excreted. The dichotomy between ruby-colored nutriment and clear or whitish

18 NOLLE (1655), 47.

19 NOLLE (1655), 49: "These Salts (believe me) doe better expresse and discover unto us the essences and distinctions of Tartareous or saltish diseases, then those four humours which are commonly termed the Sanguine, the Phlegmatic, the Bilious, and the Melancholy, both because that these latter termes, signifie nothing unto us of the essence or matter of the Disease, and also because that those Dogmatists themselves, Hallucinate and stagger very much both in the formation or aptnesse, and in the application of their said termes."

20 NOLLE (1655), 52. See also 67: "The Stars also doe frequently powre down into the Aire, and upon the Earth, certain Astral Emunctions, and Arsenical vapours, with other noxious Excretions and Exudations. [...]. Hence proceed Distraction, Phrensies, Plurisies, the Plague, and frequent, suddaine Dysenteries."

waste provides the logical basis for chemical uroscopy, but is also grounded in Galenic coction theory. According Nolle, tartarous mucilage, a reddish and sandy tartar, is present in all our food and drink. It is the function of the stomach,

> which is an instrument of the Archaeus of man, or an internall, innate Chymist [...] to separate out the tartar impurity, sending the pure part to nourish and preserve the body. But [...] if the stomack be weake, the impure portion is through the Mesaraic veins conveyd to the Liver, where a second digestion or separation is made. Here the Liver separates againe the pure from the impure, the Rubie from the Chrystall, that is to say, the Red from the White: The Red is the nutriment of all the members the heart, the brain, &c. The white, or that which is no nutriment, is driven by the Liver to the Reyns and it is Urine, which is nothing else but Salt.[21]

This salt is separated from the mercurial part of the blood and forced to dissolve in water by the liver before being passed on to the kidneys. The kidneys again separate it and send it on to the bladder. If the kidneys are malfunctioning, the tartar salts coagulate and form a mucilage, gravel, or stone, which can obstruct the passages. Thus, the connection between astral medicine and tartar theory, and the logical foundations for why Paracelsian digestions and therefore tartar diseases might be reflected in the excreted urine, are evident in Nolle's system.

Nolle's treatise establishes that Paracelsus' tartar theory was already developed to include astral and meteorological causes of disease by the early seventeenth century and points to uroscopy as a possible diagnostic tool. De Benneville's actual source, however, was not Nolle's work, but a now rare text, printed under the title *Drey unterschiedliche neue Tractätlein* and attributed by its editor to a little-known German medical writer named Johann Hayne.[22] My English translation of the title of Hayne's book, which was written and published in Germany during Nolle's lifetime, makes plain the commonality between it and de Benneville's treatise: *Three diverse new treatises. The first on astral diseases [...] the second on tartar diseases [...] the third comprehends the foundation and the true basis for how one can judge man's urine*. Indeed, the three segments of

21 NOLLE (1655), 50–51.

22 Johann Hayne, *Drey underschiedliche newe Tractätlein. Deren Erstes von astralischen Kranckheiten Das Andere, von tartarischen Kranckheiten [...]. Das Dritte, begreifft in sich das Fundament [...] wie man die Urinen des Menschen [...] künstlich iudiciren erkennen möge* (Frankfurt am Main: Paul Jacob and Johan Dreutels, 1620). The book was published in three later editions, 1663, 1683, and 1700, the last two with title *Trifolium medicum, oder: Drey höchst- nützliche Tractätlein deren Erstes von astralischen Kranckheiten [...] Das Andere, von tartarischen Kranckheiten [...] Das Dritte vom rechten Fundament und Grund wie man die Urinen [...] erkennen möge* (Frankfurt a. M.: George Heinrich Oehrling, 1683 and 1700). Renate Wilson found this title at the Wellcome Library and brought it to my attention. Through the generosity of Harold Cook and the Wellcome Library, who provided us with a microfilm of the 1663 Thomae Matthiae edition Frankfurt a. M. (HAYNE 1663), we were able to compare de Benneville's text directly with Hayne's, with the result that it is now clear that de Benneville in the main followed Hayne's organizational scheme and selectively copied practical applications from his book, or possibly from an unknown intermediary text. All citations to Hayne's book in this paper are to this second edition. Translations into English are mine.

the *Medicina Pensylvania* that I identified above, although not contiguous in de Benneville's compilation, were taken quite literally from the three *Tractätlein* that constitute Hayne's book, but selectively, with a much diminished emphasis on theory. The German title of the first segment under consideration here, "Von Astralischen Kranckheiten ins gemein," is taken from the heading of the first of Hayne's *Tractätlein.*[23] However, where Hayne explained the concepts of astral diseases more fully and grounded them in theory, de Benneville seems to have been more interested in applications; he selected remedies from Hayne – sometimes modifying them – and eschewed the theoretical considerations that bound this therapeutics into a general framework of Paracelsian tartar theory.[24]

Similarly, de Benneville's "Part Second, Of Astralis or Astrabolismus Tartarous Diseases" (in the facing German text "Der 2te Theil. Von Tartarischen Kranckheiten") is drawn from Hayne's second treatise, *Das andere Tractätlein von Tartarischen Krankheiten.* De Benneville begins this segment with a little over a page of theory that is extracted from the first ten pages of Hayne's text: Tartar is an impurity found in food and drink that we take from the earth and water, and if it is not properly separated and excreted, it coagulates in the body in various forms, giving rise to a class of diseases called "tartarous diseases." Tartar is coagulated by spirit of salt, and these coagulations may occur in various forms. Tartar that can be coagulated is separated from nutriments in any of three sequential digestive processes: in the stomach, where sulphurous substances are separated from the nutriment; in the liver or the associated mesaraic veins, where saline substances are separated; and in the veins in general, where the mercurial substances are separated. Tartars resulting from deficiencies in these digestions or separations are distributed to the body and may, along with the spirit of salt, be excreted in sweat, stool, or urine.[25] The similarities between Hayne's (and de Benneville's) medicine and Nolle's are plain, and we can assume that much of this tartar theory was common to Paracelsian medicine as it was developed and

23 Compare DE BENNEVILLE (2005), fol. 66 [171]: "Erster Theil. Von Den Astralischen Kranckheiten ins gemein, darinn feuer und lufft [...]" and HAYNE (1663), 1: "Cap. I. Von Astralischen Kranckheiten in gemein, darinn Feuer und Lufft begriffen." Since *Medicina Pensylvania* is a bilingual text, with generally correlated facing-page English and German text, it is possible to compare Hayne's published text with de Benneville's German text (accessible on line, see n. 1 above). That de Benneville appropriated text wholesale from another book without citation is not to be wondered at. Early Modern authors often made liberal use of others' work, and citation practices varied considerably. See more recently HABERMANN (2001). For example, a generation before de Benneville, Cotton Mather freely used information from printed sources, sometimes with citation and othertimes not. See BEALL & SHRYOCK (1954), 63.

24 Tracing recipes is problematic, since in many instances ingredients are added or dropped, quantities and proportions vary, and languages differ. However, for the recipe on fol. 71 [180] ("When the Tartar Causes an Obstruction in the Liver [...]. For this take Carduus, Betony each one hand full, Chicorium leaves [...]"), it is apparent that this is a close variant of the remedy for "Verstopffung der Leber," HAYNE (1663), 75 ("Rx. Herb. Chic. mj Card. benedicti [...]").

25 DE BENNEVILLE (2005), fol. 69–70 [176–179]; HAYNE (1663), 45–54.

flourished in the late sixteenth and seventeenth centuries. However, where Nolle's book stopped short of describing Paracelsian uroscopic theory, Hayne presents this uroscopy as an integrated part of tartar theory and Paracelsian practice.

Hayne's Chemical Uroscopy as Paracelsian Diagnostic Practice

Johann Hayne is an obscure historical figure. We would know little about his existence had not Georg Faber, the editor of 1620 edition of Hayne's *Drey unterschiedliche neue Tractätlein*, translated a Latin text into German and published the treatise that he attributed to Hayne in his introduction. Three later editions, 1663, 1683, and 1700, feature the *Ad lectorem benevolum* by the editor of the 1663 edition, Johann Schröder (1600–1664).[26] Despite the four editions of this work, which argue for Hayne's significance in seventeenth century medicine, he was not much noticed by posterity and is almost wholly unknown today. A Latin version of Hayne's treatises is not in evidence at this point, and it may be that the Latin text mentioned by Faber and Schröder was a manuscript. Although it is possible that Faber came up with the *Drey unterschiedliche neue Tractätlein* elsewhere, or that he composed them himself and attributed them to Johann Hayne, we must proceed on the assumption that the editors' attribution of the treatises to Johann Hayne, physician to the Pomeranian court in Stettin, is sincere and that the texts took shape sometime in the decades just before or after 1600.[27] That Johann Hayne was a real physician at work in Stettin as noted by these editors is corroborated by another Paracelsian physician, Leonhard Thurneisser (1531–1596), who dedicated his 1571 treatise on chemical uroscopy, the *Praeoccupatio*, to his good friend Johann Hayne.[28] Thurneisser's dedication, dated Berlin, August 6, 1571, places Hayne in Stettin as a municipal physician. Thurneisser goes on to say that Hayne is sure to know the patients whom he discusses anonymously in the *Praeoccupatio,* and that although Hayne is already con-

26 Johann Schröder studied medicine in northern Germany and in Copenhagen and served as a surgeon in the Swedish army before gaining European fame as a publisher of a chemical pharmacopeia that was republished several times and translated into other languages. It is on the title page and in Schröder's *Ad lectorem* to the second (1663) edition of Hayne that we learn of Faber's German translation and publication of Hayne's original Latin version. Schröder's *Ad lectorem* is reprinted with the third and fourth editions of *Drey unterschiedliche neue Tractätlein.*

27 Johann Schröder's *Ad lectorem* to HAYNE (1663), sig. b3r–4v: "Diese mit andere ihren Kranckheiten, neben auch einem sonderbahren Iudicio Vrinae, hatt vor etliche Jahren vnternommen zubeschreiben und in Lateinischer Sprache auszgehen zulassen, der Vornehme D. Iohan Hayne &c. welches Tractaetlein also angenehm gewest, dasz es folgents D. Faber in die Teutsche Sprache zuübersetzen, und in Truck zugeben bewogen hatt."

28 THURNEISSER (1571), I (sig. Aiij r.): "Dem Wolgelehrten und Achtbarn Herrn Johann Heynen, der freyen Künsten Magistro, unnd bestelten Physico zu Stettin in Pommern, seinem günstigen lieben und guten freundt."

vinced of the importance of chemical medicine, Thurneisser is writing the book in order to forestall critics who are ignorant or dismissive of it.[29] One gets the sense from this dedication that Hayne and Thurneisser were indeed good friends, perhaps sharing common background at Frankfurt an der Oder, where the physician Jodocus Willichius had practiced uroscopy. Willichius' knowledge of the subject was sufficiently well known that Hieronymus Reusner used his uroscopy manuscript as the basis for a commentary, in which we glimpse the incorporation of Thurneisser's chemical uroscopy into the traditional semiological literature.[30]

Looking ahead to the last segment of the *Medicina Pensylvania*, the uroscopy (fol. 137–149 [312–337]), we can observe here that it is the supposed excretion of tartar and salt in urine that makes uroscopy useful as a diagnostic tool for the Paracelsian physician, since it provides insight into the state of the sulphur, salt, and mercury separations in the body and in principle helps identify the chemical natures of diseases resulting from ineffective separations or digestions. As with astral diseases, de Benneville provides pages of remedies for tartar diseases that are specific to the different parts of the body in which coagulated tartar

29 THURNEISSER (1571), IX (sig. Avij v.): "Aus der ursach und darumb hab ich dieses Büchlein mit dem Griechischen Namen Prokatalepsis oder Praeoccupatio, das ist, ein vorableinung eines dings, so man einem hernach möcht fürwerffen, genennet, allein diese hochtrabende Sophisten mit jrem ludibrio und gespött abzuwiesen. Und ich hab auch derhalben dises Büchlein [...] zum ersten an tag kommen und ausgehn lassen wollen, dieweil darin 12 Proben (die ich zu Franckfurt an der Oder der zeit, wie bey jeder verzeichnet stehet, gemacht hab) beschrieben sind [...] dieweil auch jhr dieselbigen allesampt wol kennet, und den mehrern theil vorhin inn ewer Cur gehabt habendt."

30 Willichius' uroscopy was based on the late medieval elaboration of humoral uroscopy by the Byzantine physician Johannes Actuarius. We see the integration of this medieval uroscopy with Thurneisser's Paracelsian chemical uroscopy especially in the section of Reusner's commentary called "On the Spagyricists' utterly new examination of urine; which is done by means of the separation and resolution of Mercury, Sulphur, and Salt." REUSNER (1582), 286: "De spagyricorum nova prorsus urinae probatione: quae sit per separationem & resolutionem Mercurij, Sulphuris, & Salis." BLEKER (1976), 73, argued that Thurneisser took over the idea of associating the urine glass with the human body from Actuarius and that Thurneisser's subdivision of the cucurbit into twenty four zones was a doubling of Actuarius' twelve-zone inspection glass. This does not account for the application of color semiology in chemical uroscopy, however, since Thurneisser believed such direct qualitative observations to be undependable. Thurneisser regarded the visual, qualitative inspection of urine, the primary method of medieval uroscopy, to be of limited usefulness, owing to the weakness and unreliability of the human sense of sight. He thought that one ought rather to base a scientific assessment on quantitative measurement of urine and its fractions. See BLEKER (1976), 71; THURNEISSER (1571), I–II (sig. Aiij r–v). Despite their commonalities, Hayne did not follow Thurneisser in discarding traditional uroscopy as useless and erecting a sophisticated and expensive instrument-dependent diagnostic scheme. Instead he elaborated a qualitative chemical uroscopy that yoked the qualitative observations of traditional late medieval uroscopy to Paracelsian tartar theory, making the practice of uroscopy a truly Paracelsian diagnostic tool, able to guide the Paracelsian iatrochemical practitioner in arriving at a diagnosis in terms of Paracelsian pathology. Hayne's method did not depend directly on the laboratory, but rather was as portable as his book, explaining perhaps how it ended up in de Benneville's manuscript.

might lodge, from the teeth and brain to the joints and "private parts" (fol. 70–76 [178–191]). The remedies that de Benneville offers for astral and tartar diseases are straightforwardly therapeutic in nature and assume that an appropriate diagnosis has already been made. But in one case, tartar settled in the blood, he notes that the disease is "very ketching" and that "the colour of the urin is of a dark brown."[31] These evidently characteristic signs remind us that there is a diagnostic side to this medicine, too, thus the uroscopy.

De Benneville's Uroscopy

Compared to the rest of the *Medicina Pensylvania*,[32] the uroscopy section is poorly rendered in English, becoming somewhat incoherent and difficult to construe at points, unless one is equipped with Hayne's German text. It is clear from the opening lines of this portion that inspection of the urine can reveal the condition of the digestions in the stomach, where topaz-coloured sulphur is separated, and in the liver, where salts are separated. This is taken over directly from the beginning of Hayne's third *Tractätlein*, although truncated to leave out specifying the third digestion (namely the separation of mercurial substances) in the kidneys.[33] De Benneville was clearly aiming to eliminate unessential theory or condense it into a table as much as possible and get on with the diagnostic details. He skimmed over Hayne's explanation of how examination of the urine can reveal the operations of the four elements and associated four "seeds," which are concocted in the Paracelsian three primary substances, although he alluded to it in the subsequent table. He simplified all this, stating only that it is useful to know the working of the four elements by their influences and "to know the foundation of such contents, the humours of the brains, the scum and bula of the urine."[34] This terse, confused prose – at least in its English translation – presents something of a bare outline of Hayne's fuller and systematic breakdown of diseases into those that arise from stony matter, astral diseases, diseases coming

31 DE BENNEVILLE (2005) fol. 74 [186].

32 For the use of language and the sources for the portions of this ms. dealing with pharmaceutical manufacture, see WILSON, in this volume.

33 DE BENNEVILLE (2005), fol. 137 [312], here quoting HAYNE (1663), 194–195: "Der Medicus soll am aller ersten die geschaffenheit eines Menschens Urin wissen, und derhalben in derselben die gute Dauung dess Menschen Magens, oder aber Fäulnuss im Magen, an Sulphuris scheidung von Topasii Farben erkennen, darneben die scheidung an der Leber, dess Saltzes an hypostasi, wann die beysammen auffgespitzet stehen, und wenig Tartar Saltz sich hin und wider angehengt hat: vor gesund ermessen: Also auch, wann das Sedimentum unter liegt, die Mercurii scheidung davon vollkömlich vor gesund judiciren, und nicht die Zufälle der Kälte und Hitze allein ansehen."

34 DE BENNEVILLE (2005), fol. 137 [312]; HAYNE (1663), fold-out table between 194–195; the heading reads "Der Grund solcher Contenten zu wissen, soll verstanden werden, was im Gehirn vor eine Materia liegt, die Schaum, Jest und Bullen mache, ist alles in Contenten auss nachfolgender Figur zu ersehen."

naturally from the four elements, or from arsenic, orpiment, and mercury, and diseases caused by *semina* or seeds. Hayne's presentation reflects a broader Paracelsian scope, reminiscent of Paracelsus' disease categories *elemental, astral,* and *poisonous*.[35]

Eliminating theoretical detail, de Benneville's text launches into a series of definitions of the various distinct parts of the urine in the inspection flask (the urine glass, or *matula*). These definitions are not quite orthodox, and they are condensed from Hayne's text, as are the various terms for forms of tartar. Similarly, de Benneville's list of nine aspects of urine to be examined and the correspondence between the regions of the urine glass and the regions of the human body mirror Hayne's discussion.

Much of fol. 139 [316] (in German fol. 137 [313]) of the *Medicina Pensylvania* is taken up with a table that combines various tables appearing in the 1663 Hayne edition. There, one table summarizes signs observable in the urine, how they should be interpreted, and what diseases they indicate. Other tables list various components or factors that make up the human body, which taken together describe an early modern version of the medieval *res naturales*, the seven kinds of natural things that govern physiology.[36] Another table correlates the four basic complexions with the four Galenic qualities and with the four Hippocratic flavors or powers, which are labeled humors here, namely the salty, the sweet, the bitter, and the sour.[37]

De Benneville's English explanation of these tables identifies the stomach as "the greatest digestor," which separates the sulphurous humors and passes the excrement to the intestines for elimination. If it is working well, the urine should be a golden color, presumably because of the sulphur. The liver is the next, and it separates salts. When it is functioning properly, a fine sediment "like fine lights" of a transparent yellow color should appear on the bottom of the urine glass, which is evidence that the vital balsam is being maintained and that the impure tartar is being excreted. The third digestion (located in the kidneys here) separates mercury, and when this is healthy, the uroscopist should see a heavy sediment on the bottom of the urine glass and no froth or scum on the surface of the urine. This indicates that the tartarous wastes of the third digestion are being sweated out through the pores of the skin. All three digestions separate what is called "external tartar," which is evident in "external urine," and all three must be working properly for the body to be healthy.[38]

35 *Ens naturale*, *ens astrale* or *ens astrorum*, and *ens veneni* were three of the five categories of diseases (which included also spiritual and divine diseases) that were identified by Paracelsus in his early work *Volumen medicinae paramirum* (ca. 1520), PARACELSUS (1929), 173–174. See PARACELSUS (1990), 45.

36 The seven naturals are elements, qualities, humors, spirits, powers, members, faculties.

37 On the Paracelsians' reshaping of Hippocrates as a forerunner of chemical medicine, see SHACKELFORD (2002a), and SHACKELFORD (2004), 157–158.

38 DE BENNEVILLE (2005), fol. 139–140 [316, 318] (in German fol. 138 [315]); HAYNE (1663), 203–204: "Der Magen, als der erste und gröste Topff, scheidet durch seine Perfect Fäulung

De Benneville following Hayne next turns to signs of failed digestions, and here we leave theory and get into practical diagnosis. If the urine is pale and cloudy, it indicates a bad first digestion and that tartar is passed into the body with the nutriments. Foam on the urine then indicates heartburn, stomach problems, vomit, daily fevers, and rheumatism. If the second digestion is failing, one finds a "hypostasis," and the urine is red. This, along with a hard liver, indicates that the tartar is fixed in the liver as well as spreading over the whole body, occasioning pleurisy on the right side, tertian fevers, and dropsy. Faulty third digestion results in an absence of sediment and hypostasis in the urine glass, the presence of a whitish grey color at the top, a thick foam, and small grains in the urine. These signs indicate palsy, convulsions, fits, and "very dangerous catarrhs."[39]

For diagnosis to be most meaningful, one needs to distinguish external urine, which results directly from the three digestions acting on what we eat and drink, from internal urines, which derive from the parts of the body and flow to the bladder as vapors. One can discover by experiment whether these three digestions are healthy or corrupted by examining the urine: if it is clear, transparent, and golden, the body is in perfect health; if it "grows suddenly gloomy" it is a sign of poorly digested spirit of sulphur or vitriol; if it remains clear, it is a sign of salts predominating; gloomy urine with sediment indicates poisonous vapors in the body.[40]

Different colors of urine have specific semiological value, as itemized in a fold-out table by Hayne (1663) and replicated in prose by de Benneville: Black urine without sediment, but with hypostasis of equal thickness and gloomy, is a

und Digestion den Sulphur [...]. Die Leber ist der ander grosse Topff, dieser scheidet und digerirt den Saltz [...]. Der dritte Topff sind die Nieren, da wird digerirt unnd unterscheiden der Mercurius [...]. Auss diesen 3 vornembsten Dawungen, digestionen und separationen wird die Vrina exterior und Tartarum exterum geheissen, und muss also der dreyer Ampt unnd Arbeit den Cörpern zur Gesundheit dienen."

39 De Benneville (2005), fol. 140 [318] (in German fol. 138 [315]); Hayne (1663), 204–205: "Wann aber solchen digestiones und separationes nicht recht vollkommen [...] unnd wann sich Tartarum als ein Schaum oder Jest auffhebet, wircket er das Sodbrennen am boden dess Magens [...] Hiervon Febres Cottidianae [...] So aber die Leber ihre digestion unnd separation nicht vollkommen verrichtet [...] darauss dreytäglich Feber [...] darauss Wassersucht [...]. Wenn aber der Mercurius ubel digerirt unnd separirt wird, so ist kein Sediment noch hypostasis zu finden, und ist Vrina weises und gräwlecht [...] die bedeuten den Schlag, Paralysin, schwere Kranckheit, fallende Sucht, zukünfftig alle im Häupt herkommende gefährliche Flüsse."

40 De Benneville (2005), fol. 141 [320] (in German fol. 140 [319]); Hayne (1663), 215–17: "Zum Beschluss dieses Capitels, soll man mercken, dass zweyerley Vrina sey: Eusserliche Vrina, die da kömpt von aussen hinein, als von Speysen und Trincken [...]. Die innerliche Vrina geht auss allen andern innerlichen Gliedern zusammen, zur Blasen zu, wie ein Dunst oder Vapor, wie im 3. Tractat zu finden. [...]. Wenn die Vrina bald bricht, ist ihr spiritus Sulphur. oder Vitriol. nicht recht fertig, vollkommen, bereit oder digerirt worden, sondern wird von widerwertigen dingen, als Tartaro, Fäulnuss, Wind oder Gifft zerstört, und trüblecht zerbrochen gesehen."

sign of death; urine turning blackish and without both sediment and hypostasis is a sign of grave danger to life; brown, gloomy urine with black and reddish sediment indicates tartar in the liver, spleen, and blood, resulting in dangerous fevers, jaundice, scurvy, and dropsy; tile-colored urine with hypostasis points to lung disease; green hypostasis is a sign of jaundice, pleurisy, and obstructions of the heart, resulting from tartar in the gall bladder; red urine with thick hypostasis is a sign of fevers with high heat; and so on.[41]

Basically what we have here in Hayne's text and epitomized by de Benneville is a semiology based on close examination of the color and consistency of the urine, its contents, and any sediments, but one that yields results expressed in terms of a distinctly Paracelsian pathology. This is in fact a chemical uroscopy, but one that resembles antecedent medieval uroscopy and does not, by itself, demand fractional distillation or quantitative measures, which historians have typically associated with the proto-urology of Leonhard Thurneisser, some 30 years after Paracelsus' death. Indeed, Walter Pagel attributed to Paracelsus a rather dim view of traditional uroscopy.[42] So in what sense is Hayne's uroscopy Paracelsian? A closer look at Paracelsus' teaching reveals that the basic components of chemical uroscopy were already a part of his medical thinking in the 1520s and can be seen as fundamental to his medical development. It is necessary to establish this connection in order to understand how uroscopy developed as a key component of Paracelsian practice.

41 DE BENNEVILLE (2005), fol. 142 [322] (in German fol. 141 [321]); HAYNE (1663), fold-out table between 218–219, with the title "Tabella der Farben, was in der Urin darauss zu erkennen." The reference to brown urine indicating tartar in the spleen, here in the uroscopy section of the Medicina Pensylvania, echoes de Benneville's mention of brown urine as a diagnostic sign in the "other diseases" section, fol. 74 [186], which was noted above. This suggests that he was in fact using uroscopy as a diagnostic tool in his practical medicine, knitting together the Paracelsian chemical semiology and the therapeutic indications of his practical medicine.

42 Walter Pagel mentions Paracelsus' criticism of uroscopy in PAGEL (1962), 19 and PAGEL (1982), 190–192, noting that Paracelsus thought that distillation of urine would reveal information of use in diagnosing abnormal amounts of salt, sulphur, and mercury. Pagel's assessment is repeated by MURPHY & DESNOS (1972), 124: "During the Renaissance, this method of uroscopy was challenged and discredited by Paracelsus." These leading scholars ignore or diminish Paracelsus' dependence on and development of medieval uroscopy. Instead, they highlight only his suggestion that fractional distillation of urine might permit chemical diagnosis, an idea they recognized as one root of modern urinalysis when more fully developed by Leonhard Thurneisser.

Chemical Uroscopy as Paracelsian Practice

Despite Paracelsus' widespread reputation as a medical iconoclast, core elements of his teaching derive from traditional antecedents. Relevant to the present argument is his approach to medical uroscopy, which he chose as the subject of his first public lecture on medicine, following his appointment as municipal physician in Basel in 1527.[43] Examination of this lecture material clearly reveals his chemical interpretation of traditional medieval uroscopy as the basis for later incorporation of chemical uroscopy – as a diagnostic semiology cast in terms of chemical medicine – into chemiatric therapy.

Traditional instruction in the Middle Ages typically involved the oral reading (*lectio*) of a particular text or texts on a specific topic, combined with commentary or discussion that aimed to elucidate the texts' meanings and compare them with other teachings. Despite flouting tradition by lecturing in vernacular German, Paracelsus appears in 1527 to have followed the traditional scholastic pedagogical form of reading and explaining a Latin text. The treatise he chose to present was not a classic, or even a well-known contemporary authority, but a short work that he, Paracelsus, was in the process of writing. According to its title, it was a treatise comprising two subjects: first, the judgment of urines and pulses; and second, physiognomy insofar as it pertained to the physician. He did not publish this text, but various notes survived and were published by Johann Huser, and from these we can reconstruct something of his teaching.[44] Paracelsus' choice to lecture on diagnosis by examining a patient's urine and pulse –

43 Paracelsus' fame as a revolutionary is emblematized by the possibly spurious story that he cast a valuable copy of Avicenna's Canon, still the premier medical textbook in the early sixteenth-century university, into one of the bonfires that are customarily lighted on St. John's Eve – barely two months before he began lecturing on uroscopy. This alleged act symbolized for modern historians Paracelsus' total rejection of over thirteen centuries of medical tradition and earned him a reputation among modern scholars as a revolutionary iconoclast – someone who caused a rupture in medical history, not a contributor to a continual, progressive development of late medieval medicine. It may therefore come as a surprise to some readers that Paracelsus began his brief teaching career with a series of lectures on uroscopy, perhaps the most defining aspect of traditional medieval medical diagnosis.

44 "De urinarum ac pulsuum judiciis libellus, item De physiognomia, quantum medico opus est," PARACELSUS (1931), 549–579, and accompanying notes "In librum de urinarum ac pulsuum iudiciis: item de physiognomia medica, aliae quaedam annotationes," 583–595. Sudhoff noted in his introduction (xxxii–xxxviii), that the published lecture and notes mainly stem from a copy written down by one of Paracelsus' students, but are supported by autographical fragments, and that Paracelsus appears to have followed the traditional scholastic lecture format of reading a text and then commenting on it as he went through it. Johann Huser published the uroscopy lecture in the Basel quarto collected works of Paracelsus, which served as the basis for republication and edition by Benedictus Figulus in 1608: Paracelsus, *Zween underschiedene Tractat. I. von desz Harns und Puls Vrtheil[...] II. von den Gradibus unnd Compositionibus der Recepten und natürlichen dingen. Aus dem Fünfftem und Siebendem Theyl seiner operum in quarto zu Basel getruckt* (Strassburg: Lazarus Zetzner, 1608) (after Sudhoff).

two components of basic medical instruction that went back to the twelfth-century Salernitan *Ars medicinae* or *Articella* – does not strike one as the choice of a revolutionary.[45] It was rather a choice to lecture on a topic that was still fundamental to a medical degree and therefore would attract a broad audience. It was also Paracelsus' opportunity to expound his theories of health and disease within a traditional framework.

As it appears in the modern printed edition, Paracelsus' treatise on urines and pulses is divided into books, "tractates," and chapters, with annotations to the chapters, and includes several outlines or tables, which were typical of the humanist uroscopy genre. The text is in Latin, interspersed with occasional German words and phrases. The sentences are usually readable, grammatically simple, and often short. They do not always present a clear and eloquent thesis, but they do clearly indicate the fundamentals of Paracelsus' theory. The text begins by defining urine as either external, internal (of the blood, *cruor*), or a mixture of these two; external urine comes rather directly from what we eat and drink and is nothing else but salt that has been separated from ingested nutriment by digestions that take place in the three principal organs, namely the stomach, liver, and kidneys.[46] It therefore reveals only the condition of these three digestions.[47] If one wishes to evaluate the condition of the other parts of the body, one must obtain internal urine, the urine of the blood. One does this by having the patient refrain from eating and drinking, which produces the external urine, and then collect a urine sample after midnight.[48] This is an important distinction. If, for example, the uroscopist is examining the "circle" of the urine glass (the upper surface of the urine sample) to see if a headache is indicated, he must be looking at internal urine, because the external urine yields diagnostic information about the digestions of the nutriment, but not about diseases of the head.[49] In other words, Paracelsus taught that the excreted urine sample mirrored the condition of the blood, which reflected both the state of the principal digestive processes (producing external urine) and the general condition of the body's parts, which produce internal urine. Both could be diagnostically useful, but needed to be distinguished.

The details of Paracelsus' uroscopy are difficult to comprehend and quite involved, but one can make several observations from these lecture notes. First, much of Paracelsus' approach and terminology is either traditional or is drawn

45 O'BOYLE (1998), 83 and 92, notes that the treatises on urines and pulses were part of the *Articella*, which became a stabile curriculum early in the 12th century. Uroscopy remained part of the core curriculum into the late Middle Ages.

46 Paracelsus, *De urinarum ac pulsarum iudiciis libellus* and notes, PARACELSUS (1931), 550, 583.

47 PARACELSUS (1931), 553: "Exterior urina provenit ex iis, quae aut comedimus aut bibimus, id est ex nutrimentis, nec quidquam aliud indicat, quam quod ad stomachum, hepar aut renes attinet."

48 PARACELSUS (1931), 553.

49 PARACELSUS (1931), 554.

from traditional uroscopy with some alterations in meaning. Second, he believed that what one sees in the urine glass reflects the condition of the body's interior, but interpreted in terms of his own ideas about nutrition. The three principal organs, the stomach, liver, and kidneys, are responsible for three distinct digestions, by which sulphur, mercury, and salt are separated from the nutriment and kept in harmonious balance in the healthy individual. The results of these separations are evident in various parts of the urine in the inspection glass, the *hypostasis, fundus,* and *circulus*, by examining their colors, thicknesses, and other specific qualities, which are therefore useful in diagnosis.[50]

When a person's digestive processes are awry, the urine in the inspection glass will show the presence of tartar. Paracelsus took this material to be a basic component of many foodstuffs, particularly those with a mucilaginous content, and based his pathology of tartar diseases on this. Tartar in urine indicates a congelation, putrefaction, or obstruction in the body; a reddish substance – nutriment – indicates that good nutriment is being erroneously separated and expelled from the body.[51] Here we see the root of the idea that Heinrich Nolle would later express, that the function of the liver is to separate the red or ruby-colored from the white or crystal and that the presence of these tinctures in the urine glass is semiologically significant. The astute reader will recognize in this teaching the fundamental elements of Johann Hayne's theory, which was the basis for chemiatric diagnosis and therapeutics in the *Medicina Pensylvania.* But what is especially interesting is that in these Basel lectures we see clearly the defining features of Paracelsian medicine already applied to uroscopy, notably Paracelsus' elaboration of a tartar theory of pathogenesis.

De Benneville as Chemiatric Physician – Some Conclusions and Speculations

Of course, a vestigial presence of Paracelsian uroscopy in an eighteenth-century text does not by itself shed much light on the nature of George de Benneville's Pennsylvania practice. Nor is there an obvious reason why a well established bilingual dispensatory apparently intended for colonial pharmacists should include this type of discourse. Clearly, his drug lists and therapies, which make up the largest portions of the compilation (the *materia medica* [015–037]; the preparations fol. 1–65 [040–169]; the main diseases fol. 76–117 [190–273]; and the

50 Paracelsus' use of the terms hypostasis and fundus are somewhat different from the typical uses in medieval uroscopy. "Hypostasis" refers to what settles on the bottom of the matula and is usually the same as sediment. The body of the urine is usually called the enaeorema or swim. Here Paracelsus is distinguishing "hypostasis" and "fundus" from each other and from the basic color of the urine: "hypostasis enim salis qualitatem, tinctura [qualitatem] sulphuris, fundus [qualitatem] mercurii denotat;" PARACELSUS (1931), 554. If he is following Actuarius and other medieval uroscopies, the hypostasis should be the lower part of the urine and the fundus the bottom of the urine glass.

51 PARACELSUS (1931), 558.

appendix on women's diseases fol. 122–132 [282–303]), point to an eclectic medicine that followed standard eighteenth-century practice in employing chemiatric drugs (see Crellin in this volume). But the surviving elements of Hayne's medicine in the *Medicina Pensylvania*, especially when viewed against other manuscript material attributed to de Benneville that is of clear alchemical and chemiatric origin, suggest de Benneville's serious immersion in transmutational alchemy and Paracelsian chemical medicine. Although no compelling proof of de Benneville's authorship of these manuscripts has been found, the striking similarity in tone and content of the first paragraph of the *Ad lectorem benevolum* of the *Medicina Pensylvania* and the beginning of the short *Ad lectorem benevolum* in Schwenkfelder ms., *Tinctura Universalis*, strongly suggests their common authorship. The latter begins on the back of the title page of this manuscript and briefly introduces a 33 folio treatise on the transmutation of metals that covers the basic alchemical laboratory procedures. Appended is a list of chemicals, apparatus, etc. in Latin and German, with corresponding symbols, from *acetum* to *urina*.[52]

These two introductions are by no means identical and in fact serve very different purposes. The first paragraph of the *Ad lectorem* to the *Medicina Pensylvania* begins an almost four-page introduction to astral and tartar medicine, which provides the theoretical explanation for uroscopy as a diagnostic semiotics. This material is taken wholesale from Johann Schröder's 1662 introduction to the 1663 edition of Hayne's *Drey unterschiedliche neue Tractätlein*, much of it verbatim with some large lacunae and occasional rephrasings to economize and omit identifications of particular scholarly traditions. For example, the fourth to the last paragraph of the *Ad lectorem benevolum* [011], which copies Schröder's account of Paracelsus' classification of diseases,[53] omits mention of Paracelsus in connection with the classes of diseases, ending with "diesen ursprung nennet man so Ens venenatum, nicht das alle diese in specie gifftig sondern in genere schädlich und kranckIich seyn" as a replacement for "Diesen Ursprung nennet P. [Paracelsus] Ens Venenatum, nicht dass alle diese in specie gifftig, sondern, in genere schädlich und kräncklich seyn."[54] De Benneville's use of Schröder is clear; he copied entire paragraphs with minor changes.

52 This and other manuscripts attributed in the cataloging records to George de Benneville reside at the Schwenkfelder Library and Heritage Center, Pennsburg, Pennsylvania. SCHWENKFELDER MS. VR 42–42, *Tinctura Universalis*, begins on folio 1 recto; "*Ad Lectorem Benevolum*" is on fol. 1v–2r; fol. 2v is blank; and *Transmutation der metallen* begins on fol. 3r and continues to fol. 35v. Folios 27r–35v comprise an alphabetical list of chemical procedures from *amalgamatio* to *trituratio*. Folios 36r–39r are blank, and a final section fol. 39v–41v is the alphabetized list of chemicals.

53 Hayne (1663), b2v–b3v.

54 De Benneville's *Ad lectorem benevolum* adds an initial and ultimate paragraph to a text that is otherwise drawn from Schröder's *Ad lectorem benevolum* to his edition of Hayne's text. Following the initial paragraph, de Benneville begins where Schröder does, HAYNE (1663), a1r, but breaks off at the top of a2r, where Schröder begins to provide scholarly background in chemical philosophy as the basis for astrological medicine, discussing the generation of

The apparent purpose of this *Ad lectorem* is to present the diverse parts of the *Medicina Pensylvania* as constituting a coherent medicine based on the chemical foundations that Schröder had identified as having been established by Paracelsus and elaborated by his seventeenth-century followers, but without identifying these authors, as Schröder had done. The purpose of the *Ad lectorem* to the *Tinctura universalis* is far different. It is composed as a short and personal message to a friend, Jacob Brown, intended to accompany a treatise that might help him achieve the universal tincture, the elixir that might be prepared by an adept who has been graced by God (receiving the *donum Dei*), and which then may be used for metallic transmutation and as a powerful medical panacea.[55] As such, the style of this *Ad lectorem* is personal missive rather than academic introduction, and the choice of pronouns and verb forms reflects this.

Nevertheless, despite these very different styles and genres, the two *Ad lectorem* prefaces begin almost identically and follow a similar pattern for several lines of text, suggesting either a very normative prosody or a close connection between these texts, perhaps common authorship.[56] If the latter is the case, then the first and final paragraphs of the *Medicina Pensylvania*'s *Ad lectorem benevolum* must have been penned much later, or perhaps modified by a compiler, since the handwriting is not identical to that of the Tinctura Universalis and the orthography suggests a more modern standard, more in keeping with Schröder's German *Ad lectorem*, which constitutes the bulk of the *Ad lectorem* in the *Medicina Pensylvania.* Clearly much closer philological and historical scholarship needs to be brought to bear on these colonial German manuscripts in order to determine their connections, if any, and identify the historical circumstances of

the macrocosm, the generation of plants, and the generation of animals in turn. It is not until Schröder reaches the generation of humans (a7v) that de Benneville resumes copying and follows it through the penultimate paragraph, with a couple of omissions and minor rewordings. De Benneville then replaces Schröder's ultimate paragraph (where Schröder identifies the text as Hayne's) with a conclusion praising the creator in his Trinitarian glory, announcing his own humility "als der aller unwürdigster wurm," and concluding with an Amen and Hallelujah – none of which we find in Schröder's introduction. By this bowdlerization, the compiler of *Medicina Pensylvania* effectively effaced his dependence on Schröder, Hayne, and Paracelsus' medicine.

55 SCHWENKFELDER MS. VR 42–42, Tinctura Universalis, fol. 1v–r.

56 DE BENNEVILLE (2005) begins: "*Ad Lectorem Benevolum.* Es ist ein edler Stand, was in dem gebrechlichen Leben des menschlichen Geschlechte, [...] nemlich Kranckheiten der Kayser wie der Betler haben eine Gleichformigkeit, in Kranckheiten, wie im Sterben. Zur Zeit der Schmertzen seufftzet ein jeder nach voriger Gesundheit [...]. Keine Mühe wird geachtet, kein geld gesparet umb nur sein zweck zu erreichen und wenn der Herr und höchster Artzt [...]." Compare this with the beginning to SCHWENKFELDER MS. VR 42–42, Tinctura Universalis, fol. 1v: "*Ad Lectorem Benevolum.* Mein ins besonder geliebter Jacob Brown. Es ist ein edler stand, was in dem gebrechlichen leben, des menschlichen geschlechte, ein jeder erfahren müssen, ohne ausnahme wer sie auch seie, von dem kayser bis auff dem betler, nemlich kranckheiten, zu solcher zeit, seufftzet ein jeder mit recht nach der gesundheit, da wendet man sein alles an, umb solches zu erlangen, diesen zweck recht zu erreichen, [...] ob der herr und artz, [...]." Both end with the word "Hallelujah." The similarity is manifest.

their composition and intellectual traditions. In the case of the *Medicina Pensylvania*, the circumstances of composition are only beginning to be illuminated, in part through the revelation that the compiler has drawn very heavily from standard eighteenth-century formularies, the use of elaborate chemically prepared drugs, and an underlying diagnostic and therapeutic procedure that is based on Paracelsian chemical and astral medicine.

In conclusion, I speculate that chemical uroscopy, created by Paracelsus and elaborated by his sixteenth-century followers Hayne and Thurneisser, and perhaps others, helped enable Paracelsian chemiatric practice and gave it a utility among seventeenth-century healers and a longevity into eighteenth-century medicine that is not understood or appreciated in today's history of medicine, which often regards Paracelsian medicine as having been fundamentally transformed in the early seventeenth century, by van Helmont for example, and subsequently found application mainly in an eclectic polypharmaceutical Galenism. For these reasons, historians have preferred the term Helmontian for later chemical medicine, arguing that the essential identity of Paracelsian medicine vanished as it became absorbed and diluted in seventeenth-century eclecticism. But we know that Paracelsian theory retained followers into the late seventeenth and eighteenth centuries – perhaps for religious and other cultural reasons – so why not also a Paracelsian practical medicine that was grounded in that theory? Indeed, I claim that Hayne's medicine is a prominent example of the process by which Paracelsian chemical theory was translated into a functional Paracelsian clinical medicine, which persisted in practice in de Benneville's eighteenth-century medicine.

Unpublished Sources and References

Schwenkfelder Ms. VR 42–42
Tinctura Universalis. Transmutation der metallen. Schwenkfelder Library & Heritage Center, Pennsburg, PA, VR 42–42.

Beall & Shryock (1954)
Beall, Jr., Otho T.; Shryock, Richard H.: Cotton Mather. First Significant Figure in American Medicine. Baltimore: Johns Hopkins Press, 1954.

de Benneville (2005)
de Benneville, George: Medicina Pensylvania Or The Pensylvania Physician. In: Eighteenth-century Colonial Formularies. The Manuscripts of George de Benneville and Abraham Wagner. The College of Physicians of Philadelphia Digital Library.
Recent website address (access date: June 23, 2008): http://www.accesspadr.org/cpp/.

Bleker (1976)
Bleker, Johanna: Chemiatrische Vorstellungen und Analogiedenken in der Harndiagnostik Leonhard Thurneissers (1571 und 1576). In: Sudhoffs Archiv 60 (1976), 66–75.

Gevitz & Sullivan-Fowler (1995)
Gevitz, Norman; Sullivan-Fowler, Michaela: Making Sense of Therapeutics in Seventeenth-Century New England. In: Caduceus. A Museum Quarterly for the Health Sciences 11 (1995), 87–102.

Gilly (1998)
Gilly, Carlos: 'Theophrastia Sancta' – Paracelsianism as a Religion, in Conflict with the Established Churches. In: Ole Grell (Ed.): Paracelsus. The Man and His Reputation, His Ideas and Their Transformation. Leiden: Brill, 1998, 151–185.

Habermann (2001)
Habermann, Mechthild: Deutsche Fachtexte der frühen Neuzeit. Naturkundlich-medizinische Wissensvermittlung im Spannungsfeld von Latein und Volkssprache. Berlin: de Gruyter, 2001.

Hayne (1663)
Hayne, Johann: Drey underschiedliche newe Tractätlein. Deren Erstes von astralischen Kranckheiten Das Andere, von tartarischen Kranckheiten [...]. Das Dritte, begreifft in sich das Fundament [...] wie man die Urinen des Menschen [...] künstlich iudiciren erkennen möge. Frankfurt/Main: Thomae Matthiae, 1663.

Moran (1991)
Moran, Bruce T.: The Alchemical World of the German Court. Occult Philosophy and Chemical Medicine in the Circle of Moritz of Hessen (1572–1632). Stuttgart: Franz Steiner, 1991.

Murphy & Desnos (1972)
Murphy, Leonard J. T.; Desnos, Ernest: The History of Urology. Springfield, IL: Charles C. Thomas, 1972.

Newman (2001)
Newman, William R.: Experimental Corpuscular Theory in Aristotelian Alchemy. From Geber to Sennert. In: Lüthy, Christoph; Murdoch, John; Newman, William (Eds.): Late Medieval and Early Modern Corpuscular Matter Theory. Leiden: Brill, 2001, 291–329.

Newman (1994)
Newman, William R.: Gehennical Fire. The Lives of George Starkey, an American Alchemist in the Scientific Revolution. Cambridge, MA: Harvard University Press, 1994.

Nolle (1655)
Nolle, Heinrich: Hermetical Physick. Or, the right way to preserve, and to restore health. Trans. Henry Vaughn. London: Moseley, 1655.

O'Boyle (1998)
O'Boyle, Cornelius: The Art of Medicine. Medical Teaching at the University of Paris, 1250–1400. Leiden: Brill, 1998.

Pagel (1982)
Pagel, Walter: Paracelsus. An Introduction to Philosophical Medicine in the Era of the Renaissance. Rev. ed. Basel: Karger, 1982.

Pagel (1962)
Pagel, Walter: Das medizinische Weltbild des Paracelsus. Seine Zusammenhänge mit Neuplatonismus und Gnosis. Wiesbaden: Franz Steiner, 1962.

Paracelsus (1990)
Paracelsus: Essential Readings. Ed. and trans. Nicholas Goodrick-Clarke. Wellingborough, England: Aquarian Press, Crucible, 1990.

Paracelsus (1931)
Paracelsus: Sämtliche Werke. Ed. Karl Sudhoff. I. Abteilung I, Bd. IV. München: R. Oldenbourg, 1931.

Paracelsus (1929)
Paracelsus: Sämtliche Werke. Ed. Karl Sudhoff. I. Abteilung I, Bd. I. München: R. Oldenbourg, 1929.

Pumfrey (1998)
Pumfrey, Stephen: The Spagyric Art; Or, The Impossible Work of Separating Pure from Impure Paracelsianism. A Historiographical Analysis. In: Grell, Ole (Ed.): Paracelsus. The Man and His Reputation, His Ideas and Their Transformation. Leiden: Brill, 1998, 21–51.

Reusner (1582)
Reusner, Hieronymus: Urinarum probationes D. Iodoci Wilichii Reselliani illustratae scholis medicis, Hieronymi Reusneri Leorini D. Med. in quibus principia solidae uroscopiae, ad solidae philosophiae fontes revocantur multique medicorum errores deteguntur. His accessere variae matularum delineationes atque genuini urinarum colores. Remedia item plurima ex urina desumpta maxima vero ex parte chemica. Basel: Sebastian Henricpetri, 1582.

Schneider (1972)
Schneider, Wolfgang: Chemiatry and Iatrochemistry. In: Debus, Allen (Ed.): Science, Medicine and Society in the Renaissance. Essays to honor Walter Pagel. New York: Science History Publications, 1972, 141–50.

Shackelford (2004)
Shackelford, Jole: A Philosophical Path for Paracelsian Medicine: The Ideas, Intellectual Context, and Influence of Petrus Severinus (1540/2-1602). Copenhagen: Museum Tusculanum Press, 2004.

Shackelford (2002a)
Shackelford, Jole: The Chemical Hippocrates: Paracelsian and Hippocratic Theory in Petrus Severinus' Medical Philosophy. In: David Cantor (Ed.): Reinventing Hippocrates. Aldershot, Hampshire: Ashgate, 2002, 59–88.

Shackelford (2002b)
Shackelford, Jole: To Be or Not to Be a Paracelsian. Something Spagyric in the State of Denmark. In: Scholz Williams, Gerhild; Gunnoe, Charles D., Jr., (Eds.): Paracelsian Moments. Science, Medicine, and Astrology in Early Modern Europe. Kirksville, MO: Truman State University Press, 2002, 35–69.

Thurneisser (1571)
Thurneisser zum Thurn, Leonhard: Prokatalepsis. Oder Praeoccupatio, Durch zwölff verscheidenlicher Tractaten, gemachter Harn Proben. Frankfurt/Oder: Johan Eichorn, 1571.

THE CIRCULATION OF THE BLOOD AND VENESECTION: ON THE RELATION BETWEEN MEDICAL THEORY AND PRACTICE IN THE EARLY EIGHTEENTH CENTURY

Marion Maria Ruisinger

Some 150 years after William Harvey (1578–1657) published his treatise on the circulation of the blood,[1] Johann Wolfgang von Goethe (1749–1832) wrote his famous novel of sensitivity, *The Sorrows of Young Werther* [*Die Leiden des jungen Werther*], an epistolary novel that ended with the suicide of the protagonist and a final phlebotomy:

> At six in the morning, his servant comes in with a lamp. He finds his master on the floor, the pistol, and blood. He calls out, he grasps him. No answer, only a rattle. He runs for the doctors, [...]. When the doctor came to the unfortunate man he found him on the floor, beyond help, his pulse still beating, all his limbs paralyzed. He had shot himself in the head above the right eye, the brain was protruding. Pointlessly [*zum Überfluss*], a vein was opened in his arm, the blood flowed, he was still gasping for breath. [...] Werther died around noon.[2]

In these memorable closing lines, Goethe devoted three sentences to the medical attendant, offering an external perspective on Werther's body, a cool and distanced medical gaze undistorted by the emotions coloring the perceptions of the bystanders. At the same time, he characterized the medicus as representative of a therapeutic world which was still alive though it already belonged to the past, a living anachronism. The medicus administered venesection to the young Werther, who had already lost considerable blood and was in mortal agony. In other words, Werther was subjected to a final emergency procedure based on humoral pathology that by the eighteenth century had been superseded by a fuller understanding of human physiology.[3] To put it in Goethe's own, somewhat ambiguous formulation: the venesection was undertaken here "*zum Überfluss,*" as a last, possibly superfluous measure to relieve the plethora or excess of blood.

When Goethe let the medicus perform venesection on an already bleeding person, he hinted at the crisis faced by contemporary medicine. This therapeutic procedure, perhaps more than any other, highlights a striking gap between medi-

1 HARVEY (1628).

2 GOETHE (2001), 152–153: "Morgens um sechse tritt der Bediente herein mit dem Lichte. Er findet seinen Herrn an der Erde, die Pistole und Blut. Er ruft, er fasst ihn an; keine Antwort, er röchelte nur noch. Er läuft nach den Ärzten [...]. Als der Medicus zu dem Unglücklichen kam, fand er ihn an der Erde ohne Rettung, der Puls schlug, die Glieder waren alle gelähmt. Über dem rechten Auge hatte er sich durch den Kopf geschossen, das Gehirn war herausgetrieben. Man ließ ihm zum Überfluss eine Ader am Arme, das Blut lief, er holte noch immer Atem. [...]. Um zwölfe mittags starb er." The translation is based on a recent English edition of *The Sorrows of Young Werther* by Burton Pike (2004).

3 Bloodletting as a treatment for the wounded had been questioned well before Harvey, among others by the Zurich surgeon Felix Würtz, based not on physiological theory but rather his own rich concrete experience as a physician, see WÜRTZ (1687), chapter V.

cal theory and medical practice.[4] The present paper[5] will explore this gap in four stages: First it presents the Galenic interpretation of venesection, followed by an overview of the changes in this interpretation as a result of Harvey's model of circulation. The paper then examines the extent to which modifications in theory had led to a change in the actual practice of bloodletting, based on selected surgical texts and manuals of the early modern period. A final section then turns to another source: the letters and recommendations of the consultations of Lorenz (Laurentius) Heister (1683–1758), the famous physician and surgeon.

Venesection in the Framework of Galenic Physiology

The Galenic theory of the four humors and their associated four qualities remained the medical canon until well into the early modern period, as was true for his physiology, which was especially important for the question of bloodletting.[6] It offered a coherent explanatory model for the movements of the organs and for the flow of the blood, which was conceived as a unidirectional streaming from the liver to the periphery.

On the basis of this model, three different effects were attributed to venesection: a quantitative effect as a result of the removal of excessive blood (the "plethora"), which posed a burden for the body; a qualitative effect by draining off harmful moistures that manifested themselves in the form of eczema, running sores, abscesses or open ulcers; and finally, a dynamic impact on the internal circulation of the humors. To achieve this last effect, to reestablish the flow of the stagnant humors or to divert them to other areas of the body, the choice of vein to be opened was decisive. Central here was the notion of a specificity of individual veins for certain parts of the body. Thus, the *Vena cephalica* on the inside of the elbow was associated with the head, and the *Vena splenica* in the left arm with the spleen. A competing theory was the concept of *repulsio* and *derivatio*, the repulsion and redirection of the blood to a specific part of the body by means of venesection. Here the choice of the vein to be opened was important not so much in terms of a specific vein, but rather of the body part to be targeted.

4 The history of phlebotomy has been a topic of the medical literature since the late eighteenth century and has been viewed from a variety of different perspectives. But the question of the relation between theory and practice has not been explicitly investigated; see inter alia MEZLER (1793), BAUER (1870), RISSE (1979), MAIBAUM (1983), KURIYAMA (1995).

5 The paper is based on an inaugural lecture by the author on June 7, 2005 to conclude her Habilitation (venia legendi); the lecture was entitled *Aderlass und Blutkreislauf. Kontinuitäten und Brüche in der frühneuzeitlichen Medizin* (Phlebotomy and the Circulation of the Blood. Continuities and Discontinuities in Early Modern Medicine). In the present paper, translations into English of German citations are provided by the author, unless otherwise indicated.

6 SCHÖNER (1964). For a recent English summary of humoralism in medical history, see NUTTON (1993).

For example, in a blocked menstruation, venesection was performed at the foot; in the case of excessive menstrual bleeding, the procedure was performed at the arm in order to redirect the blood away from the lower body.

The dynamic effect of bloodletting was only considered if there was some disturbance in the internal flow of the humors. Therefore, it was always linked to a therapeutic objective. By contrast, the quantitative and qualitative regulative potential of bloodletting could also be utilized as a preventive measure. As will be shown, this was of special importance for the social context of the practice of venesection.

Venesection in the Context of the Circulation of the Blood

While venesection enjoyed continuing popularity, its basis in the Galenic theory of the genesis and motion of the blood had gradually begun to weaken since the Renaissance. One small shock to the theoretical edifice followed upon the other, until William Harvey's *De motu cordis et sanguinis*[7] in 1628 upset it entirely. The only gap in Harvey's model of circulation, the missing link between the arteries and veins, was closed by Marcello Malpighi (1628–1694) in 1661 with his discovery of the capillary vessels, which offered final proof for the circulation of the blood.[8] But what did this new theory of the circulation of the blood mean for the time-honored theory of venesection and its threefold principal effects? [9]

To summarize, the quantitative effect retained its importance even in connection with new ideas on circulation. True, the doctrine of a plethora of blood inimical to health was closely associated with Galenic physiology, but it did not necessarily become obsolete with the adoption of a model in which the blood circulated throughout the body. In addition, the hydraulic model of circulation which Harvey had developed provided new physical arguments for the therapeutic and preventive utility of reducing the volume of circulating blood. Something similar also held in connection with the qualitative effect. The presence of deleterious or spoiled humoral fluid was regarded as an indication for venesection even in the framework of the circulation model. By contrast, Harvey's model had rendered obsolete the long-held conception of the unidirectional internal flow of the humors. Now the blood circulated ceaselessly through the body. The often hotly contested choice of the appropriate vein had become meaningless. Thus, acceptance of the circulation of the blood did not mean a general break with the practice of bloodletting but only with the previous, elaborate system of differentiating among the sites of the body to be cut – the location of venesection. Theoretically at least, the principle of organ specificity, *derivatio* and *repulsio*, had been washed away by the new conception of blood flow throughout the entire

7 HARVEY (1628).
8 MALPIGHI (1661).
9 For the early reception of Harvey's theory, see BRÖER (1994), 113–117.

body. We are now able to better reformulate our question as to the relation between medical theory and medical practice by focussing on that aspect of venesection where the model of the circulation of the blood was most influential: the importance accorded to the anatomical site of venesection.

Venesection in the Medical Practice of the Early Eighteenth Century

If we look more closely at the social context in which venesection took place, we find two persons at center stage: the patient who allowed his or her vein to be opened and the person performing the venesection. There might be additional individuals at the scene: physicians, other trained providers of medical care, or lay persons. There are many issues in terms of how and by whom medicine in general and venesection in particular was practiced; here we will restrict ourselves to two aspects that relate to the pair seated at the center:

> How was the theory of the circulation of the blood received by those performing venesections, in general non-academic barber surgeons (*Handwerkschirurgen*),[10] in the early eighteenth century?
>
> In what way was the practice influenced by the men and women who offered their veins to these practitioners?

The reception of the circulation of the blood by these surgeons and barber surgeons will be assessed by looking at surgical texts available in the German technical vernacular by the early eighteenth century. Our selection is based on a comprehensive list in the most influential German surgical text of the period, the 1719 *Chirurgie*, a textbook by the physician, surgeon, anatomist and botanist Lorenz Heister.[11]

In the introduction to his *Chirurgie*, Heister presents a historical overview, followed by a list of the 35 best-known "moderns,"[12] who either "wrote entire surgery texts, or the greater part of them, and which are available in German, not to include others here."[13] Heister also mentions specialized topics in surgery,

10 SANDER (1989). – In German-language areas, surgery including venesection was shared by three different groups of medical providers until well into the eighteenth century: the dominant and large group of *Handwerkschirurgen* or barber-surgeons, who were craftsmen with artisanal but no academic training; a small group of academic physicians, like Lorenz Heister, who performed surgery themselves; and a varied group of empirics and other healers like stone-cutters.

11 Heister's solid knowledge of the surgical literature of his time is evident from the 45-page bibliography he published in HEISTER (1739).

12 The term "Of the Moderns" is from a 1748 English translation (HEISTER 1748), 6. In his 1719 *Chirurgie*, the reference is to "Von den neuern Chirurgischen Scribenten," 1719, 7–9.

13 "[...] welche entweder gantze Chirurgien, oder doch die gröste Theil davon geschrieben, und in teutscher Sprach zu haben, anderer hier nicht zu gedencken," HEISTER (1719), 7–8. – The authors listed by Heister were Hieronymus Fabricius ab Aquapendente, Paul Barbette,

including three treatises on venesection.[14] By the beginning of the eighteenth century, their works were available in German and represented more or less the entire canon of knowledge available to these practitioners. Had circulation as postulated by Harvey in 1628 then found its way into the manuals of surgery by the end of the seventeenth century?

The time elapsed since Harvey's seminal treatise would make its reception appear possible: half of the works cited by Heister had been published after 1700, and another 25 percent were from the 1690s (Figure 1).[15] Thus, most of the commercially available German editions of the writers in Heister's catalogue were actually quite recent and two generations beyond Harvey's publication. We will investigate in the following the extent to which his theory of circulation had penetrated the surgical writing during this period.

Of the 38 works mentioned, 36 were available for inspection.[16] Thirteen proved to be of little relevance for the question at hand. These were books on military surgery and surgical techniques or treatises on *Chirurgia theoretica*, where venesection was only mentioned tangentially or not at all.[17]

In the remaining 23 works, we note a basically positive view of the practice

Johan van Beverwijck, Steven Blanckaert, Cornelis Bontekoe, Peter Bürger, Charles G. LeClerc, Giovanni Andreas dalla Croce, Ludwig Cron, Pierre Dionis, Wilhelm Fabry, Yves Gaukes, Georg Gelman, Cornelius Herls, Johann von Jessen, Franz Joël, Philibert Jondot, Johann Helfrich Jüngken, Joseph de LaCharrière, Frideric de Leauson, Johann Munniks, Johann von Muralt, Carolus Musitanus, Erhardt Norren, Antonius Nuck, Jan Palfijn, Ellis Prat, Matthäus G. Purmann, Joseph Schmid, Tobias Schütze, Johannes Scultetus, Cornelius Solingen, Johann Verbrug, Jean Baptiste Verduc, Johann Jacob Woyt, Felix Würtz.

14 HEISTER (1719), 8. – The three authors were Ludwig Cron, Philibert Jondot and Joseph Schmid. If one takes into account the fact that Joseph Schmid, who wrote both a surgical textbook and a treatise on bloodletting, is mentioned twice, a total of 37 writers on surgery are cited by Heister.

15 The surgical works cited by Heister were examined using the Karlsruhe Virtual Catalogue (www.ubka.unikarlsruhe.de/kvk.html). The German language editions available in 1719, when the *Chirurgie* was published, were the following, listed in chronological order: Dalla Croce (1607), Fabry (1652), Schmid (1653), Beverwijck (1674), Jessen (1674), Schmid (1675), Scultetus (1679), Gelman (1680), Joël (1680), Würtz (1687), Prat (1690), Muralt (1691), Blanckaert (1692), Bürger (1692), Herls (1692), Bontekoe (1697), LeClerc (1699), Munniks (1700), Horlacher (1701), Musitanus (1701), Purmann (1705), Gaukes (1709), Leauson (1709), Nuck (1709), Jondot (1710), Dionis (1712), Solingen (1712), Verduc (1712), Schütze (1714), LaCharrière (1715), Verbrug (1715), Woyt (1715), Fabricius ab Aquapendente (1716), Cron (1717), Norren (1717), Palfijn (1717), Barbette (1718), Jüngken (1718).

16 The copies examined were all from the holdings of the Erlangen-Nuremberg University Library, especially from the special private library of the Nuremberg physician Christoph Jacob Trew (1695–1769), housed at the University Library; see KEUNECKE (1995).

17 These are BONTEKOE (1697), GAUKES (1709), HERLS (1692), HORLACHER (1701), LEAUSON (1709), MUNNIKS (1700), MUSITANUS (1701), PALFIJN (1717), PURMANN (1705), SCHÜTZE (1714), SCULTETUS (1679), VERBRUG (1715), WÜRTZ (1687).

of venesection. The only physicians to express a critical view were Johann Helfrich Jüngken (1648–1726)[18] and Steven Blanckaert (1650–1702).[19] They argued for greater caution and reserve in utilizing bloodletting as a therapy. But they did not go so far as to exclude it totally from their textbooks, for practical rather than theoretical reasons: "[…] due to the use of this practice, which is still possible here or there."[20]

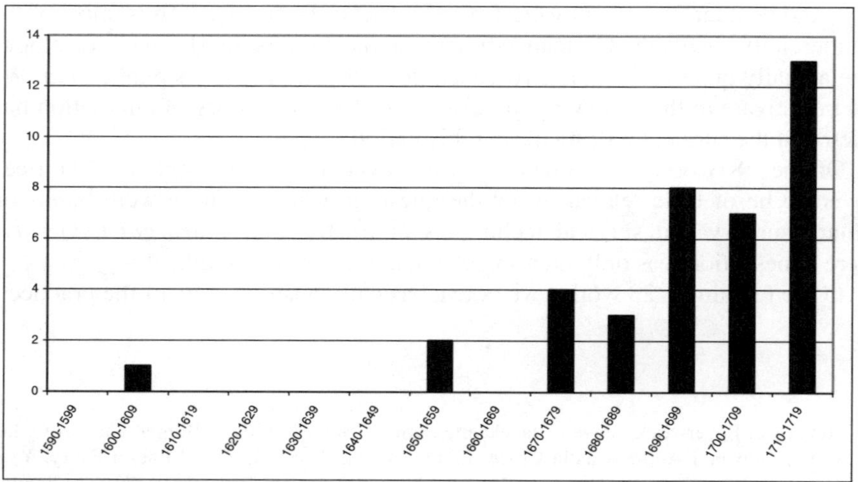

Fig. 1: Lorenz Heister recommended in his *Chirurgie* (1719) 38 textbooks of 37 "modern" surgical authors. The graph shows the publication date of the latest German editions available in 1719.

What was the significance of bloodletting in these works? Were their authors still adherents of the Galenic tradition, or had they already embraced Harvey's model of the body? As noted, the new theory departed most markedly from the old model with respect to the influence of bloodletting on the internal flow of the humors. Here, the question of site differentiation – which vein to strike – became crucial for the surgeons: should they, as before, accord the selection of the correct vein great weight, or should they, in accordance with Harvey, simply open the best and most visible vein?

This delicate question was dealt with in different ways in the works examined, regardless of their date of publication. A number of authors omitted all mention of the topic,[21] or referred to older works such as *De efficaci medicina* of

18 JÜNGKEN (1691), "Von der Ader-Oeffnung oder Aderlassen," 332–341.

19 BLANCKAERT (1692), "Von der Venaesectione, Phlebotomia oder Aderlassen," Vol. II, 30–37.

20 "[...] des Gebrauchs halber, der hie oder da noch statt finden könnte," BLANCKAERT (1692), 30.

21 Such as BARBETTE (1694), NUCK (1709) and WOYT (1715).

Marco Aurelio Severino (1580-1656), published in 1646.[22] Others rejected the traditional practice of site differentiation as totally antiquated, relying in part on the model of circulation,[23] in part on vascular anatomy.[24] Still others, indifferent to anatomical and physiological evidence, remained adherents of the pre-Harveyan tradition as late as 1700, relying on classical authorities and describing a large number of specific venesection sites.[25] The circulation of the blood was mentioned by only seven of the works examined.[26]

It seems reasonable to assume on this basis that the authors cited resisted embracing Harvey's model or at least were reluctant to apply it to surgical practice. Yet such an interpretation would overlook an important point: namely that the first edition of a work could far predate its first printing in the German language. That in turn would mean that some of the authors Heister mentions were perhaps not at all behind their times, but rather were survived by their writings, so to speak, which were published posthumously. Such was the case of Franz Joël (1508–1579), for example, who died in 1579, but whose medical writings, *Opera medica*, were not published even in Latin until 1631, including some material on surgery, which was printed in German as late as 1680, well over 100 years after the author's death.[27] Almost a century elapsed between the first edition of the *Wund-Artzney* by Felix Würtz in 1596 and its reprint in 1687.[28] These

22 "Die, welche die Circulation, oder Umblauff des Geblütes nicht annehmen, und Lust haben andere und unterschiedliche Adern zu lassen, die können den Marcum Severinum Aurellium de Efficaci Medicina nachlesen [...] allwo sie genug von dieser Materie finden werden," SOLINGEN (1693), 555.

23 CRON (1717).

24 Abandoning the idea that venesection is organ specific is only a limited indicator for how Harvey's theory was received and accepted, since it was based in part on the observations of older generations of anatomists. Thus, the Augsburg surgeon Joseph Schmid noted in 1653 in his *Examen phlebotomicum* that there was "no difference in the veins," ["Hie merck, daß kein unterscheid der Adern sei"] and that from neighboring veins, it was best to open the one which was most prominent to the eye, see SCHMID (1653), 63. – The argument put forward by Steven Blanckaert four decades later sounds fairly similar: "There are some who make a big mistake when they think that one or another vein in the arm has a special connection with certain internal organs, such as the liver, spleen, etc., since the anatomists can readily see that all such veins in the arms derive from the same trunk" ["Einen grossen Fehler begehen einige, indem sie vermeynen, daß diese oder jene Ader des Arms mit denen innerlichen Theilen, als der Leber, Miltz, etc. eine sonderliche Verwandnisse habe, da doch die Anatomici mit ihren Augen sehen, daß alle solche Adern eben am Arm aus einem Stamme gleichsam entspringen"], BLANCKAERT (1692), 33. – Using vascular anatomy, the Königsberg surgeon Peter Bürger also argued against the organ specificity of venesection; see BÜRGER (1692), 537.

25 As, for example, NORREN (1693) and JONDOT (1710).

26 In BEVERWIJCK (1674); BÜRGER (1692); CRON (1717); JÜNGKEN (1718); SOLINGEN (1712); WOYT (1715); VERBRUG (1715).

27 JOËL (1680).

28 WÜRTZ (1687).

were not isolated cases, as is evident from a listing of the first editions in Latin or a national vernacular of the 38 works examined (Figure 2).[29]

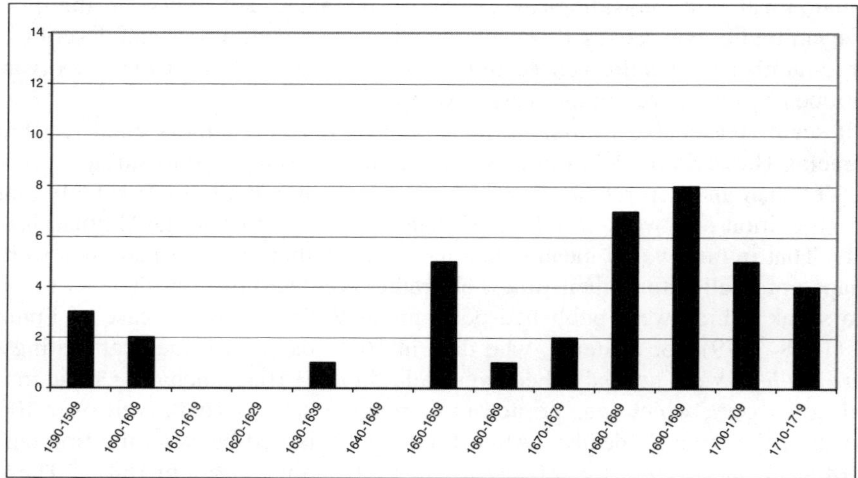

Fig. 2: The graph is based on the same 38 surgical textbooks as Figure 1, but uses the publication date of the first edition, irrespective of language.

When the profiles in Figures 1 and 2 are compared, there is a clear shift to the left that flattens the curve: Among the German editions available in the eighteenth century, 18 were printed after 1700, but only nine were first editions. Thus, the median date of publication shifts back from 1700 to 1685. If we use Harvey's work as a watershed, 5 first editions in fact appeared before 1628, the year of publication of *De motu cordis et sanguinis*, and another six were published prior to 1661, when Malpighi closed the last gap in the chain of evidence. Thus, the work of about a third of the authors Heister described as "the moderns" actually antedates the general acceptance of Harvey's theory.

These findings on the lag between theory and reception show that Harvey's discovery did not in fact constitute a watershed in early modern surgical literature. Evidently, well into the eighteenth century, there was a market for textbooks on surgery in the German technical vernacular that presented a pre-

29 The earliest extant editions in Karlsruhe Virtual Catalogue were used for this list. According to date of publication: Fabricius ab Aquapendente (1592), Dalla Croce (1596), Würtz (1596), Jessen (1601), Fabricius Hildanus (1606), Joël (1631), Gelman (1652), Schmid (1653), Scultetus (1655), Schmid (1656), Barbette (1657), Beverwijck (1672), Herls (1663), Bürger (1674), Blanckaert (1680), Bontekoe (1681), Purmann (1684), Norren (1684), Solingen (1684), Schütze (1687), Munniks (1689), Prat (1690), Jüngken (1691), Muralt (1691), LaCharrière (1692), Nuck (1692), Verduc (1694), LeClerc (1695),Musitanus (1698), Gaukes (1700), Horlacher (1701), Dionis (1708), Leauson (1709), Palfijn (1710), Jondot (1710), Woyt (1715), Verbrug (1715), Cron (1717).

Harveyan, humorally oriented surgical practice. The market must have been sufficiently strong to make reprints of older works potentially lucrative. Indeed, even after 1700, surgical texts continued to be written and published that adhered to the traditional practice of bloodletting. This suggests that these procedures continued to be of everyday relevance for the barber surgeon who still had to be able to open veins in the "old style." In part this demand may well have been due to the wishes of the patients or, in more market-oriented terms, the customer.

Surgical handbooks where venesection was only one topic among many did not make explicit mention of customer demand as a factor. But the three special works on venesection mentioned by Heister took a different approach. Ludwig Cron can serve as a representative source here. He was the personal surgeon of the Prinz zu Schwartzburg und Rudolstadt and author of an instructional manual on venesection published in 1717. He complained copiously about the still widespread belief that venesection was organ specific:

> And there is such a degree of election or selection so deeply entrenched in the thinking of people, both those from a high station and those of a lower estate, that, in the thinking of some patients, the surgeon would almost be committing a crime of lèse-majesté were he to open a vein different from the one deemed specifically appropriate for this sickness.[30]

Cron concludes by assigning to the barber surgeon the role of a subordinate who must carry out instructions, even if that contradicts his own convictions:

> So you have to cut the vein and perform a venesection when the attending physician, patient or those gathered around so desire, and as reluctant as one may be, often open that vein on that specific member where they demand and desire that it be done, although that may be virtually impossible.[31]

Heister's *Chirurgie* (1719) also refers to the discrepancy between the wish of the layman and the more solid knowledge base of the surgeon. Heister here recommended that barber surgeons respond very pragmatically to what the client wanted. Since it was unimportant which vein was cut, one might just as well use the one that the person desiring the venesection preferred.[32]

In the great emporium of bloodletting, demand determined supply, and demand in turn determined the educational and informational needs of the barber surgeon. An author on surgery who dealt with venesection had to address this

30 "Und ist solche election oder Erwehlung noch bey den meisten so wohl hohes als niedrigen Standes-Leuten, so tieff eingewurtzelt, daß auch derjenige Chirurgus fast ein crimen laesae majestatis, bey manchen Patienten, in seinen Gedancken begienge, wann er eine andere Ader für diejenige, so zu dieser Kranckheit gewidmet wäre, [...] liesse," CRON (1717), 38–39.

31 "[...] und sage nur noch kürtzlich dieses man müsse Aderlassen, wann es der Medicus, oder der Patient, oder die umstehenden haben wollen, und offt so ungern als man es auch thut, diejenige Ader und an dem Glied, wo sie es verlangen und haben wollen, wann es schon fast unmöglich ist," CRON (1717), 61.

32 "Man pfleget auf der Hand zwo Adern zu lassen [...] und muß ein Chirurgus solche öffters lassen, [...] weil manche Leut auf diese sonderlich ihr Vertrauen haben," HEISTER (1719), 357–358; HEISTER (1748), 279–280.

need, in doubtful cases even against his better judgment. Ludwig Cron solved this dilemma for himself in a very pragmatic manner – and he was not the only one to do so. As mentioned, in his tractate on bloodletting, he severely criticized the idea that the procedure could be specific to a given organ. In order nonetheless to provide his readers with knowledge that was relevant for their practice, even if outdated, he supplemented his text by an appendix of almost 30 pages.[33] This appendix contains not just a highly detailed list of all veins that were amenable to venesection and their respective specific effect, but also a skinless venesection model body covered with veins, as an anatomical illustration (Figure 3). Both the text and the copperplate etching were taken by Cron from a treatise on venesection published about 60 years earlier by the Augsburg barber-surgeon and municipal surgeon Joseph Schmid. Schmid had been openly opposed to the notion of organ specificity, but he too made concessions to the needs of his co-practitioners by his decision to present this annex.[34]

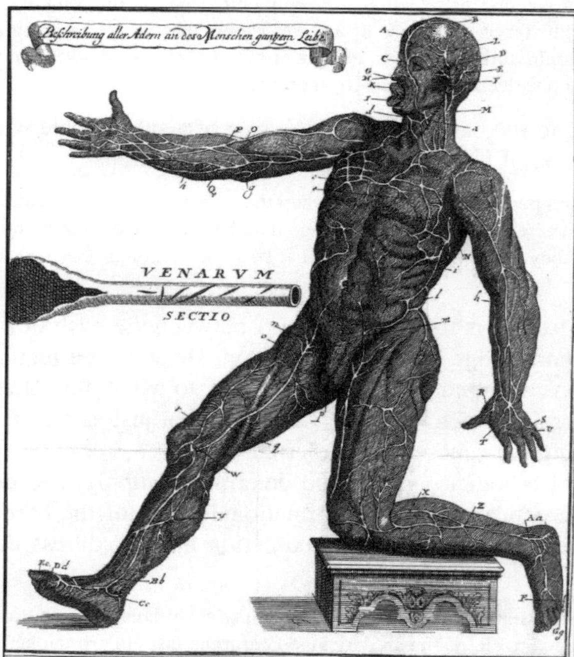

Fig. 3: Accurate Abbildung aller Adern, an des Menschen gantzen Leibe, und wofür eine iede zulassen sey, welches vor diesem von unsern Altvätern gar sonderlich ist observiret worden [Accurate representation of all veins throughout the entire human body, and for which each might be cut, as our ancestors specially observed]. In Cron (1717), p. 199.

To explore the importance of patient preferences for the practice of bloodletting we must consult sources closer to the therapeutic realities than printed textbooks. One such source is the patient letters found in the medical consultation correspondence of the period. Here, I will briefly examine the correspondence of Lo-

33 CRON (1717), 199–228.
34 SCHMID (1653).

renz Heister to shed some light on the practice of venesection from the patient's point of view.[35]

Lorenz Heister's Consultations

Lorenz Heister's written consultations are today located in the Trew letter collection at the University Library of Erlangen-Nuremberg.[36] It comprises 888 documents, both letters to Heister and answers drafted by him, which mainly date from the period 1730–1758. They reflect a total of 304 medical histories, with males twice as frequent as females.[37] Among both sexes and where stated, the average age is about 35, with a wide range from infants to old age.[38]

A statistical analysis of this correspondence with regard to venesection indicates that in two of three histories, the patient neither reported a previous venesection, nor did Heister in his response address this possibility. At least in this correspondence, therefore, venesection did not occupy the dominant position within the therapeutic arsenal that was suggested by some contemporary critics of the practice. Interestingly, the 114 "phlebotomy-positive" case histories do not indicate any gender bias, nor dependence on a surgical option. Women and men, surgical and medical patients all were equally prepared to expose their veins to the surgeon's lancet. The difference was found only at the two ends of the age range, following the customary recommendation never to open the vein of children, and to do so only in special cases when it came to the elderly. Discussion of venesection was by far most frequent in the age group 45 to 54.

Next, we turn to what the 114 phlebotomy-positive medical histories tell us about the way in which phlebotomy was carried out, how its effect was interpreted and who ultimately initiated the procedure. It is notable that venesection, if referred to in patients' letters, was not necessarily connected to a specific treatment. About every fifth correspondent simply informed Heister that he or she, quite apart from the present complaints and malady, was accustomed to a regular venesection at specific intervals and noted the last time one had been performed.[39]

35 See PORTER (1985).

36 SCHMIDT-HERRLING (1940); SCHNALKE (1997). – On the relevance of Heister's correspondence for patient histories, see RUISINGER (2001, 2002, 2005, 2007).

37 In one case, gender was not indicated. Of the 303 remaining correspondence patients, 94 were female and 209 male.

38 In the case of 47% of the women and 40% of the men, there is no indication of age or it is at best far too vague ("junger Herr," "Demoiselle Tochter") to allow for a statistical evaluation.

39 Thus, in 1741 Major von Vegesack reported to Heister that he was "very plethoric, which is why I must have a phlebotomy two or three times a year" ["Ich bin sehr vollblütig, weswegen mich des Jahres 2 auch wohl 3 mahl in die Ader laßen mus"], Vegesack to Heister, October 12, 1741 (UBE BT, Vegesack 1, Annex).

The site of the venesection evidently no longer was of much importance for the patients; for the most part they did not even indicate whether the veins on the arm or the leg or foot had been opened.[40] Only in one case is there any discussion of which veins were opened in relation to a specific organ. Significantly, this is in the earliest letter of the entire correspondence: in December 1716, Esther Lucia von Lindenfels contacted Heister. She stated that because of unspecified female complaints but apparently related to her womb ("*Mutter-Zufälle*"), she had been bled three times, first "on the foot, initially in the saphenous vein, and then in the cephalic vein," and a few months later she had her "median vein on the arm" opened.[41] Mrs von Lindenfels used a terminology rooted in the conception of organ specificity, but here the concepts appear to have already been emptied of their conceptual basis and serve only for topographic orientation in the network of veins – just as when we today still speak of the *vena basilica* and *vena cephalica*. While this assumption does not conclusively indicate that Heister's patients truly rejected the notion of organ specificity, it might suggest that they were aware that their eminent correspondent rejected this notion and knew how to phrase their letters accordingly.

Interestingly, the patients' letters addressed not only when and how they had been bled or were being bled on a customary schedule, but they also mentioned the previous neglect of bleeding or else their total rejection of the practice. In the case of omission, this was important information for the etiological interpretation of the complaint, such as when "for several years running, the otherwise customary venesections had been neglected," and this had caused plethora and related complaints.[42] Those who rejected bloodletting hoped that Heister would recommend a therapy that did without this procedure. Thus, a consistory director Schlüter from Wolfenbüttel let the professor know in no uncertain terms that he "was unaccustomed to venesection and cupping [...], and disinclined to any such procedure."[43] And the report about the Freifrau von Werthern, who at age 28 had already given birth to ten children, noted that she "had never had undergone ve-

40 The formulation in the case of the Landdrostin von Oldershausen, of whom it is reported that she "was bled at the feet in the spring and autumn" ["sie laßen Frühling und Herbst auff den Fußen zur Ader"] is an exception, and the venesection site is probably mentioned mainly in order to get some explanation for the later obstipation (intestinal blockage) which developed; see Naumann, on behalf of the patient, to Heister, May 10, 1754 (UBE BT, Oldershausen 1, Annex).

41 "[...] ich habe zwar schon vergangenen Frühling angefangen mit einer Aderlaß auf dem Fuß, und zwar anfangs in der rosen – hernach in der Haupt Ader [...]. Im vergangenen August Monath habe ich [...] auch die median Ader auf den Arm gelaßen," Esther Lucia von Lindenfels to Heister, December 14, 1716 (UBE BT, Lindenfels 1).

42 "[...] daß d[er] H[err] Patient einige jahre hindurch die sonst gewöhnliche Aderlasse versäumet, wodurch Vollblutigkeit verursacht worden," consultation letter by Heister to Pastor Guthe in Dielmissen, September 25, 1752 (UBE BT, Heister 127).

43 "Zum Aderlaß u. Schröpffen ist Patient nicht gewohnt, auch nicht geneigt," Franz Ernst Brückmann to Heister, June 23, 1752 (UBE BT, Brückmann, F. E. 18).

nesection and was in no way inclined to being bled."[44] A *Medicus ordinarius* noted that his patient, himself an apothecary, had an especially "great aversion to venesection," and that he "had never had a vein opened, [...] and as soon as the snapper or lancet was raised, he would promptly fall into a swoon."[45]

For his part, Heister had a high opinion of the therapeutic utility of venesection. He stood for an iatromechanically reformulated humoral pathology, and used bloodletting in order to influence the quantity and quality of the mixture of humors. On the other hand, the concept of organ specificity had long since become obsolete in the eyes of an accomplished anatomist like Heister. But he considered the local obstruction and blocking of the humors to be an important cause of disease and was convinced that in these cases it was possible to provide relief by properly placed venesection. As a rule, Heister limited himself to naming the half of the body where pressure on the blood should be relieved, and he recommended venesection at the foot, hand or the "healthy side."[46] Only in the case of especially serious local changes did he deviate from this rule, recommending that blood vessels be opened close to the affected body part. In the case of a tumor on the tongue, he suggested the jugular vein be opened in order to "draw off the thick stagnant blood."[47] In the case of a heavy flow from the eye, he recommended opening the temporal artery.[48] On such occasions he even gave a detailed explanation of the effect of bloodletting, as in his answer to a letter from the Hamburg merchant Petrus van Spreckelsen, who had contacted him in the case of a fellow Hamburg burgher suffering from a cataract:

> Although now is not a usual time for venesection, the patient has great discomfort from the *haemorrhoidibus*, which appears not to have sufficient opening to drain. And the nasty plethoric blood in such subjects, as oftentimes observed, presses to the head and brain and often even to the eyes, where it settles and stagnates, blocking the visual nerves and the crystalline corpus, a cause for debility and even blindness in the eyes. Thus, I consider it necessary after giving a [...] footbath to then open a vein in the patient's foot. And after assessing the strength of the patient, left to the judgment of the attending physician, a substantial quantity

44 "Die Patientin hat sein [!] tage nicht Adergelaßen, will sich auch keines weges dazu resolviren," annex by an unnamed writer, attached to the letter by Adolph Georg Freiherr von Werthern to Lorenz Heister, November 4, 1734 (UBE BT, Werthern 1, Annex).

45 "Eine venae sectionem habe [weil] der Herr Patiente eine große aversion für das Ader laßen haben, wordurch es den auch geschehen, daß Sie noch nie mahlen zur Ader gelaßen, [nicht] instituiren können, und bekommen dieselben so bald nur der Schnepper oder Lancet gerühret wird, eine Ohnmacht," postscript by Gustav Adolph Volckmar to his letter to Heister, January 16, 1752 (UBE BT, Volckmar 3, Annex).

46 Draft of Heister's answer to the letter by E. Rischmüller, February 6, 1740 (UBE BT, Rischmüller 3).

47 "Um das dicke stockende geblüt von der Zunge abzuziehen, rath ihm die Halsadern, vena jugularis genannt, welche man am besten sehen kan, [...] zu laßen und ohngefehr 6 Untzen blut wegzulassen," from draft of Heister's answer, March 5, 1750, to the letter of Johann Peter Lorang under the same date (UBE BT, Lorang 1).

48 "Man solle ihm [dem Patienten] auch in 8 Tagen die Schlagader am schlafe öffnen und [...] Blut weglaßen," draft of Heister's answer, December 1, 1752, to the letter of Friedemann Adolf Starck, November 26, 1752 (UBE BT, Starck, F. A. 1).

> of blood should be taken in order that the head, which in such cases tends to be heavy, can be relieved of the excessive plethoric blood, so that afterward the remaining blood can circulate all the more easily.[49]

Nowhere in his letters or in his *Chirurgie* does the anatomist Heister relate venesection to the anatomy of the venous system, the circulation of the blood or the principle of venous drainage. Whenever he explains to his correspondent the mechanism and effect of a recommended venesection, he refers to the humors instead of the solid organs of the body – not only in relation to his patients' letters, but also with regard to his own health. Because Heister, the physician, also emerges in his medical correspondence as Heister, the patient. In his youth, as a result of frequent periods spent in damp dissection rooms, he had "lost his hearing completely for an extended period."[50] The remedies that brought him relief at the time were ones he later recommended to his patients – above all else, venesection at the foot twice a year, in order "to draw the flows away from the region of the head and ears."[51]

Where the localization of the vein to be opened was not indicated by the complaint, Heister left it up to the patient to decide whether he or she preferred the arm or the foot. Venesection of the cubital veins in the bend of the elbow was more risky because here, unlike on the lower extremity, there was danger of injury to the sinews, arteries or nerves.[52] Nonetheless, the arm was the most frequent site chosen, perhaps because the patient was able to maintain better control over the procedure if carried out on the arm and its veins, rather than in the case of manipulation at the foot. But there may have been another reason: the blood

49 "Ob schon eben jetzo keine Gewöhnliche Aderlaß Zeit ist, der Herr Patient aber sehr starck an denen haemorrhoidibus laborirt, welche nicht genugsammen fortgang zu haben scheinen, das üble überflüssige geblüt aber bey solchen subjectis, gleich wie offters observirt, nach dem Haupt und Gehirn und gar offt nach den Augen dränget, sich daselbsten setzet und stocket, die SeeNerven und das crystallinische corpus verstopffet, als wodurch schwachheiten oder gar völlige blindheiten an den Augen entstehen, als halte vor nöthig fodersamst nach vorher gebrauchten [...] Fußbad eine Ader auf dem Fuß zu öffnen, und nach befinden der Kräfften des Herrn Patientens, als welches dem Herrn Medico ordinario zu beurtheilen überlaße, eine gute quantitaet geblüt abzapffen zulaßen, auf daß dadurch das Haupt, das ordentlich bei dergleichen Zufällen schwer zu seyn pfleget, von dem überflüßigen geblüt wohl erleichtert werde, und das übrige hernach desto leichter circuliren möge." Heister to P. van Spreckelsen, February 4, 1738 (UBE BT, Heister 44).

50 "[...] daß ich in meinem jungen Jahr von etlich und 20 Jahren als ich in Holland Audirte und viel im kalten anatomirte mein gehör gantz (und lang) verlohren hatte." Draft of Heister's answer to the letter of Johann Hermann Jacob Glaser, July 7, 1754 (UBE BT, Glaser, J. H. J. 1).

51 "[...] um die Flüße von dem Kopff und Ohren abzuziehen," draft of Heister's answer to the letter of Johann Hermann Jacob Glaser, July 7, 1754 (UBE BT, Glaser, J. H. J. 1).

52 The French surgeon Charles G. LeClerc refers in this connection to the apothegm: "Your arm, you should best entrust, for purposes of phlebotomy, to no one other than a master. But your foot you may give to an apprentice" ["daß man seinen Arm, zum Aderlassen, keinem andern, als nur einem Meister vertrauen soll: Den Fuß aber einem Lehr-Jungen hinrecken mag"], LECLERC (1699), 273.

left the body more rapidly from the large veins in the arm compared to the thinner veins in the foot, and people therefore believed bleeding a vein in the arm offered a more effective influence on the internal flow of the humors.

In conclusion, I want to look once again at this correspondence and focus only on those letters that are both "venesection-positive" and were actually written by the affected persons themselves. These criteria are met by 36 histories in the correspondence. How do patients position themselves in the social setting of a venesection? What respective role do they assign to themselves and their practitioner in this process? What are the dynamics of power between the patient and the barber-surgeon?

First, we note that the patient correspondents act with considerable assurance in the market of medical possibilities, making their selection from the abundance of available options or, to use the language of the time, they "medicated themselves" ("*medicinirten*")[53] and "used medications."[54] That is most especially true for those medical-surgical services which were part not only of therapy but of improving overall health, in particular venesection. In preventive venesection, the "patient" was not the passive recipient of an intervention but a customer who expected his or her instructions to be followed. This role relationship was reproduced and codified in regular venesection in the spring and fall. It continued even after the aim of the surgical procedure shifted when the "customer" fell ill and became a "patient," with preventive care turning into treatment. This lay autonomy is evident in the discourse of Heister's correspondents. Catharina Wackershagen, for instance, informed Heister that "she had opened the vein the past autumn."[55] She chose an active voice, rather than an impersonal formulation (she had a vein opened). The writer did not frame herself as the object of the barber-surgeon and his lancet, but rather retained control over the situation. This turn of phrase is characteristic for patient letters, along with the fact that Mrs Wackershagen made no mention whatsoever of the surgeon who had opened her vein. In her eyes, he was completely interchangeable, and thus non-descript as a person: he simply followed the orders and instructions she had given him, providing a specified service. He remains almost invisible, becoming comprehensible for us in a sense only in the end through the traces which he left on the body of the patient.

53 Thus, when his complaints and difficulties temporarily receded, Stambke observed that "for almost an entire year, he had not been allowed to think of any medicining" ["daß fast ein gantzes Jahr an kein mediciniren gedencken dürffen"] (UBE BT, Stambke 1). Brauer by contrast reported he "had to date not stopped with medicining" ["nun habe mit Medicinniren nicht auf gehert"] (UBE BT, Brauer 1).

54 "God only knows that enough medications have been utilized, but unfortunately this has not been to any avail" ["Gott weiß daß bißhero genung gebrauchet, aber leider keine Hülffe kriege"] (UBE BT, Oelsnitz 1). Heydecke experienced no improvement, though he "used the medications prescribed for this" ["ob ich wohl die hierzu verordneten Medicamente gebrauchte"] (UBE BT, Heydecke 1).

55 "[...] zur Ader habe mich verwichenen Herpst gelaßen," Catharina Wackershagen to Heister, January 10, 1754 (UBE BT, Wackershagen 1).

Conclusion

The theory of the circulation of the blood posed a major challenge to the Galenic interpretation of venesection by breaking with the principle of organ specificity. But the new, modified theory of venesection was accepted only slowly by the textbooks written for the practicing barber-surgeon. This temporal difference in reception of a new theory by scholarly knowledge on the one hand and practical textbook knowledge on the other hand can be explained by reference to the needs of surgical practice. In large part, patients continued to demand venesection in accordance with pre-Harveyan methods. They insisted on personally selecting the specific vein to be opened, in this way maintaining some measure of control over the events within their body. To forego the notion of organ specificity in selecting the site for a venesection would have meant, quite importantly, a potential loss of autonomy. In addition, as a result of regular venesection, a hierarchy of power was generated between the healthy customer and the surgeon. That hierarchy then played a role in actual treatment. The rooting of venesection in a context that was largely external to therapy thus probably contributed significantly to the continuation and survival of pre-Harveyan principles.

Unpublished Sources and References

UBE BT
Lorenz Heister's consultation letters. Trew Collection, University Library of Erlangen Nürnberg. UBE BT (letters from Brauer, Brückmann, Glaser, Heydecke, Lindenfels, Lorang, Oelsnitz, Oldershausen, Ritschmüller, Stambke, Starck, Vegesack, Volckmar, Wackershagen, Werthern; one letter by Heister).

Barbette (1657)
Barbette, Paul: Chirurgie, nae de hedendaeghsche Practijck. (2nd ed.), Amsterdam: Lescaille, 1657.

Barbette (1694)
Barbette, Paul: Chirurgische und Anatomische Schrifften. (3rd printing), Frankfurt: Johann Melchior Bencard, 1694.

Barbette (1718)
Barbette, Paul: Medicinische, Chirurgische und Anatomische Schrifften. (5th printing), Leipzig: Kloß, 1718.

Bauer (1870)
Bauer, Josef: Geschichte der Aderlässe. (2nd printing), München: Gummi, 1870 (reprinted by Werner Fritsch. München, 1966).

Beverwijck (1672)
Beverwijck, Johan v.: Chirurgia oder Heyl-Kunst. Frankfurt/Main: Fievet, 1672.

Beverwijck (1674)
Beverwijck, Johan v.: Allgemeine Artzney. Part 3: Von der Wund-Artzney. Frankfurt/Main: Fievet, 1674.

Blanckaert (1680)
Blanckaert, Steven: Nieuwe konst-kamer der chirurgie ofte heel-konst. Amsterdam: ten Hoorn, 1680.

Blanckaert (1692)
Blanckaert, Steven: Neue Kunst-Kammer der Chirurgie oder Heil-Kunst. Hannover, Hildesheim: Heinrich Grentz, 1692.

Bontekoe (1681)
Bontekoe, Cornelis: Niew Gebouw van De Chirurgie of Heel-Konst. s'Gravenhage: Hagen, 1681.

Bontekoe (1697)
Bontekoe, Cornelis: Neues Gebäude der Chirurgie. Frankfurt, Leipzig: Gottfried Freytag, 1697.

Bröer (1994)
Bröer, Ralf: Grenzüberschreitender wissenschaftlicher Diskurs im Europa der Frühen Neuzeit. Der gelehrte Brief im 17. Jahrhundert. In: Eckart, Wolfgang; Jütte, Robert (Eds.): Das europäische Gesundheitssystem. Gemeinsamkeiten und Unterschiede in historischer Perspektive. Stuttgart: Steiner, 1994, 107–121 (Medizin, Gesellschaft und Geschichte, Beiheft 3).

Bürger (1674)
Bürger, Peter: Candidatus chirurgiae, das ist kurtze doch gründliche Erörterung aller [...] anatomischer und chirurgischer Fragen. Königsberg: [Selbstverlag],1674.

Bürger (1692)
Bürger, Peter: Candidatus chirurgiae. Das ist kurtz doch gründliche Erörterung, aller und jeder fast erdencklichen anatomischen und chirurgischen Fragen. Hannover, Wolfenbüttel: Gottlieb Heinrich Grentz, 1692.

Cron (1717)
Cron, Ludwig: Der bey dem Ader-lassen und Zahn-ausziehen sicher, geschwind, glücklich und recht qualificirte Candidatus Chirurgiae oder Barbier-Geselle. Leipzig: Friedrich Groschuff, 1717 (Reprint by BEGO. Bremen, 1989).

Dalla Croce (1596)
Dalla Croce, Giovanni A.: Chirurgiae universalis opus absolutum. Venezia: Meiettus, 1596.

Dalla Croce (1607)
Dalla Croce, Giovanni A.: Officina aurea. Das ist, güldene Werckstatt der Chirurgy oder Wundt-Artzney. Frankfurt/Main: Jonas Rhodius, 1607.

Dionis (1708)
Dionis, Pierre: Cours d'opération de chirurgie. Bruxelles: Les Frères t'Serstevens et Antoine Claudinot, 1708.

Dionis (1712)
Dionis, Pierre: Chirurgie. Augsburg: Paul Kühtze, 1712.

Fabricius ab Aquapendente (1592)
Fabricius ab Aquapendente, Hieronymus: Pentateuchos Cheirurgicum. Frankfurt: 1592.

Fabricius ab Aquapendente (1716)
Fabricius ab Aquapendente, Hieronymus: Chirurgische Schrifften. Nürnberg: Johann Daniel Taubers seel. Erben, 1716.

Fabry (1606)
Fabry, Wilhelm: Observationum et curationum chirurgicarum centuriae. Basel: Regis, 1606.

Fabry (1652)
Fabry, Wilhelm: Wundt-Artzney. Frankfurt/Main: Beyer, 1652.

Gaukes (1700)
Gaukes, Yves: Praxis medico-chirurgica rationalis. Groningen: Barlinck-Hof, 1700.

Gaukes (1709)
Gaukes, Yves: Wohlgegründete Praxis der Chirurgie und Artzeney-Kunst. Dresden: Joh. Christoph Zimmermann, 1709.

Gelman (1652)
Gelman, Georg: Chirurgiae Tripartita Flora. Das ist, dreyfache chyrurgische Blumen. Frankfurt: Joh. Kempffern, 1652.

Gelman (1680)
Gelman, Georg: Chirurgiae Tripartita Flora. Das ist, dreyfache chyrurgische Blumen. Frankfurt, Jena: Johann Meyer, 1680.

Goethe (2001)
Goethe, Johann Wolfgang v.: Die Leiden des jungen Werther. Stuttgart: Reclam, 2001 (Universal-Bibliothek 67) [Original published in 1774 by Weygand, Leipzig].

Goethe (2004)
Goethe, Johann Wolfgang v.: The Sorrows of Young Werther (new transl. and introd. by Burton Pike). New York: Modern Library, 2004.

Harvey (1628)
Harvey, William: Exercitatio anatomica de motu cordis et sanguinis in animalibus. Frankfurt/Main: Fitzer, 1628.

Heister (1719)
Heister, Lorenz: Chirurgie. In welcher Alles, was zur Wund-Artzney gehöret, Nach der neuesten und besten Art, gründlich abgehandelt, und In vielen Kupffer-Tafeln die neu-erfundene und dienlichste Instrumenten, Nebst den bequemsten Handgriffen der Chirurgischen Operationen und Bandagen deutlich vorgestellet werden. Nürnberg: Johann Hoffmanns seel. Erben, 1719.

Heister (1739)
Heister, Lorenz: Bibliotheca chirurgica, sive Scriptores mei chirurgici. In: Heister, Lorenz (Ed.): Institutiones Chirurgicae. Amsterdam: Janssonio-Waesbergios, 1739, 3–48.

Heister (1748)
Heister, Lorenz: A General System of Surgery in Three Parts. (3rd printing), London: W. Innys, 1748.

Herls (1663)
Herls, Cornelius: Examen der chyrurgie. Middelburgh 1663.

Herls (1692)
Herls, Cornelius: Examen Chirurgiae oder der Wund-Artzney. Nürnberg: Johann Hoffmann, 1692.

Horlacher (1701)
Horlacher, Conrad: Chirurgus extemporaneus per tractationem generalem et specialem enucleatus. Das ist, der mit wenig Artzneyen gründlich und unverzüglich heilende allzeit-fertige Wund-Artzt. 2 parts, Frankfurt, Leipzig: Georg Wilhelm Kühn, 1701.

Jessen (1601)
Jessen, Johann v.: Institutiones chirurgicae, quibus universa manu medendi ratio ostenditur. Wittenberg: Seuberlich, 1601.

Jessen (1674)
Jessen, Johann v.: Anweisung zur Wund-Artznei. Nürnberg: Tauber, 1674.

Joël (1631)
Joël, Franz: Methodum universales curandi morbos. Chirurgi manu utplurimum [!] tractandos. Rostock: Hallervordius, 1631.

Joël (1680)
Joël, Franz: Chirurgia oder Wund-Artzney. Nürnberg: Johann Daniel Tauber, 1680.

Jondot (1710)
Jondot, Philibert: Vollständige Nachricht vom Aderlassen. Regensburg: Hagen, 1710.

Jüngken (1691)
Jüngken, Johann H.: Compendium chirurgiae manualis absolutum. Oder vollkommener doch kurtzer Begriff aller Hand-Arbeiten oder Operationen der Chirurgie. Frankfurt, Nürnberg: Johann Zieger, 1691.

Jüngken (1718)
Jüngken, Johann H.: Chirurgia manualis. Oder kurtzer doch vollkommener Begriff, derer zur der Chirurgie in speciè gehörigen Operationen oder Hand-Arbeiten. Nürnberg: Rüdiger, 1718.

Keunecke (1995)
Keunecke, Hans-Otto: Die Trewschen Sammlungen in Erlangen. In: Schnalke, Thomas (Ed.): Natur im Bild. Anatomie und Botanik in der Sammlung des Nürnberger Arztes Christoph Jacob Trew. Erlangen: Universitätsbibliothek, 1995, 131–164 (Schriften der Universitätsbibliothek Erlangen-Nürnberg 27).

Kuriyama (1995)
Kuriyama, Shigehisa: Interpreting the History of Bloodletting. In: Journal of the History of Medicine and Allied Sciences 50 (1995), 11–46.

LaCharrière (1692)
LaCharrière, Joseph de: Nouvelles opérations de chirurgie. Paris: Horthemels, 1692.

LaCharrière (1715)
LaCharrière, Joseph de: Tractatus operationum chirurgicarum. Oder Abhandlung chirurgischer Hand-Griffen. (2nd printing), Frankfurt/Main: Margar. Gertr. Isingin, 1715.

Leauson (1709)
Leauson, Frideric de: Operationes chirurgicae oder Manualcuren. Dresden: Johann Jacob Winckler, 1709.

LeClerc (1695)
LeClerc, Charles G.: La Chirurgie Complète. Paris: Michallet, 1695.

LeClerc (1699)
LeClerc, Charles G.: Vollkommene Chirurgie. (2nd printing), Dresden: Johann Jacob Winckler, 1699.

Maibaum (1983)
Maibaum, Elke: Der therapeutische Aderlaß von der Entdeckung des Kreislaufs bis zum Beginn des 20. Jahrhunderts. Herzogenrath: Murken-Altrogge, 1983 (Studien zur Medizin-, Kunst- und Literaturgeschichte 2).

Malpighi (1661)
Malpighi, Marcello: De pulmonibus observationes anatomicae. Bologna, 1661.

Mezler (1793)
Mezler, Franz X.: Versuch einer Geschichte des Aderlasses. Ulm: Wohler, 1793.

Munniks (1689)
Munniks, Johann: Cheirurgia. Trier: Franciscus Halma, 1689.

Munniks (1700)
Munniks, Johann: Praxis Cheirurgica oder Wund-Artzney. Frankfurt: Kühn, 1700.

Muralt (1691)
Muralt, Johann v: Chirurgische Schrifften. Basel: Emanuel and Joh. Rudolph Thurneysen, 1691.

Musitanus (1698)
Musitanus, Carolus: Chirurgia theoretico-practica seu trutina chirurgico-physica. 4 vols. Leiden: Cramer and Perachon, 1698.

Musitanus (1701)
Musitanus, Carolus: Chirurgische und Physicalische Schrifften. Frankfurt, Leipzig: Johann Jost Erythropel, 1701.

Norren (1684)
Norren, Erhardt: Chirurgischer Wegweiser. Nürnberg: Johann Hoffmann, 1684.

Norren (1693)
Norren, Erhardt: Chirurgischer Wegweiser. Nürnberg: Johann Hoffmann, 1693.

Norren (1717)
Norren, Erhardt: Chirurgischer Wegweiser. Nürnberg: Johann Hoffmann, 1717.

Nuck (1692)
Nuck, Antonius: Operationes et experimenta chirurgica. Leiden: Boutesteyn, 1692.

Nuck (1709)
Nuck, Antonius: Chirurgische Handgriffe und Experimenta. Lübeck, Wismar: Johann Christian Schmidt, 1709.

Nutton (1993)
Nutton, Vivian: Humoralism. In: Bynum, W.F.; Porter, Roy (Eds.): Companion encyclopedia of the history of medicine, Vol. 1, London, New York: Routledge, 281–291.

Palfijn (1710)
Palfijn, Jan: Nauwkeurige Verhandeling van de voornaemste handwerken der heelkonst zoo in de harde, als sagte deelen van's menschen lichaem. 2 parts. Leiden: Vermey, 1710.

Palfijn (1717)
Palfijn, Jan: Ausführliche Abhandlung, der vornehmsten Chirurgischen Operationen, so wohl an den harten: als weichen Theilen, des Menschlichen Leibes. Part 1. Frankfurt, Leipzig: Johann Jacob Wolrab, 1717.

Porter (1985)
Porter, Roy: The Patient's View. Doing Medical History from Below. In: Theory and Society 14 (1985), 175–198.

Prat (1690)
Prat, Ellis: Vade Mecum Chirurgicum. Oder nothwendiges Handbuch eines Wund-Artztes. (2nd printing), Hamburg: Schultz, 1690.

Purmann (1684)
Purmann, Matthäus G.: Neu herausgegebener Lorbeer-Krantz oder Wund-Artzney. Halberstadt: Johann Erasmo Hynitzsch, 1684.

Purmann (1705)
Purmann, Matthäus G.: Grosser und gantz neugewundener Lorbeer-Krantz oder Wund-Artzney. Frankfurt, Leipzig: Rohrlach, 1705.

Risse (1979)
Risse, Günter: The Renaissance of Bloodletting. A Chapter in Modern Therapeutics. In: Journal of the History of Medicine and Allied Sciences 34 (1979), 3–22.

Ruisinger (2001)
Ruisinger, Marion M.: Auf Messers Schneide. Patientenperspektiven aus der chirurgischen Praxis des 18. Jahrhunderts. In: Medizinhistorisches Journal 36 (2001), 309–333.

Ruisinger (2002)
Ruisinger, Marion M.: Lorenz Heister and the Challenge of Trepanation. A Neurosurgical Case Study from the 18th Century. In: Journal of the History of the Neurosciences 11 (2002), 286–300.

Ruisinger (2005)
Ruisinger, Marion M.: „Mit vielen Trännen schreibe ich dieses“. Ein Beitrag zur Patientinnen-Geschichte des 18. Jahrhunderts. In: Stahnisch, Frank; Steger, Florian (Eds.): Medizin, Geschichte und Geschlecht. Körperhistorische Rekonstruktionen von Identitäten und Differenzen. Stuttgart: Franz Steiner, 2005, 83–101 (Geschichte und Philosophie der Medizin 1).

Ruisinger (2007)
Ruisinger, Marion M.: Patientenwege. Die Konsiliarkorrespondenz Lorenz Heisters (1683–1758) in der Trew-Sammlung Erlangen. Stuttgart: Franz Steiner, 2007 (Medizin, Gesellschaft und Geschichte, Beiheft 28, in print).

Sander (1989)
Sander, Sabine: Handwerkschirurgen. Sozialgeschichte einer verdrängten Berufsgruppe. Göttingen: Vandenhoeck & Ruprecht, 1989 (Kritische Studien zur Geschichtswissenschaft 83).

Schmid (1653)
Schmid, Joseph: Examen Phlebotomicum. Das ist: Gründliche Erforschung unnd Underweisung von dem Aderlassen unnd Schrepffen. Augsburg, Ulm: Johann Görlin, 1653.

Schmid (1656)
Schmid, Joseph: Speculum chirurgicum oder Spiegel der Wund-Artzney. Ulm: Wehe, 1656.

Schmid (1675)
Schmid, Joseph: Speculum chirurgicum oder Spiegel der Wund-Artzney. Nürnberg: Michael und Johann Friderich Endter, 1675.

Schmidt-Herrling (1940)
Schmidt-Herrling, Eleonore: Die Briefsammlung des Nürnberger Arztes Christoph Jacob Trew (1695–1769) in der Universitätsbibliothek Erlangen. Erlangen: Universitätsbibliothek, 1940 (Katalog der Handschriften der Universitätsbibliothek Erlangen 5).

Schnalke (1997)
Schnalke, Thomas: Medizin im Brief. Der städtische Arzt des 18. Jahrhunderts im Spiegel seiner Korrespondenz. Stuttgart: Franz Steiner, 1997 (Sudhoffs Archiv, Beiheft 37).

Schöner (1964)
Schöner, Erich: Das Viererschema in der antiken Humoralpathologie. Wiesbaden: Franz Steiner, 1964.

Schütze (1687)
Schütze, Tobias: Chyrurgischer Handleiter. Leipzig, Frankfurt: Rupert Völcker, 1687.

Schütze (1714)
Schütze, Tobias: Chyrurgischer Handleiter (2nd printing). Berlin: Papen, 1714.

Scultetus (1655)
Scultetus, Johannes: Armamentarium chirurgicum. Ulm: Kühne, 1655.

Scultetus (1679)
Scultetus, Johannes: Wund-Artzneyisches Zeug-Hauß. Frankfurt: Gerlin, 1679.

Solingen (1684)
Solingen, Cornelius: Manuale operatie der Chirurgie. Amsterdam: Jan Bouman, 1684.

Solingen (1693)
Solingen, Cornelius: Hand-Griffe der Wund-Artzney. Frankfurt/Oder: Jeremias Schrey und Henrich Joh. Meyers Erben, 1693.

Solingen (1712)
Solingen, Cornelius: Hand-Griffe der Wund-Artzney. (2nd printing), Wittenberg: Zimmermann, 1712.

Verbrug (1715)
Verbrug, Johann: Examen chirurgicum oder vollkommene Praxis chirurgico-medica. Dresden: Zimmermann, 1715.

Verduc (1694)
Verduc, Jean B.: Les opérations de la chirurgie. Paris: Laurent d'Houry, 1694.

Verduc (1712)
Verduc, Jean B.: Chirurgische Schrifften. 2 parts. Leipzig: Gleditsch, 1712.

Woyt (1715)
Woyt, Johann J.: Die curiöse Chirurgie. Dresden: Johann Jacob Wincklern, 1715.

Würtz (1596)
Würtz, Felix: Practica der Wundartzney. Basel: Henricpetri, 1596.

Würtz (1687)
Würtz, Felix: Wund-Artzney. Basel: Emanuel und Johann Georg König, 1687.

EXPERIENCE, EXPERIMENT AND THEORY: JUSTIFICATIONS AND CRITICISMS OF PHARMACOTHERAPEUTIC PRACTICES IN THE EIGHTEENTH CENTURY

Andreas-Holger Maehle

The eighteenth century is a particularly exciting period for studying the various factors that have an impact on therapeutic practices. This is not only true for social and religious influences but also for conceptual changes within medicine itself.[1] The eighteenth century is known as an age of medical systems or theories which claimed to overcome and supersede the Galenism of the previous centuries.[2] Traditional medical historiography, however, has tended to dismiss these theoretical efforts as exaggerated speculations that were lacking solid empirical foundations, failed to effect a true reform of conventional methods of treatment, and constituted at best rationalizations of therapeutic preferences and practices.[3]

In this contribution I intend to qualify this view by demonstrating how some eighteenth-century therapeutic methods and theories of pharmacological action were actually supported, or at least influenced, by evidence from contemporary therapeutic trials and experiments with drugs.[4] I do not wish to suggest that such supporting evidence should be understood in a modern sense, implying that experiments were used to verify or falsify clearly defined hypotheses. Rather, in order to do justice to the meaning and status of pharmacological and therapeutic experiments in the eighteenth century, one has to let oneself in for their use in this historical period itself. They served as arguments, as it were, in a general European discourse which was concerned with the justification or critique of specific pharmacotherapeutic practices, and which aimed at a rational understanding of the mode of action of medicines.

In the following sections I will illustrate this point through three case studies: on trials with opium, with Peruvian bark, and with medicines for dissolving urinary stones, the so-called lithontriptics. These examples have not been chosen arbitrarily. They represent medical issues that generated numerous publications in the late seventeenth and eighteenth centuries, thus reflecting strong contemporary interest.[5] Furthermore, the choice of these three examples permits discussion of contemporary uses of a traditional medicine (opium), of a relatively new drug (Peruvian or Jesuit's bark), and of so-called secret remedies (lithontriptics).

1 For links between pharmaceutical trade and Pietism, see WILSON (2000); for physico-theological interpretations of drugs, see DEHMEL (1996).

2 See for example RISSE (1992) and PORTER (1995).

3 Cf. KOELBING (1985), 114; ACKERKNECHT (1973), 78; ACKERKNECHT (1962), 395, 408.

4 A full exposition of my argument can be found in MAEHLE (1999). – The research underlying this paper was supported by the Wellcome Trust, London.

5 For a quantitative analysis of the pharmacological and therapeutical contents of relevant eighteenth-century periodicals, see MAEHLE (1999), 9–35.

Opium

Let us start with a quotation from the *Lectures on the Materia Medica* of Charles Alston (1683–1760), who taught botany in the medical school of the University of Edinburgh around the middle of the eighteenth century. He summarized contemporary views of the nature and mode of action of opium as follows:

> [...] some strenuously maintain that opium is cold in the fourth degree; other[s] that it is hot, yea caustic; some that it is an alcali, others an acid; some that it rarefies the blood, other[s] that it coagulates it; some think that its virtues are lodged in its sulphureous, and other[s] in its gummy parts, etc. each accounting for its effects from his own opinions in their own way, though none of them are founded on experience, and easily confuted.[6]

Alston's account not only reflected the parallel existence of Galenist, iatrochemical and iatromechanist views but also of completely contrary positions within these medical systems or theories. However, his contention that none of these different opinions were founded on experience was arguably wrong.

Opium had been known since antiquity as a drug for the relief of pain and for induction of sleep. According to Dioscorides (fl. 40–80) and Galen of Pergamon (129–c. 200) it had a cooling and drying effect on the body's humours.[7] In the seventeenth century iatrochemical authors, such as Michael Ettmüller (1644–1683) in Leipzig and Georg Wolfgang Wedel (1645–1721) in Jena, conceptualized this classical view in a new way. The chemically active substance contained in opium was now believed to bind, fixate, condense, coagulate or even destroy the animal spirits (*spiritus animales*) in the nervous system, thus removing pain and causing sleep.[8] However, at the new medical school in Halle and the older university of Wittenberg (Wittenberg was joined with Halle only under the 1817 medical reforms in Prussia), this interpretation was criticized with reference to clinical and post-mortal symptoms of patients and findings in animal experiments.

A doctoral student of the iatromechanist Friedrich Hoffmann (1660–1742) in Halle, Jacob Descazals, pointed in 1700 to the clinical appearance of patients who had taken opium. Their faces went red, the blood vessels of the head appeared swollen, and sometimes nosebleeds occurred. Moreover, clotted blood was detected in the cerebral ventricles of individuals who had died from narcotics poisoning. Descazals explained these phenomena by assuming a "resolvable and evaporable sulphur" in the opium, which rarefied the blood. This resulted in overfilling of the blood vessels and in slowing, and eventually stagnation, of the circulation of the blood, especially in the brain. With the help of such mechanis-

6 ALSTON (1770), Vol. 1, 40.

7 RIDDLE (1985), 38; SCARBOROUGH (1995), 7; KREUTEL (1988), 24–28; HARIG (1974), 130–131.

8 WEDEL (1674), 35–41; ETTMÜLLER & ACOLUTH (1679), chapters 1 and 2.

tic interpretations this disciple of Hoffmann felt confident to explain all the known effects of opium.[9]

Three years later, the Wittenberg professor of medicine, Johann Gottfried Berger (1659–1736), and his doctoral student, Christoph Fimmler, provided evidence from animal experimentation in support of this mechanist theory. When dissecting cats which had been poisoned orally with opium, they found that the blood was "never clotted, but rather dissolved, serous and fluid." Berger and Fimmler also opened the skulls of dogs that had been stupefied by intravenous injection of opium solutions. The blood vessels of their brains appeared "swollen and dilated," and when they were cut, "bright red, thin and serous blood" flowed out. On the basis of these findings the two Wittenberg authors assumed that the effects of opium were produced through blood vessels, overfilled with thinned blood, pressing on the brain and neighbouring nerves.[10]

In the early 1740s Charles Alston turned especially against such a mechanist understanding of the mode of action of opium. In his experiments on animals and *in vitro* on blood he could not confirm a rarefying effect of the drug. Referring to his therapeutic experience, he pointed out that taking a few drops of *Liquid Laudanum* (opium in alcohol) could remove a violent tenesmus (painful urge for passing stools or water) "in a Moment" and stopped vomiting, eased pain, and induced sleep "almost as soon." He therefore suggested that opium acted directly on nerves, i.e. in case of oral administration on nerve endings in the stomach walls and from there by sympathy or "by Consent" on the whole nervous system.[11] Such a theory of drug action had been propagated, on the basis of many animal experiments with various plant poisons, by the Swiss physician Johann Jakob Wepfer (1620–1695), whom Alston cited in this context. Vivisecting poisoned animals, Wepfer had found that grave symptoms of intoxication such as convulsions already occurred while the drugs had apparently not yet left the stomach and not visibly altered the blood.[12]

These few examples may suffice to show that physiological or pharmacological theories of the eighteenth century were not mere speculations but drew also upon clinical and experimental observations. But, how, if at all, did the formation of such theories affect therapeutic practices? On the basis of the pharmacological and therapeutic literature of the eighteenth century that I have examined, this question can only be answered to a certain extent, namely at the level of therapeutic recommendations made in this literature. Other sources, such as contemporary collections of recipes, doctors' consultation letters or case histo-

9 HOFFMANN & DESCAZALS (1700), 20–23. On Hoffmann's iatromechanism see MÜLLER (1991).

10 BERGER & FIMMLER (1703), 10–13.

11 ALSTON (1742), 160, 165, 168–170.

12 ALSTON (1742), 165; WEPFER (1679). For a detailed discussion of Wepfer's animal experiments and his theory of the action of drugs and poisons see MAEHLE (1987).

ries, and students' notes, can shed additional light on the complex relationship between medical theory and therapeutic practices in the eighteenth century.[13]

Regarding therapeutic recommendations, links with empirically and experimentally supported pharmacological theories can indeed be demonstrated – at least for some cases. For instance, adherents of the mechanist theory that opium thinned the blood regarded conditions such as plethora, apoplexy, paralysis and acute inflammations as absolute contraindications for giving opium.[14] For an advocate of the concept of direct nervous action of the drug, such as Alston, administering opium preparations to plethoric patients was not necessarily forbidden. He, in turn, feared that those who believed in the blood rarefaction theory of opium were making a serious mistake if they treated – according to their logic – opium poisoning with bloodletting. Alston made reference to a case in which a short interval between ingestion of opium and bloodletting had apparently led to the patient's death. Based on his theory of a direct action of opium on the nervous system he recommended the drug particularly for treating "Disorders of the Nerves."[15] This was also true for his Edinburgh colleague, the professor of medicine, Robert Whytt (1714–1766), who believed to have confirmed the theory of the immediate nervous action of opium in numerous animal experiments, especially on frogs. Whytt used opium above all for the treatment of "violent disorders of the nervous and hysteric kind."[16]

The link between pharmacological experimentation and therapy in the eighteenth century can also be demonstrated in the opposite direction, i.e. from therapy to experiment. An example for this is provided by the therapeutic system of Brunonianism, in which opium and alcohol were used as stimulants in treating so-called asthenic diseases. In his *Elements of Medicine* (1788), John Brown (c. 1735–1788) had referred to opium as the strongest stimulant.[17] The question whether opium was primarily a sedative or primarily a stimulant (and only secondarily sedating) led to numerous experimental investigations, especially also because it was still connected with a famous older controversy between Albrecht von Haller (1708–1777) and Robert Whytt on the relationship between sensibility and irritability.[18] Against this background, Alexander von Humboldt (1769–1859), for example, examined the effect of alcoholic solutions of opium on the vagus nerve of a dog, the ischiadic nerve of a lamb, on the axillary nerves of

13 See for example LANZ (1995), 174–176, who sees a connection between Friedrich Hoffmann's mechanistic pharmacological concept and his preference for treatments with simple evacuant and stimulant drugs; and by contrast, RISSE (2005), 11, who identifies a "deep chasm between eighteenth-century medical theories and practices" with reference to Edinburgh physicians such as William Cullen and James Gregory.

14 HOFFMANN & DESCAZALS (1700), 22; HOFFMANN & MULLER (1702), 29–31.

15 ALSTON (1742), 161–162, 171–172, 176.

16 WHYTT (1768), 494, 643–644.

17 BROWN (1788), Vol. 1, 103–104. On Brunonianism see for example BYNUM & PORTER (1988).

18 For a discussion of these experiments see MAEHLE (1995), 60–63. For a recent summary of the Haller-Whytt controversy see STEINKE (2005), 190–193.

frogs, and on isolated frog hearts. Von Humboldt reported that he found in these experiments an initial increase of electrical excitability followed by a stage of atony and lack of irritability, which he attributed to over-stimulation.[19] He regarded these experimental findings as providing confirmation of the Brownian system, or, as he put it in 1797:

> These facts and experiences now convince me completely that opium [...] weakens, sedates, or acts as a narcotic only through over-stimulation. What I have observed in cold- and warm-blooded animals, in voluntary and involuntary muscles, confirms the doctrines of the Brownian school [...].[20]

Peruvian Bark

Having reviewed, through the example of opium, the change of interpretations of a traditional remedy, I would like to turn now to the Peruvian Bark – a drug that was still relatively new in early eighteenth-century European medicine. Peruvian bark, i.e., the quinine containing bark of South American Cinchona trees, began to be shipped to Europe more regularly from the 1640s. It served as a so-called specific medicine against intermittent fevers (malaria). Central to the early imports were South American missionaries of the Jesuit order and the Jesuit cardinal, Juan de Lugo (1583–1660), and the physician to Pope Innocent X, Gabriele Fonseca (d. 1668). It has been suggested in some of the secondary literature that this religious connection promoted the spread of Peruvian bark treatment in Catholic countries, whereas anti-Catholicism may have hindered the acceptance of the drug elsewhere, particularly in England.[21]

The primary literature on Peruvian bark that I have examined points to another, probably more important, obstacle: the fact that the efficacy of the bark in fevers could not be reconciled with Galenist doctrine.[22] The latter required that an effective febrifuge had an evacuant (purging, diaphoretic, or diuretic) action, in order to remove the "matter" that caused the fever from the patient's body. Peruvian bark, by contrast, suppressed fits of fever without having a visibly evacuant effect. Some critics suspected that the bark fixed harmful humours inside the body, thus making the disease even worse in the long run.[23]

Against the background of these difficulties, experimental work on the mode of action of Peruvian bark had been carried out since the late seventeenth century. The Paris physician Jacques Minot, for example, was an adherent of the iatrochemical view that intermittent fevers arose from an excess of acid in the blood and chyle, which could be neutralized by taking Peruvian bark. In order to

19 HUMBOLDT (1797), Vol. 2, 407–414.

20 Cf. HUMBOLDT (1797), Vol. 2, 408. My translation.

21 Cf. JARCHO (1993), 214.

22 This point is also made by JARCHO (1993), 214.

23 See for example the criticism by the Louvain professor of medicine, Vopiscus Fortunatus Plempius (1601–1671), in PROTIMUS [Plempius] (1655), 5–6.

prove that this theory was correct, he performed in the 1680s a series of controlled *in vitro* experiments, testing the effect of the bark on blood and milk (as an analogue to chyle). Minot found that Peruvian bark inhibited the coagulation of these fluids or even rarefied them.[24] This observation did clearly not support the fears of Galenist critics. Johann Balthasar Schondorff, another doctoral student of Friedrich Hoffmann in Halle, reported similar trials in his thesis of 1694. Hoffmann and Schondorff had found, however, an increased coagulation of blood and milk if Peruvian bark was admixed. Nevertheless they arrived, on the basis of mechanist considerations, at a positive assessment of the bark as an astringent and tonic medicine.[25]

This assessment, in turn, was diametrically opposed to that of the followers of Georg Ernst Stahl (1659–1734). For the adherents of Stahl's animism, fever (as well as pain) was a natural reaction of the soul-guided body to "harmful matter." In 1706 Stahl had this theory defended by his Halle doctoral student R. Gottfried Meyer. Peruvian bark was accordingly rejected in this dissertation as a "suppresser of rising nature." Instead, Meyer recommended digestive salts and absorbents in order to help nature in removing the pathogenic matter.[26] In a historical account of the Peruvian bark, the Göttingen professor of the practice of medicine, Ernst Gottfried Baldinger (1738–1804), attributed a delayed acceptance of the bark in the German countries to the resistance of Stahlians. Baldinger wrote that he had still witnessed himself "the hatred against the bark in Halle," and he declared:

> Peruvian bark was in the schools of Hoffmann and Stahl the sibboleth and shibboleth [i.e. password] by which the two parties could be distinguished. The devotionists hate the devil less than the Stahlians the Peruvian bark, and the sight of water shatters the hydrophobe less than the name of Peruvian bark the true follower of Stahl [...].[27]

Despite this resistance of an important school of physicians, the therapeutic use of Peruvian bark was gradually accepted throughout Europe in the course of the eighteenth century. Remarkably, during this process the spectrum of indications for the use of the drug was broadened, so that Peruvian bark developed from a specific against intermittent fevers to a universal remedy.[28] Also in this process therapeutic experience as well as pharmacological experimentation and theories played a role.

24 MINOT (1691), 320–338.

25 HOFFMANN & SCHONDORFF (1704), 9–14.

26 STAHL & MEYER (1706). For recent discussions of Stahlian medicine see HELM (2000), GEYER-KORDESCH (2000) and CHANG (2004).

27 My translation. BALDINGER (1778), 1054: "Chinarinde war in Hoffmanns und Stahls Schule das Sibolet und Schibolet, wodurch beyde Partheyen kenntlich waren. Die Andächtler hassen den Teufel nicht so, als die Stahlianer die Chinarinde, und der Anblick von Wasser, erschüttert den Hydrophobum nicht so, als der Name Chinarinde den ächten Anhänger Stahls [...]."

28 For full discussion of this transition see MAEHLE (1999), 223–309.

Based on therapeutic experience, several British surgeons introduced in the 1730s the internal use of Peruvian bark for the treatment of external diseases, in particular gangrenous leg ulcers.[29] This therapeutic innovation was linked with some scornful comments about the abilities of academic physicians who were officially in charge of prescribing internal remedies.[30] Yet, regardless of professional rivalries, this "surgical" area of bark treatment soon became widely accepted. In the German-speaking countries, this kind of therapy was especially promoted by the Nuremberg physician Georg Leonhart Huth (1705–1761).[31]

In the early 1750s, the British Physician-General, John Pringle (1707–1782), examined in numerous *in vitro* experiments on pieces of meat, egg yolk and blood, whether Peruvian bark and other substances (e.g., snakeroot, chamomile flowers, and sea salt) prevented putridity. The bark turned out to be an effective "antiseptic" (i.e. anti-putrid) substance in these trials, and Pringle therefore supported its use not only as a remedy for intermittent fevers, but also in so-called putrid fevers and in gangrenes – diseases that were relevant to military medicine.[32]

In times of war, shortages of Peruvian bark and rises in its price led to some statistical comparisons with other forms of treating fevers. During the American War of Independence the British naval surgeon Robert Robertson (1742–1829), for example, compared the mortality of sailors suffering from ship fever (probably typhus) who had either been treated with Peruvian bark or with antimony compounds and camphor.[33] The mortality of the sailors who received the bark treatment was lower, a result that made Robertson become a passionate advocate of Peruvian bark therapy for almost all kinds of fevers. Looking back in 1789, he wrote:

> The danger which some theorists threaten us with, from an early and liberal use of the [Peruvian] bark in fever, strikes me with the same idea as if they told me, I should possibly fall, if they saw me running out of a magazine of [gun] powder, which I knew was immediately to blow up by a train leading to it being lighted.[34]

Moreover, following on from Hoffmann's views, the Edinburgh professor of chemistry and medicine, William Cullen (1710–1790), and his students propagated the use of Peruvian bark as a general tonic.[35] Alexander von Humboldt sought experimental proof that this practice was justified. In experiments on isolated nerve-muscle preparations he observed that extract of Peruvian bark re-

29 See RUSHWORTH (1732); DOUGLAS (1732); SHIPTON (1732).

30 DOUGLAS (1732), 14, 33, 41.

31 HUTH (1760).

32 PRINGLE (1753), 309–403.

33 ROBERTSON (1807), Vol. 2, 176–177, 233. For a general discussion of therapeutic trials in the British army and navy during the eighteenth century, see TRÖHLER (2000).

34 ROBERTSON (1789), 371–372.

35 CULLEN (1827), Vol. 1, 639–640; WARREN (1770); BROWN (1779).

stored the tonus and irritability of relaxed muscle fibres. In his view this confirmed Cullen's doctrine.[36]

The example of the Peruvian bark has illustrated processes of appropriation of a new remedy by the European medicine of the late seventeenth and eighteenth centuries. It showed how therapeutic experience, experiments and theoretical considerations interlinked in legitimizing an initially controversial drug treatment. My third case study looks into the adoption of an empirical secret remedy by regular physicians and surgeons in the eighteenth century.

Lithontriptics

So-called dissolvents for urinary stones (in particular bladder stones) or "lithontriptics" had been known since antiquity. Dioscorides, for example, listed as medicines of this type several plant drugs, such as cardamom, laurel, lithospermon, and saxifrage, as well as mineral substances, such as Lapis Judaicus (fossil sea urchin spines) and stones found in sea sponges.[37] Through medieval Arabic authors this knowledge was passed on to the early modern period.[38] From their place in domestic health manuals, lithontriptics appear to have been a popular choice for sufferers from the stone. Taking such an oral medicine, even if its efficacy was doubted, seemed preferable to lithotomy, which was not only painful and dangerous, but could have unpleasant long-term consequences, such as fistulas, incontinence, and impotence.[39] Unsurprisingly, therefore, news of an apparently effective, secret "medicine against the stone," prepared by the English empiric Joanna Stephens (d. 1774), received much public attention.

Supported by the physician and clergyman David Hartley (1705–1757), Mrs Stephens petitioned Parliament for a £5,000 reward for revealing the composition of her secret remedy. A Parliamentary commission of seventeen, including aristocrats, clergymen, physicians and surgeons, came to a positive conclusion about the efficacy of her "medicine against the stone," and after its recipe had been published in 1739, the reward was paid out to Mrs Stephens in 1740.[40] Her secret remedy turned out to be a mixture of calcined eggshells and snails, soap, honey, and various herbs. The proof of efficacy that had convinced the commission consisted of a trial on four patients who had all been catheterized in order to confirm that they had a bladder stone. After several months' treatment with Mrs Stephens's remedy, during which they excreted stony material with their urine,

36 HUMBOLDT (1797), Vol. 2, 421–422.

37 DIOSCORIDES (1902), 28, 100, 108, 141, 355, 374–375, 420, 549–550, 553; RIDDLE (1985), 39, 67, 162,

38 RHAZES (1896), 17–23, 240–241, 246–256; LAUREMBERG (1610), 345–346.

39 See WILSON (1992); COOK (1994), 76–105.

40 VISELTEAR (1968).

the patients were catheterized again: in none of them the stone could be found any longer.[41]

Mrs Stephens's medicine did not only attract much attention in England, but was also made quickly known on the European continent, e.g. by the Halle professor of medicine, Johann Heinrich Schulze (1687–1744), and by the Académie Royale des Sciences in Paris.[42] Numerous experiments with the remedy or its components were carried out on patients as well as *in vitro* on urinary stones. Especially influential were the trials performed by two Fellows of the Royal Society of London, the Reverend Stephen Hales (1677–1761) and the physician James Jurin (1684–1750), and by Robert Whytt in Edinburgh.[43] The results of their experiments indicated that the efficacious components of Mrs Stephens's medicine were the lime from burnt eggshells and snail shells and the soap. Limewater and diluted soap-lye became the two most important lithontriptics in the eighteenth century. They were thought to act by alkalizing the patients' urine. Accordingly, alkaline mineral waters, both artificially produced and natural ones (e.g., Carlsbad water), were also used in treating patients suffering from bladder or kidney stones.[44] Only around the turn to the nineteenth century, when analytic chemistry enabled the distinction between different chemical types of urinary stones, did this therapy become more differentiated.[45]

The process of appropriation of Mrs Stephens's empirical remedy by the regular medicine of her time had some remarkable features. This applies first of all to the efforts to objectivize the efficacy of her remedy in therapeutic and chemical experiments, which led to a debate on the validity of the produced evidence. Another Fellow of the London Royal Society, the physician James Parsons (1705–1770), voiced particularly pertinent criticisms in this regard. Collections of case histories of subjectively cured patients were in his view too unreliable, and even a second catheter examination after treatment was insufficient for excluding with certainty that the bladder stone was still present. He also thought that the results of chemical *in vitro* experiments on urinary stones could not simply be transferred to the conditions in the human body. Especially alarming was Parsons' suspicion that the stony material excreted with the patients' urine did not come from their bladder stones at all but was actually produced by Mrs Stephens's medicine itself.[46]

Besides such awareness of methodical problems and of fallacies of medical evidence, the appropriation of Mrs Stephens's lithontriptic remedy reflected also two other, general phenomena in eighteenth-century therapeutics. One was the reduction of contemporary pharmacopoeias by eliminating very complex com-

41 D'ESCHERNY (1755), 11–20; VISELTEAR (1968), 201–206.

42 SCHULZE AND JETZKE (1739); GEOFFROY (1739); MORAND (1740).

43 HALES (1740); JURIN (1745); WHYTT (1752).

44 See for example SPRINGSFELD (1756); FALCONER (1789).

45 See for example FOURCROY (1804), Vol. 10, 330–343, 352–366; MARCET (1819).

46 PARSONS (1742), 70–92, 111–115, 121–124, 188.

pound and magic remedies.[47] Such simplifications of pharmacotherapy did not necessarily, however, prevent commercialization. James Jurin, for example, had his diluted soap-lye sold through two London apothecaries as a specific remedy called Jurin's *Lixivium lithontripticum.*[48] Secondly, the increasing influence of chemistry on medical therapy became apparent in the eighteenth-century debate on lithontriptics. This influence increased considerably in the early nineteenth century when alkaloids were isolated from medicinal plants and drugs and identified as the physiologically active substances.[49]

Conclusion

This contribution has illustrated through case studies of three types of drugs how pharmacotherapeutic practices became the subject of a European discourse in the eighteenth century. Therapeutic observations and trials, experiments on animals and *in vitro* tests were all used to provide arguments in discussions about the justification of certain forms of treatment. These discussions were not only about the efficacy (or lack of efficacy) of the drug concerned, but also about a rational understanding of its mode of action and, linked with this, about its correct and differentiated therapeutic use. New therapeutic indications for a particular remedy sometimes emerged from such investigations and discussions. Thus, in the eighteenth century a kind of "protopharmacology" emerged as a developing science that increasingly informed therapeutic preferences and choices.[50]

47 See on this phenomenon MATTHEWS (1962), 74–83, and KÜHN (1976).
48 JURIN (1745), 20–21.
49 See LESCH (1984).
50 This term was introduced by LEAKE (1975), 118, and taken up by ESTES (1990).

References

Ackerknecht (1962)
Ackerknecht, Erwin H.: Aspects of the History of Therapeutics. In: Bulletin of the History of Medicine 36 (1962), 389–419.

Ackerknecht (1973)
Ackerknecht, Erwin H.: Therapeutics from the Primitives to the 20th Century. New York: Hafner Press, 1973.

Alston (1742)
Alston, Charles: A Dissertation on Opium. In: Medical Essays and Observations 5/1 (1742), 110–176.

Alston (1770)
Alston, Charles: Lectures on the Materia Medica. Published by J. Hope. 2 vols. London: E. and C. Dilly, 1770.

Baldinger (1778)
Baldinger, Ernst Gottfried: Geschichte der Chinarinde und ihrer Wirkungen. In: Magazin vor Aerzte 2 (1778), 993–1030, 1049–1067.

Berger & Fimmler (1703)
Berger, Johann Gottfried; Fimmler, Christoph: De vi opii rarefaciente, a qua ostenditur omnia illius effecta in homine proficisci. Wittenberg: Gerdesianus, 1703.

Brown (1779)
Brown, George: De usu corticis Peruviani in febribus intermittentibus. Edinburgh: Balfour and Smellie, 1779.

Brown (1788)
Brown, John: The Elements of Medicine; or a Translation of the Elementa Medicinae Brunonis. 2 vols. London: J. Johnson, 1788.

Bynum & Porter (1988)
Bynum, William F.; Porter, Roy (Eds.): Brunonianism in Britain and Europe. London: Wellcome Institute for the History of Medicine, 1988.

Chang (2004)
Chang, Ku-Ming (Kevin): Motus Tonicus. Georg Ernst Stahl's Formulation of Tonic Motion and Early Modern Medical Thought. In: Bulletin of the History of Medicine 78 (2004), 767–803.

Cook (1994)
Cook, Harold J.: Trials of an Ordinary Doctor. Joannes Groenevelt in Seventeenth-Century London. Baltimore: Johns Hopkins University Press, 1994.

Cullen (1827)
Cullen, William: The Works of William Cullen, M.D. Edited by J. Thomson. 2 vols. Edinburgh: W. Blackwood, 1827.

Dehmel (1996)
Dehmel, Gisela: Die Arzneimittel in der Physikotheologie. With a preface by Fritz Krafft. Münster: Lit, 1996.

D'Escherny (1755)
D'Escherny, David: A Treatise of the Causes and Symptoms of the Stone and of the Chief Remedies now in Use to cure this Distemper. London: J. Haberkorn, 1755.

Dioscorides (1902)
Dioscorides: Arzneimittellehre in fünf Büchern. Translated and edited by J. Berendes. Stuttgart: F. Enke, 1902 (reprint Graz: Akademische Druck- und Verlagsanstalt, 1988).

Douglas (1732)
Douglas, John: A Short Account of Mortifications, and of the Surprising Effect of the Bark, in Putting a Stop to their Progress, etc. London: J. Nourse, 1732.

Estes (1990)
Estes, J. Worth: Dictionary of Protopharmacology. Therapeutic Practices, 1700–1850. Canton, MA: Science History Publications, 1990.

Ettmüller & Acoluth (1679)
Ettmüller, Michael; Acoluth, Johannes: Virtutem opii diaphoreticam examini publico exponunt. Leipzig: Brand, 1679.

Falconer (1789)
Falconer, William: An Account of the Aqua Mephitica Alkalina; or, Solution of Fixed Alkaline Salt, Saturated with Fixible Air, in Calculous Disorders, and Other Complaints of the Urinary Passages (3rd ed.). London: T. Cadell, 1789.

Fourcroy (1804)
Fourcroy, Antoine François: A General System of Chemical Knowledge; and its Application to the Phenomena of Nature and Art. Translated by W. Nicholson. 11 vols. London: Cadell and Davies, 1804.

Geoffroy (1739)
Geoffroy, Claude-Joseph: Sur le Remède Anglois pour la Pierre. In: Histoire de l'Académie Royale des Sciences, année 1739, 275–297; 441–446.

Geyer-Kordesch (2000)
Geyer-Kordesch, Johanna: Pietismus, Medizin und Aufklärung in Preußen im 18. Jahrhundert. Das Leben und Werk Georg Ernst Stahls. Tübingen: Max Niemeyer Verlag, 2000 (Hallesche Beiträge zur Europäischen Aufklärung 13).

Hales (1740)
Hales, Stephen: An Account of Some Experiments and Observations on Mrs. Stephens's Medicines for Dissolving the Stone. London: T. Woodward, 1740.

Harig (1974)
Harig, Georg: Bestimmung der Intensität im medizinischen System Galens. Ein Beitrag zur theoretischen Pharmakologie. Berlin: Akademie-Verlag, 1974.

Helm (2000)
Helm, Jürgen: Das Medizinkonzept Georg Ernst Stahls und seine Rezeption im Halleschen Pietismus und in der Zeit der Romantik. In: Berichte zur Wissenschaftsgeschichte 23 (2000), 167–190.

Hoffmann & Descazals (1700)
Hoffmann Friedrich; Descazals, Jacob: De opiatorum nova eaque mechanica operandi ratione. Halle: C. Henckel, 1700.

Hoffmann & Muller (1702)
Hoffmann, Friedrich; Muller, Friedrich Christian: Opii correctionem genuinam et usum [...] proponit. Halle: C. Henckel, 1702.

Hoffmann & Schondorff (1704)
Hoffmann Friedrich; Schondorff, Johann Balthasar: De Chinae Chinae modo operandi, usu et abusu [1694]. Halle: C. A. Zeitler, 1704.

Humboldt (1797)
Humboldt, Friedrich Alexander von: Versuche über die gereizte Muskel- und Nervenfaser nebst Vermuthungen über den chemischen Process des Lebens in der Thier- und Pflanzenwelt. 2 vols. Posen: Decker und Compagnie, 1797.

Huth (1760)
Huth, Georg Leonhart (Ed.): Sammlung verschiedender die Fieberrinde betreffender Abhandlungen und Nachrichten. Nürnberg: J. M. Seligmann, 1760.

Jarcho (1993)
Jarcho, Saul: Quinine's Predecessor. Francesco Torti and the Early History of Cinchona. Baltimore, MD: Johns Hopkins University Press, 1993.

Jurin (1745)
Jurin, James: An Account of the Effects of Soap-Lye Taken Internally, for the Stone, in the Case of James Jurin, M.D. Written by Himself (2nd ed.). London: R. Manby and H. S. Cox, 1745.

Koelbing (1985)
Koelbing, Huldrych M.: Die ärztliche Therapie. Grundzüge ihrer Geschichte. Darmstadt: Wissenschaftliche Buchgesellschaft, 1985.

Kreutel (1988)
Kreutel, Margit: Die Opiumsucht. Stuttgart: Deutscher Apotheker Verlag, 1988.

Kühn (1976)
Kühn, Jochen: Untersuchungen zur Arzneischatzverringerung in Deutschland um 1800. Braunschweig: Technische Universität, 1976.

Lanz (1995)
Lanz, Almut: Arzneimittel in der Therapie Friedrich Hoffmanns (1660–1742) unter besonderer Berücksichtigung der Medicina Consultatoria (1721-1723). Braunschweig: Deutscher Apotheker-Verlag, 1995.

Lauremberg (1610)
Lauremberg, Wilhelm: Epistolica dissertatio, continens historiam curationis calculi vesicae (1610). In: Haller, Albrecht von (Ed.): Disputationes chirurgicae selectae. 5 vols. Lausanne: M.-M. Bousquet, 1755–1756, Vol. 4, 336–346.

Leake (1975)
Leake, Chauncey D.: An Historical Account of Pharmacology to the 20th Century. Springfield, Illinois: Charles C. Thomas Publisher, 1975.

Lesch (1984)
Lesch, John E.: Science and Medicine in France. The Emergence of Experimental Physiology, 1790–1855. Cambridge, MA: Harvard University Press, 1984.

Maehle (1987)
Maehle, Andreas-Holger: Johann Jakob Wepfer (1620–1695) als Toxikologe. Die Fallstudien und Tierexperimente aus seiner Abhandlung über den Wasserschierling (1679). Aarau: Verlag Sauerländer, 1987.

Maehle (1995)
Maehle, Andreas-Holger: Pharmacological experimentation with opium in the eighteenth century. In: Porter, Roy; Teich, Mikuláš (Eds.): Drugs and Narcotics in History. Cambridge: Cambridge University Press, 1995, 52–76.

Maehle (1999)
Maehle, Andreas-Holger: Drugs on Trial. Experimental Pharmacology and Therapeutic Innovation in the Eighteenth Century. Amsterdam: Rodopi, 1999 (Clio Medica 53).

Marcet (1819)
Marcet, Alexandre: An Essay on the Chemical History and Medical Treatment of Calculous Disorders (2nd ed.). London: Longman, Hurst, Rees, 1819.

Matthews (1962)
Matthews, Leslie G.: History of Pharmacy in Britain. Edinburgh: E. and S. Livingstone, 1962.

Minot (1691)
Minot, Jacques: De la Nature, et des Causes de la Fièvre. Du Légitime Usage de la Saignée et des Purgatifs. Avec des Expériences sur le Quinquina, et des Réflexions sur les Effets de ce Remède (2nd ed.). Paris: L. d'Houry, 1691.

Morand (1740)
Morand, Sauveur-François: Examen des Remèdes de Mademoiselle Stephens pour dissoudre la Pierre. In: Histoire de l'Académie Royale des Sciences, année 1740, 177–200.

Müller (1991)
Müller, Ingo W.: Iatromechanische Theorie und ärztliche Praxis im Vergleich zur galenistischen Medizin (Friedrich Hoffmann – Pieter van Foreest – Jan van Heurne). Stuttgart: Franz Steiner, 1991 (Historische Forschungen 17).

Porter (1995)
Porter, Roy (Ed.): Medicine in the Enlightenment. Amsterdam: Rodopi, 1995.

Pringle (1753)
Pringle, John: Observations on the Diseases of the Army, in Camp and Garrison (2nd ed.). London: A. Millar and D. Wilson, 1753.

Protimus [Plempius] (1655)
Protimus, M. [Plempius, Vopiscus Fortunatus]: Antimus Conygius, Peruviani pulveris defensor, repulsus. [No place], 1655.

Rhazes (1896)
Rhazes: Traité sur le Calcul dans les Reins et dans la Vessie. Translated and edited by P. de Koning. Leyden: E. J. Brill, 1896.

Riddle (1985)
Riddle, John M.: Dioscorides on Pharmacy and Medicine. Austin: University of Texas Press, 1985.

Risse (1992)
Risse, Guenter B.: Medicine in the Age of Enlightenment. In: Wear, Andrew (Ed.): Medicine in Society. Historical Essays. Cambridge: Cambridge University Press, 1992, 149–195.

Risse (2005)
Risse, Guenter B.: New Medical Challenges During the Scottish Enlightenment. Amsterdam: Rodopi, 2005 (Clio Medica 78).

Robertson (1789)
Robertson, Robert: Observations on Jail, Hospital, or Ship Fever, from the 4th April, 1776, until 30th April, 1789, Made in Various Parts of Europe and America, and on the Intermediate Sea (New, enlarged edition). London: Printed for the Author by G. G. J. and J. Robinson, 1789.

Robertson (1807)
Robertson, Robert: Observations on Fevers which Arise from Marsh Miasmata, and from Other Causes, in Europe, Africa, the West Indies, and Newfoundland; with Occasional Remarks on the Principal Diseases Incident to Seamen. 4 vols. London: T. Cadell and W. Davies, 1807.

Rushworth (1732)
Rushworth, John: The Great Advantage of the Use of the Bark in Mortifications. With Several Additions. London: L. Gilliver, 1732.

Scarborough (1995)
Scarborough, John: The Opium Poppy in Hellenistic and Roman Medicine. In: Porter, Roy; Teich, Mikuláš (Eds.): Drugs and Narcotics in History. Cambridge: Cambridge University Press, 1995, 4–23.

Schulze & Jetzke (1739)
Schulze, Johann Heinrich; Jetzke, Georg Ludwig: De lithontriptico nuper in Britannia publici juris facto (1739). In: Haller, Albrecht von (Ed.): Disputationes chirurgicae selectae. 5 vols. Lausanne: M.-M. Bousquet, 1755–1756, Vol. 4, 373–393.

Shipton (1732)
Shipton, John: De usu corticis Peruviani ad gangrenam et sphacelum. In: Philosophical Transactions 37 (1732), 434–443.

Springsfeld (1756)
Springsfeld, Gottlob Carl: Commentatio de praerogativa thermarum Carolinarum in dissolvendo calculo vesicae prae aqua calcis vivae. Leipzig: J. C. Langenheim, 1756.

Stahl & Meyer (1706)
Stahl, Georg Ernst; Meyer, R. Gottfried: De tertiana febris genium universum manifestante (1706). In: Haller, Albrecht von (Ed.): Disputationes ad morborum historiam et curationem facientes. 7 vols. Lausanne: Bousquet & Socior., 1757–1760, Vol. 5, 1–39.

Steinke (2005)
Steinke, Hubert: Irritating Experiments. Haller's Concept and the European Controversy on Irritability and Sensibility, 1750–1790. Amsterdam: Rodopi, 2005 (Clio Medica 76).

Tröhler (2000)
Tröhler, Ulrich: "To Improve the Evidence of Medicine." The 18th Century British Origins of a Critical Approach. Edinburgh: Royal College of Physicians of Edinburgh, 2000.

Viseltear (1968)
Viseltear, Arthur J.: Joanna Stephens and the Eighteenth Century Lithontriptics; a Misplaced Chapter in the History of Therapeutics. In: Bulletin of the History of Medicine 42 (1968), 199–220.

Warren (1770)
Warren, John: Dissertatio de cortice Peruviano. Edinburgh: Balfour, Auld, and Smellie, 1770.

Wedel (1674)
Wedel, Georg Wolfgang: Opiologia ad mentem Academiae Naturae Curiosorum. Jena: J. Fritsch, 1674.

Wepfer (1679)
Wepfer, Johann Jakob: Cicutae aquaticae historia et noxae. Commentario illustrata. Basel: J. R. König, 1679.

Whytt (1752)
Whytt, Robert: An Essay on the Virtues of Lime-Water in the Cure of the Stone. Edinburgh: Hamilton, Balfour, and Neill, 1752.

Whytt (1768)
Whytt, Robert: The Works of Robert Whytt, M.D. Published by his Son. Edinburgh: J. Balfour, 1768.

Wilson (1992)
Wilson, Philip K.: Acquiring Surgical Know-How. Occupational and Lay Instruction in Early Eighteenth-Century London. In: Porter, Roy (Ed.): The Popularization of Medicine 1650–1850. London: Routledge, 1992, 42–71.

Wilson (2000)
Wilson, Renate: Pious Traders in Medicine. A German Pharmaceutical Network in Eighteenth-Century North America. University Park, PA: Pennsylvania State University Press, 2000.

„WER SEINE GESUNDHEIT LIEBT, DER FLIEHE DIE MEDICOS UND ARTZNEYEN“ – ZUM VERHÄLTNIS VON MEDIZINISCHER THEORIE UND DIÄTETISCHER PRAXIS

Karin Stukenbrock

In Zedlers *Universallexikon* von 1734 findet man unter dem Begriff „Diätetica“ folgenden kurzen Eintrag:

> Diätetica heißt nicht nur das Speise-Regiment, oder vorgeschriebene Ordnung im Essen, Trincken, Schlaffen, Wachen usw. sondern bedeutet auch den Theil der Artzeney-Kunst, welcher die Erkänntniß und Gebrauch derer sechs nicht natürlichen Dinge lehret.[1]

„Diätetik“ meinte im 18. Jahrhundert demzufolge Anweisungen zur „richtigen“, sprich „gesunden“ Lebensführung. Andererseits bezeichnete der Begriff aber auch den „pädagogischen Teil“ der Medizin, dessen Aufgabe es ist, diese Kenntnisse zu vermitteln.

Die Annahme eines direkten Zusammenhangs zwischen Lebensweise und Gesundheit geht zurück bis in die Antike. Etwa seit dem 5. Jahrhundert v. Chr. hielt man es auf dieser Basis für sinnvoll, sich aktiv um seine Gesundheit zu bemühen. Das Konzept der antiken und spätantiken Diätetik gründete sich auf der hippokratisch-galenischen Lehre von den vier Körpersäften (Blut, Schleim, gelbe und schwarze Galle), die im Gleichgewicht gehalten werden sollten. Der Mensch ist am gesündesten, wenn die Säfte im richtigen Verhältnis zueinander stehen, d.h. wenn die Mischung sowohl in quantitativer als auch in qualitativer Hinsicht stimmt. Ein Ungleichgewicht der Säfte bedeutete demnach Unwohlsein und Krankheit – und das sowohl in physischer als auch in psychischer Hinsicht. Entsprechend war es von großer Bedeutung, für einen ausgeglichenen Fluss der Körpersäfte zu sorgen, ein drohendes Ungleichgewicht frühzeitig zu erkennen und gegebenenfalls gegenzusteuern.[2]

Die therapeutischen Maßnahmen zur Beseitigung dieser Ungleichgewichte richteten sich nach diesem Konzept. Sie klingen deshalb entsprechend konsequent und logisch. Das erklärte therapeutische Ziel war die Wiederherstellung eines kraftvollen Flusses. Ein Ungleichgewicht wurde behandelt durch eine geeignete Diät oder durch die Gabe bestimmter Pharmaka. Dabei wurden Nahrungs- oder Heilmitteln bestimmte Qualitäten zugeschrieben. Wenn man im Körper einen Überschuss an Warmem erkannte, empfahl man Nahrungsmittel

1 ZEDLER (1734), Sp. 734.

2 Dieses Konzept beschränkte sich nicht nur auf den Mikrokosmos des individuellen Menschen, sondern fand seine Entsprechung im Makrokosmos im Verhältnis von Mensch und Natur. Siehe dazu LEMPA (2007), 21–22; BERGDOLT (1999), 24–75; STEGER (2004), 148–149; JÜTTE (1997), 40 und ALBER (1986), 33–34.

mit einer kalten Wirkung, bestand hingegen ein Überschuss an Trockenem, gab man etwas Feuchtes.[3]

Galen hat diese Überlegungen systematisiert und differenziert. Er untergliederte die Diätetik in sechs Bereiche, die später als *res non naturales* bezeichnet wurden. Gemeint waren damit die Lebensumstände wie Luft, Speisen und Getränke, Ausschweifungen und Zurückhaltungen, Bewegung und Ruhe des Körpers, Schlafen und Wachen sowie Gemütsbewegungen. Diese Faktoren konnten stark erwärmen oder abkühlen, befeuchten oder austrocknen, die Nahrungssäfte in ein Ungleichgewicht bringen, fehlerhafte Säfte erzeugen, die Ausscheidungen von überflüssigen Stoffen behindern oder gar die Seele trüben und in Verwirrung stürzen. *Non naturales* – „nicht natürlich", wie sie auch im Eingangszitat bei Zedler erwähnt werden – wurden diese Faktoren genannt, weil sie zwar zur Natur gehörten, aber, im Gegensatz etwa zur Atmung oder zum Kreislauf, als beeinflussbar galten und insofern von den Menschen gesteuert werden konnten.[4]

Wie dargestellt, orientierte sich die Diätetik der Antike und des Mittelalters am herrschenden Medizinkonzept, der Säftelehre. Im 18. Jahrhundert wurde dieses Konzept zunehmend in Frage gestellt. Neue Erkenntnisse führten dazu, dass man nach anderen Erklärungsmustern suchte. Zu nennen sind hier beispielsweise die Entdeckung des Blutkreislaufs durch William Harvey (1578–1657), der ‚Iatromechanismus' Friedrich Hoffmanns (1660–1742), die als ‚Psychodynamismus' bezeichnete Theorie von Georg Ernst Stahl (1659–1734), das Konzept von „Sensibilität" und „Irritabilität" bei Albrecht von Haller (1708–1777) oder der nach Franz Anton Mesmer (1734–1815) benannte Mesmerismus. Gleichwohl erschienen weiterhin Bücher, die den Titel „Anweisung zur Diätetik" trugen.[5] Vor dem Hintergrund der angedeuteten theoretischen und konzeptuellen Umbrüche in der Medizin des 18. Jahrhunderts stellt sich somit die Frage, wie die Diätetik in dieser Zeit vermittelt wurde und welche Rolle dabei die medizinische Theorie spielte.

In der Folge soll daher dargestellt werden, wie sich im 18. Jahrhundert unterschiedliche theoretische Konzepte auf die diätetische Praxis auswirkten. Eigentlich – so sollte man annehmen – hätten sich die „Anweisungen zur Diätetik" aus dem 18. Jahrhundert mit den neuen medizinischen Konzepten verändern müssen. Ob dies tatsächlich so gewesen ist und welche Konsequenzen dies im Hinblick auf die konkreten Ratschläge für die Menschen hatte, soll an zwei Beispielen erläutert werden. Erkenntnisleitend soll dabei die Frage sein, wie sich theoretische Konzepte auf die Gesundheitsempfehlungen für die Bevölkerung auswirkten.

3 STEGER (2004), 148–149.

4 BERGDOLT (1999), 103–109, und VON ENGELHARDT (1996), 107–110.

5 Bereits im 18. Jahrhundert lässt sich allerdings eine Tendenz erkennen, die diesen Begriff auf Fragen der angemessenen Ernährung einschränkte. Um sich davon abzusetzen, wurde der dritten Auflage der Schrift *Die Kunst das menschliche Leben zu verlängern* von Christoph Wilhelm Hufeland (1762–1836) der Oberbegriff „Macrobiotic" hinzugefügt. Siehe dazu RIHA (2001), 80.

Diese Frage soll an zwei Beispielen, nämlich anhand von Texten von Friedrich Hoffmann und von Franz Anton Mai (1742–1814), untersucht werden. Hoffmann schrieb und lehrte in der ersten Hälfte des 18. Jahrhunderts und kann aufgrund seines medizinischen Konzepts als Vertreter einer „klassischen Diätetik im Umbruch“ gelten. Mais diätetische Texte erschienen im letzten Jahrzehnt des 18. Jahrhunderts. Er orientierte sich in erster Linie an sozialmedizinisch-politischen Vorgaben. Beiden gemeinsam ist, dass sie sich in ihren Werken die Aufgabe gestellt hatten, nicht für ein Fachpublikum zu schreiben, sondern die allgemeine Bevölkerung zu erreichen und zu belehren.

Friedrich Hoffmann (1660–1742)

Friedrich Hoffmann hatte in Jena und Erfurt Medizin studiert. Nachdem er einige Jahre in Minden und Halberstadt als praktischer Arzt tätig war, wurde er 1693 auf die erste Professur für Medizin an der neu gegründeten Universität Halle berufen. In seinen Vorlesungen las Hoffmann über Anatomie, Chirurgie, Therapie, Physik sowie Chemie. Sein Erfolg als akademischer Lehrer lässt sich daran ablesen, dass er zahlreiche Studenten nach Halle zog. Die Hallesche medizinische Fakultät wurde unter der Leitung von Hoffmann und Stahl zu Beginn des 18. Jahrhunderts zur führenden deutschen Ausbildungsstätte für akademische Ärzte.[6]

Neben Hermann Boerhaave (1668–1738) in Leiden war Hoffmann einer der konsequentesten Vertreter einer medizinischen Richtung, die die Funktionen des menschlichen Körpers ausschließlich mit Grundsätzen der Mechanik zu erklären versuchte. Der menschliche Körper galt als eine kunstvoll zusammengesetzte Maschine, deren Bestandteile sich so bewegten, wie es sich aus ihrer Form, Größe, Lage und ihrem Zusammenwirken notwendig ergab. Diese Bewegung war das wichtigste Prinzip des lebendigen Körpers. Leben bedeutete nichts anderes als beständige Bewegung; Stillstand bewirkte Verderbnis und war gleichbedeutend mit dem Tod. Krankheiten fasste Hoffmann als Störungen in den normalen Bewegungen der festen und flüssigen Teile des Körpers auf. Aufgabe des Arztes war es demzufolge, dem Organismus zu einer Normalisierung der Bewegungsabläufe zu verhelfen. Die Therapie war zurückhaltend und mild: Im Wesentlichen bestand sie in diätetischen Maßnahmen und in der Verschreibung einfacher Medikamente.[7] Hoffmann stellte mit seinem Werk zwar die theoretischen Grundlagen der Medizin in Frage, er schuf aber auch ein System, mit dem es möglich blieb, bekannte Erklärungsmodelle beizubehalten.[8]

Es verwundert also nicht, dass die Diätetik in den großen medizinischen Werken Friedrich Hoffmanns einen breiten Raum einnimmt. Kapitel zur Diätetik

6 HELM & STUKENBROCK (2006), 657–658.
7 Vgl. dazu auch den Beitrag von Almut Lanz im vorliegenden Band.
8 HELM & STUKENBROCK (2006), 657–658; LANZ (1995); MÜLLER (1991), 275–276 und MÜLLER (1996), 233.

finden sich sowohl in den *Fundamenta Medicinae*[9] von 1695 als auch in der neunbändigen Sammlung *Gründliche Anweisung wie ein Mensch vor dem frühzeitigen Tod und allerhand Kranckheiten durch ordenliche Lebens=Art sich verwahren könne*[10] von 1715 und in dem Werk *Gründlicher Unterricht, wie ein Mensch nach den Gesundheits=Regeln der Heil. Schrift und durch vorsichtigen Gebrauch weniger auserlesener Artzneyen [...] sein Leben und Gesundheit lang conserviren könne*[11] von 1722. Diese Schriften sollen allerdings nicht die Grundlage der vorliegenden Untersuchung sein. Da hier die Frage nach diätetischen Anweisungen für die Bevölkerung im Mittelpunkt steht, wird im Folgenden eine kleine im Jahr 1743 erschienene Schrift analysiert, die Hoffmann für ein breites Publikum geschrieben hat und die ein auf die wesentlichen Hinweise reduzierter Auszug der *Gründlichen Anweisungen* ist. Sie trägt den Titel *Kurzgefaßte Diätetik oder hinlänglicher Unterricht wie ein Mensch durch ordentliche Lebensart, auch wenige und wohlfeile Mittel sich lange Zeit gesund und beim Leben erhalten könne*[12]. Ausschlaggebend sind hierbei die Adressaten des Buches. Hoffmann hat dieses Werk ausdrücklich „zum besten der Unbemittelten und auf dem Lande Lebenden“[13] verfasst. In der Vorrede wird weiter ausgeführt, dass das Buch vorrangig den Menschen nützen solle, die Anfänger seien und die auf dem Lande und insofern weit entfernt von tüchtigen Ärzten lebten. Gelehrte[14] und diejenigen, „die in guter Praxi“ sind, brauchten dieses Werk nicht. Sie sollten lieber das größere, gemeint sind die *Gründlichen Anweisungen*, kaufen.[15]

Diätetische Literatur weist dem Ziel der Gattung gemäß häufig einen stark lehrhaften Zug auf. Entsprechend wird der Stoff üblicherweise in eine übersichtliche systematische Ordnung gebracht, wie etwa die Gliederung nach den *res non naturales*.[16] Dieses Prinzip kennzeichnet auch die Vorgehensweise Friedrich Hoffmanns. Die Artikel der *Kurzgefaßten Diätetic* sind wie in einem Lexikon in alphabetischer Reihenfolge angeordnet.

9 HOFFMANN (1695). Siehe dazu MÜLLER (1996).

10 HOFFMANN (1715).

11 HOFFMANN (1722).

12 HOFFMANN (1744). Eine zweite Auflage erschien bereits im Jahr 1744 und die dritte Auflage im Jahr 1751.

13 HOFFMANN (1744), Untertitel.

14 Die Auffassung, dass eine einseitig geistige Arbeit der Gesundheit schade, führte dazu, dass sich zahlreiche Schriften zur Diätetik explizit mit der Gesundheit der Gelehrten beschäftigten. Insbesondere seit dem 16. Jahrhundert ist hier ein Anstieg zu verzeichnen. Siehe dazu KÜMMEL (1984).

15 HOFFMANN (1744), Vorrede. Hoffmanns Schrift stellt somit eine frühe Form der Anleitungen zur medizinischen Selbsthilfe und -behandlung dar, die spätestens mit den Werken von Tissot und Unzer eine hohe Popularität in der Aufklärung erlangten. Zu Tissot siehe EMCH-DÉRIAZ (2007), 1229. Dort findet sich auch weiterführende Literatur. Zu Unzer siehe REIBER (1999).

16 KÜMMEL (1984), 84.

Unter dem Stichwort „Diät“[17] finden sich zunächst sieben knapp gefasste Regeln:

> 1.) Man muß alles überflüßige meiden. 2.) Man muß nicht allzugeschwind eine Veränderung vornehmen, in demjenigen, wozu man sich lange gewöhnet, weil die Gewohnheit mit der Zeit die andere Natur wird. 3.) Allezeit fröhlich und ruhigen Gemüths seyn. 4.) Sich allezeit einer reinen und temperirten Luft, so viel möglich, bedienen. 5.) Die besten Nahrungs-Mittel, welches diejenigen sind, die unsrer Natur gemäß; in den Magen sich leicht auflösen lassen, und geschwind wieder durch den Leib paßieren, gebrauchen. 6.) Die Speisen soll man nach der Bewegung und Stärke des Leibes abmessen. 7.) Und wenn man seine Gesundheit liebt, die Medicos und die Artzneyen fliehen.[18]

Es entbehrt vordergründig nicht einer gewissen Ironie, wenn Hoffmann als Mediziner mit der letzten Regel[19] den Rat gibt, ärztliche Behandlungen nach Möglichkeit zu vermeiden. Diese Empfehlung zeigt aber auch deutlich Hoffmanns grundsätzliche Einstellung. Die Diätetik ist für ihn ein ganz wesentlicher Teil der Medizin. Er weiß, dass viele Mediziner nichts davon halten, sondern – wie er es ausdrückt – mit großen Arzneien „prahlen“. Für ihn hingegen seien eine gute Diät aus Küche und Keller besser als alle Arzneien.[20] Ein solcher Rat kommt natürlich auch der Klientel entgegen, die Hoffmann ansprechen will. Er möchte Mittel empfehlen, die man sich beschaffen und auch bezahlen kann.[21]

Außerdem propagiert er einen behutsamen Umgang mit Medikamenten. Genau darauf zielt auch seine 7. Regel. In den *Gründlichen Anweisungen* kommentiert er:

> Allein dieses gilt nur für die unerfahrnen und unverständigen Medicos, die nicht vermittelst der Diät curiren wollen/ sondern starcke Artzeneyen wieder alle Kranckheiten gebrauchen oder selbigen vorzubauen gedencken. Welches sich bey verständigen Medicis gantz anders verhält.[22]

In den vorangehenden sechs Regeln fällt eine Anlehnung an die *res non naturales* auf: Hoffmann geht z. B. auf die Gemütsbewegungen, die Luft und die Nahrungsmittel ein. Diese Aspekte werden in den darauf folgenden Ausführungen

17 HOFFMANN (1744), 116–121.

18 HOFFMANN (1744), 116.

19 Hoffmann hat den Aspekt der „Diät“ und auch diese sieben Regeln bereits in seinen *Gründlichen Anweisungen* aufgegriffen. Hier bearbeitet er ihn unter dem Titel „Die ganze Diät oder Lebens=Ordnung/ in sieben Gesetzte oder Regeln eingefasset“ allerdings sehr viel ausführlicher. HOFFMANN (1715), 93–141. Die Syntax des Titels der vorliegenden Arbeit ist aus diesem Werk übernommen. HOFFMANN (1715), 136.

20 HOFFMANN (1722), 253.

21 HOFFMANN (1744), Vorrede.

22 HOFFMANN (1715), 136. In den folgenden Jahren entwickelte sich ein breiter Zeitschriftendiskurs zu diesen Themen. Er richtete sich an ein breites Laienpublikum, aber auch an Experten aus anderen Disziplinen wie Juristen und Staatsbeamte. Siehe dazu WAHRIG (2003). Zum Umgang mit Medikamenten, zur Arzneimittelanwendung und zum Arzneimittelmarkt um 1800 siehe BEISSWANGER (2003).

detailliert beschrieben. Als Voraussetzung für die Bewahrung der Gesundheit gilt eine ausgewogene, der individuellen Konstitution angepasste Lebensweise, in der Maßlosigkeiten jeglicher Art vermieden werden sollen: also nicht zu viel Essen und Trinken, nicht zu viel Gemütsbewegung und Bewegung, nicht zu viel Schlaf usw. Wenn man Lebensgewohnheiten umstelle – was allerdings auch nur in Maßen geschehen solle – könne dies jedoch durchaus kurative Wirkungen haben. Die Erhöhung der körperlichen Aktivitäten könne die Bewegung der Säfte anregen, und durch ausreichenden Schlaf könne der Fluss der Säfte verbessert werden. Sehr feste, salzige, saure, scharfe und fettige Speisen sowie ein Übermaß an weinhaltigen Getränken seien zu vermeiden. Ausgezeichnete Nahrungsmittel sind für Hoffmann Milch, Getreideprodukte, Brot und Fleisch. Gemüse, Früchte und Fisch hält er dagegen für weniger geeignet. Das beste natürliche Getränk sei reines, klares Wasser.[23]

Genauso ausführlich wie auf die Nahrung geht Hoffmann auf die Bewegung ein: Sie befördere

> den Lauf der Säfte durch alle Gänge, vermehret derselben innerliche Wärme, löset das Zähe auf, zertreibet die Feuchtigkeit [...]. Starcke Bewegung verzehret das überflüssige Geblüt so wohl als das Fett. Die Bewegung muß geschehen in einer reinen temperirten Luft, in der Morgen=Röthe, nach der Sonnen Aufgang, vor Tisch, niemahls gleich darnach. Denen so sich nicht bewegen, ist statt dessen gut das laute Lesen oder das Schreyen: auch das Reiten. Die Bewegung muß allmählich geschehen und nicht von ungewohnten allzustarck. Die von schwacher Constitution mögen sich auch mäßig bewegen und sich vor starcker und langwieriger Arbeit oder Leibes=Übung hüten.[24]

Einen ähnlich ausführlichen Eintrag findet man unter dem Stichwort „Gelehrte“. Hoffmann vertritt die Auffassung, „dass das gar zu emsige Studieren dem Gemüte und Körper schädlich sei“.[25] Die Verhaltensregeln, die er mit auf dem Weg gibt, unterscheiden sich allerdings kaum von den Ansichten, die aus dem 15. Jahrhundert bekannt sind.[26]

Außerdem gibt es spezifische Einträge für Männer und Frauen – sie fallen ebenfalls sehr knapp aus. Für den Mann findet sich nur ein einziger Verweis: Mannspersonen, die zu viel Blut haben und sich vor einem Blutsturz bewahren wollen, sollen unter dem Stichwort „Blutsturz“ nachlesen.[27] Bei den „Frauensleuten“ findet sich dagegen der Eintrag: „Sind wegen ihres weichen und schwammigen Fleisches ungesunder als die Manns-Personen.“[28] Frauen werden demzufolge lediglich in Relation zum Mann gesehen. Allerdings hat Hoffmann zu den Frauen weitere Aspekte aufgenommen. Diese handeln von den „Zufällen“

23 HOFFMANN (1744), 116–121. Siehe dazu auch LANZ (1995), 71–73.
24 HOFFMANN (1744), 19–25, hier 19.
25 HOFFMANN (1744), 145–153, hier 145.
26 Siehe dazu KÜMMEL (1984).
27 HOFFMANN (1744), 221.
28 HOFFMANN (1744), 141. Zur Berücksichtigung des Aspekts Geschlecht in der Diätetik Friedrich Hoffmanns siehe auch MÜLLER (1991), 262–263.

während der Schwangerschaft und den Frauenkrankheiten. Gemeint sind die Probleme während der „monathlichen Reinigung“, also der Menstruation. Für diese Fälle rät er, bestimmte Nahrungsmittel zu sich zu nehmen oder wegzulassen. Auch seine eigenen „Hoffmannischen Pillen“ und die Tropfen seines „Hoffmannischen Lebens-Balsams“ fehlen hier nicht. Frauen, die sehr blutreich sind, sollen nicht nur einmal, sondern etliche Male zur Ader gelassen werden.[29]

An diesen wenigen Beispielen wird deutlich, wie eng Hoffmann der Säftelehre verhaftet war. Um gesund zu sein, müssen die Säfte fließen und dürfen nicht zu dick und nicht zu dünn sein. Verstopfungen müssen gelöst und Überfluss vermieden werden. Eine ausgewogene, maßvolle Lebensweise ist die Grundlage für ein gesundes Leben. Ausdrückliche Begründungen, die auf ein theoretisches Konzept deuten, werden in der *Kurzgefaßten Diätetic* nicht gegeben. Hoffmann stellt keine expliziten Verbindungen zwischen seinen konkreten Gesundheitsvorschriften und den Grundlagen seines mechanistischen Körperbildes her. Was jedoch auffällt, ist ein häufiger Bezug zu einem bestimmten Saft, nämlich dem Blut. Hier deutet sich zumindest ein Anknüpfungspunkt zu Hoffmanns wichtigstem Prinzip des lebendigen Körpers, der Kreisbewegung des Blutes, an.[30]

Eine mögliche Erklärung für diesen Befund wird in der Vorrede angedeutet. Es geht dem Autor in dieser Schrift nicht darum, seine Meinung zu rechtfertigen oder andere zu widerlegen. Diesen Aspekt möchte er hier nicht behandeln.[31] Wie Almut Lanz in ihrer Arbeit über die Arzneimittel in der Therapie Friedrich Hoffmanns darlegt, gibt es in den systematischen großen Werken aber durchaus Bezüge, die Rückschlüsse auf sein theoretisches Konzept zulassen.[32] Für den Leserkreis der *Kurzgefaßten Diätetic* wird dies jedoch nicht ausgeführt.

Ähnlich verhält es sich auch im zweiten Beispiel, den Schriften von Franz Anton Mai, obwohl diese vor einem gänzlichen anderen Hintergrund verfasst wurden.

Franz Anton Mai (1742–1814)

Franz Anton Mai[33] wurde 1742 in Heidelberg geboren, besuchte dort das Katholische Gymnasium und studierte ab 1760 Philosophie an der Universität. Im September 1762 wurde Mai zum Doktor der Philosophie promoviert und begann anschließend am gleichen Ort das Studium der Medizin. Während dieser Zeit hatte er Kontakt zu Johann Peter Frank (1745–1821), dem Verfasser des sechsbändigen Werkes *System einer vollständigen medicinischen Policey*. In seinem

29 HOFFMANN (1744), 140–141. Zu den Schwangeren siehe HOFFMANN (1744), 268–270.

30 MÜLLER (1996), 229 und HELM & STUKENBROCK (2006), 657–658.

31 HOFFMANN (1744), Vorrede.

32 LANZ (1995), 105–107 und 172–176.

33 Zur Biographie Franz Anton Mais siehe SEIDLER (1975), 33–58. Vgl. auch LEMPA (2007), 32–34, der sich bei seinen Ausführungen zu Mai allerdings weitgehend auf Seidler stützt.

Werk weist Mai mehrfach auf die Verbindung zu Frank hin, den er als „würdigen Freund und ehemaligen Mitschüler“ ehrt, und dem er sich auch in seinem Ansinnen und seiner Zielsetzung verpflichtet fühlte.[34]

Nach dem Studium erhielt Mai eine Anstellung in der in Mannheim gerade gegründeten Hebammenschule, der eine Entbindungsanstalt für arme und ledige Mütter angeschlossen war. Wenige Jahre später wurde er zusätzlich zum Zucht- und Waisenhausphysikus ernannt. Die Zustände in beiden Institutionen hielt er für unhaltbar und äußerte dies auch. Um konstruktiv zur Verbesserung dieser Missstände beizutragen, ließ er sich 1770 in das Consilium Medicum wählen. 1785 bekam er dann an der Universität Heidelberg die „Lehrstühle der Medizinischen Institutionen und der Hebammenkunst“. Bis zu seinem Lebensende 1814 lehrte er in Heidelberg, wohnte und lebte aber weiterhin in Mannheim. In diesen Jahren entwickelte Mai – wie Seidler es beschreibt – einen „temperamentvollen Eifer“ für sozialmedizinische Fragen, was ihm allerdings nicht immer uneingeschränkte Zustimmung einbrachte.[35] Am nachhaltigsten bekannt aus diesem Engagement ist die Gründung einer Krankenwärterschule.

Mais Vorlesungen waren in der Stadt viel beachtete Veranstaltungen. Sein Ansatz dabei war nicht streng akademisch, sondern hatte einen populärmedizinischen, volksbelehrenden Charakter.[36] Das Publikum war entsprechend heterogen: Nicht nur Studenten, sondern auch Künstler, Handwerker oder Soldaten besuchten seine Vorlesungen. Auch die Kinder ab dem zehnten Lebensjahr bezog er ein. So hielt er „mittwochs Morgens von 10 bis 11 Uhr für die Mädchen, samstags um dieselbe Stunde den Knaben, ohne Unterschied der Religion, öffentliche Vorlesung über die Mittel, gesund, stark, schön und alt zu werden“.[37] Die Grundidee, die Mai in Anlehnung an Frank und die Lebens- und Ordnungsideen der Aufklärung verfolgte, war denkbar einfach: Nur wenn der Einzelne gesund und stark ist, kann auch das Staatswesen gesund und stark sein. Gesundheit als Voraussetzung und Ergebnis einer vernünftigen Lebensführung war somit nicht mehr ausschließlich eine private Angelegenheit, sondern eine gesellschaftliche Forderung geworden.[38] An diesen Maßgaben sollten sich auch die Aufgaben des Arztes orientieren. Hinter den gesundheitspolitischen Zielsetzungen lag die Vorstellung, dass Krankheiten langfristig durch pädagogische Maßnahmen zu überwinden seien, wobei sich die Ärzte als „Freunde und Erzieher des Volkes“ begreifen sollten.[39] Im Zentrum dieses Konzepts stand somit die

34 MAI (1794), Vorbericht, 7. Siehe dazu auch FREVERT (1984), 66 oder ROSEN (1993), 141–143.

35 SEIDLER (1975), 40.

36 Zu den Zielen der ärztlichen Gesundheitslehren und ihren aufklärerischen Charakter siehe auch BERGDOLT (1999), 251–276 und LABISCH (1989), 18–19.

37 Zitiert nach SEIDLER (1975), 54. Die Grundlage dieser Vorlesungen bildete zunächst der 1792 erstmals erschienene *Gesundheitskatechismus* von Bernhard Christoph Faust (1755–1842). Später verteilte Mai seine eigenen Texte an die Kinder.

38 PIEPER (1998), 104.

39 PIEPER (1998), 106.

Vorbeugung, die die eigentliche Aufgabe der Ärzte sein sollte.[40] Mit diesen Einsichten fanden sich enge Anknüpfungspunkte an die antiken diätetischen Lebensordnungslehren, nach denen ebenfalls die Harmonie des Einzelnen mit seiner Umwelt durch eine maßvolle Lebensführung erreicht werden sollte.

Mai verstand es immer wieder, dieses Gesundheitskonzept mit seinen politischen Ansichten zu verknüpfen.[41] Besonders deutlich wird dies in seinen 1793 und 1794 gehaltenen und in seiner Zeit berühmten *Medicinischen Fastenpredigten oder Vorlesungen über Körper- und Seelen-Diätetik, zur Verbesserung der Sitten.*[42] Seit 1789 war Mannheim von den französischen Revolutionskriegen betroffen, die Stadt wurde besetzt und zerstört. Mai sah sich in dieser Situation genötigt, seiner Überzeugung als Monarchist, Katholik und verantwortungsbewusster Arzt Ausdruck zu verleihen und sich gegen die Freiheitsparolen der französischen Besatzer zu stellen. Zwei Tage vor der Hinrichtung Ludwig XVI. beschloss er, „statt dem Publikum in einem gewissenlosen Club Empörungsunrath vorzulegen, öffentliche Vorlesungen über Körper- und Seelendiätetik zu halten".[43] Als Ort wählte er hierzu den Konzertsaal des Mannheimer Nationaltheaters an den von Faschingsbelustigungen freien Samstagen der Fastenzeit. Auf einem Gemälde von Johann Heinrich Wilhelm Tischbein ist Mai während einer solchen Fastenpredigt zu sehen. Neben ihm, direkt am Rednerpult, ist Pfalzgraf Max-Joseph abgebildet. Sowohl der Ort als auch der Titel „Fastenpredigten" sind sicherlich kein Zufall. Der Bezug zur Tradition der Zucht- und Bußpredigten scheint offensichtlich.[44]

Die neun Vorlesungen des ersten Bandes seiner Predigten beschäftigen sich mit den klassischen diätetischen Themen: Essen und Trinken, Ruhe und Bewegung, Ausscheidungen und Gemütsbewegungen. Es ging Mai nicht darum, etwas Neues zu erfinden, sondern darum, diese Dinge öffentlich wirksam zu verbreiten. Er bezog sich explizit auf die großen medizinischen Aufklärer seiner Zeit, wie beispielsweise Johann Peter Frank, Samuel Auguste Tissot (1728–1797) und Johann August Unzer (1727–1799), deren Werke er „erbärmlich geplündert habe".[45] Gleich in seiner ersten Vorlesung, in der es um die nötigen Kenntnisse des „schön eingerichteten Menschenkörpers" und die „altdeutschen Körper- und Seelenkräfte" geht, zeigt er, wie er sich des alten diätetischen Schemas bedient, um in seinem Sinne aufklärerisch tätig zu werden:

> Eine standhafte Gesundheit des Geistes und Körpers ist unstreitig das edelste Gut, das größte Geschenk des unendlich wohlthätigen Schöpfers. Ohne den Besitz dieser angenehmen Gesellschafterin ist unser Leben eine fortdauernde Hausplage; wir sind zum Genuße erlaubter Vergnügungen unfähige, zum Studieren unbrauchbare, und für das gesellschaftliche Le-

40 SEIDLER (1975), 66. Zum Zusammenhang von Prophylaxe und Erziehung siehe auch LEMPA (2007), 24–25.

41 BERGDOLT (1999), 271 und SEIDLER (1975), 77.

42 MAI (1793) und MAI (1794).

43 MAI (1793), Vorbericht.

44 SEIDLER (1975), 77.

45 MAI (1793), Vorrede, 3v.

> ben verlohrne Weltbürger. Gesunde Luft, Mäßigung in Speiss und Trank, in Ruhe und Bewegung, im Schlafen und Wachen, Bezähmung ausschweifender Leidenschaften, Verbannung schädlicher Vorurtheile, Hang nach Rechtschaffenheit, sind die Hülfsmittel eines zufriedenen, gesunden und langen Lebens. Aus diesen Quellen erhält der Staat gesunde Bevölkerung, thätige Staatsmänner, tapfere Soldaten, nicht mit Worten, sondern mit Beispiel predigende Seelsorger, brave Bürger und Handwerker, mit einem Wort, alles was ein Vaterland beneidenswerth machen kann.[46]

Deutlich wird hier der Zusammenhang der Gesundheit des Einzelnen mit der Gesundheit des Ganzen, des Staates. Das eine funktioniert nicht ohne das andere. Jeder einzelne hat für seine Gesundheit zu sorgen, um gesund und lange zu leben. Nur so ist ein gesundes Staatsganzes möglich. Deutlich wird aber auch, dass ein gesundes Leben an eine maßvolle Lebenshaltung in Anlehnung an die *res non naturales* geknüpft wird.

Dieses Konzept findet sich auch in der dritten Vorlesung, die „von dem Einfluß der Speisen auf die Gesundheit und die Sittlichkeit“ handelt.[47] Die enge Verknüpfung zwischen Gesundheit und pädagogischem Anspruch auf Erziehung zur Sittlichkeit sowie von Bezügen dieser beiden Aspekte zum „Nationalcharakter“ werden an diesem konkreten Beispiel offensichtlich. Mai lässt sich in dieser Vorlesung seitenlang über unterschiedliche Nahrungsmittel und deren Wirkweisen aus. Bei der Beurteilung der Eier als Nahrungsmittel beispielsweise hält er sich an den „unsterblichen Boerhaave“.[48] Eier gehören zu den leichtesten und besten Nahrungsmitteln. Besonders nahrhaft ist das Gelbe der Eier – es gibt der schwachen Galle einen guten Grundstoff. Auch schwächlichen Menschen und Menschen, die viel sitzen, wird diese Speise empfohlen, da die fehlerhafte Verdauung, die dadurch entsteht, gebessert werden kann. Als Fastenspeisen eignen sich Eier allerdings genauso wenig wie Fische. Sie reizen mehr die „Begierlichkeiten des Fleisches“, als dass sie sie eindämmen. „Junge vollblütige Geistliche“ müssen sich deshalb dieser Speisen enthalten, um dem Zölibat treu bleiben zu können.[49]

Mai bleibt den *res non naturales* und dem Ausgleich der Säfte verhaftet. Er spricht von der lebendigen Bewegung der Säfte; den Verstopfungen, die durch zu langes Sitzen entstehen und die schwarze Galle plagen; auch er hebt den Umlauf des Blutes als Quelle des Lebens hervor. Was ihn aber deutlich von Hoffmann unterscheidet, ist die Verknüpfung zur Sittlichkeit und zur moralischen Bewertung der Menschen aufgrund ihrer Art der Ernährung. Mai vertritt die Auffassung, dass die Verschiedenheit der Nahrung auf den Charakter und damit letztlich auch auf die Gesundheit der Menschen wirkt:

> Man vergleiche den Fischthran saufenden schwermüthigen Esquimeaux mit dem flüchtigen leichtsinnigen Franzosen; den Nordamerikaner mit dem Europäer; den feistgenährten Höf-

46 MAI (1793), 1. Vorlesung, 6–7. Siehe auch SEIDLER (1975), 78–79.
47 MAI (1793), 3. Vorlesung, 107–148.
48 MAI (1793), 3. Vorlesung, 128.
49 MAI (1793), 3. Vorlesung, 124–125.

> ling mit dem Tagwerker, so wird man im richtigen Verhältnis der verschiedenen Atzung von dem Unterschiede ihrer Gemüthsarten und herrschenden Leidenschaften deutlich überzeuget werden.[50]

Was bei Mai im Vergleich zu Hoffmann außerdem deutlich auffällt, ist, dass Mai in den ersten neun Vorlesungen in erster Linie den männlichen Teil der Bevölkerung anspricht. Staatsmänner, Soldaten, Bürger, Handwerker – das sind die klassischen Männerrollen im Staat. Auch die Ansprache ist deutlich, wenn er sich explizit an die „schätzbaren Jünglinge!" wendet.[51] Frauen werden nicht direkt, sondern über ihren Vater oder Ehemann vermittelt angesprochen. Diese haben dafür zu sorgen, dass jene sich gesund verhalten. So weist er beispielsweise den Hausvater zurecht, der es duldet, dass

> das Jungfer Töchterchen eine Arche Noe aus ihrem Schlafzimmer mache, einige stinkende Schooßhündchen und Katzen, eine Vogelhecke und einen Papagei im Zimmer aufbewahre und sich durch die Ausdünstung und den gröberen Unrat dieser Tiere die Luft vergifte.[52]

Auf die Frage, was Gesundheit für Frauen bedeutet, und auf die Frage, was Frauen gesund erhält, geht er im 2. Teil seiner Fastenpredigten ein. Er hat diese neun Vorlesungen untertitelt: *Vorlesungen über Körper- und Seelendiätetik zur Verbesserung der abgearteten Ehestandssitten, der ehelichen Gesundheit und Kindererziehung des deutschen Vaterlandes.*[53] In diesen Vorlesungen ist der Einfluss Johann Peter Franks deutlich zu erkennen. Im Vorbericht weist Mai selbst darauf hin, dass Frank ihm bei der Ausarbeitung „die Fackel vorgetragen" habe.[54] Die Titel der Vorlesungen klingen auch ähnlich wie die Kapitelüberschriften in Franks Werk von der „medizinischen Polizei". So werden beispielsweise folgende Themen behandelt: von glücklichen Ehen; von den menschlichen Fortpflanzungstrieben; über das Schicksal der Ausschweifungen in der Jugend; für Gattinnen und Mütter und ihre physische und moralische Glückseligkeit im Ehestand; von den Pflichten des Mutterstandes in der Schwangerschaft.[55]

Kommt man vor diesem Hintergrund auf die eingangs gestellte Frage zurück, welche konkreten Ratschläge den Menschen zur Gesunderhaltung gegeben wurden, dann zeigt sich, dass sich hier nichts Grundsätzliches geändert hatte. Die Menschen erfuhren das, was ihnen schon immer gesagt wurde, und das, was sie vielleicht schon immer wussten. Weder die theoretischen Konzepte vom Anfang des 18. Jahrhunderts noch die sozialmedizinischen und politischen Begründungen für die diätetischen Anweisungen vom Ende des 18. Jahrhunderts führten zu entscheidenden Veränderungen in der tatsächlichen Ausgestaltung der Empfehlungen. Anders formuliert: Obwohl sich die theoretischen Konzepte und Be-

50 MAI (1793), 3. Vorlesung, 121.
51 So beispielsweise MAI (1793), 1. Vorlesung, 11.
52 Zitiert nach SEIDLER (1975), 79.
53 MAI (1794).
54 MAI (1794), Vorbericht, 7.
55 Zu den Kapiteln im Werk Franks siehe FREVERT (1984), 66–67.

gründungen innerhalb des medizinischen Systems änderten, führte dies nicht unweigerlich dazu, dass sich auch die praktischen Anweisungen für die Patienten entsprechend änderten. Maßhalten in allen Lebenslagen und eine ausgewogene Lebensführung entsprechend der jeweiligen Konstitution waren dabei unabhängig von theoretischen Konzepten wesentliche Grundsätze zur Erhaltung der Gesundheit.[56] Einzig die Verknüpfung mit politischen Kategorien wie dem „Nationalcharakter" oder die Gewichtung der Kategorie Geschlecht verlieh der Diätetik am Ende des 18. Jahrhunderts eine andere Konnotation.

Eine weitere wesentliche Veränderung lässt sich auf einer anderen Ebene ausmachen. Die Verbreitung dieser populärmedizinischen Ratgeberliteratur nahm am Ende des 18. Jahrhunderts erheblich zu und in diesem Zuge auch der Zugang der Bevölkerung zu solchen Anweisungen. Allein der *Gesundheits-Katechismus zum Gebrauche in den Schulen und beym häuslichen Unterrichte* von Bernhardt Christoph Faust (1755–1842) aus dem Jahre 1794 erlebte in den acht Jahren danach insgesamt neun Auflagen und eine Verbreitung von 150.000 Exemplaren.[57]

56 Dass dieses Konzept auch bei den Menschen in dieser Weise ankam und befolgt wurde, belegt das Beispiel des Kölner Bürgers und Ratsherrn Hermann Weinsberg aus dem 16. Jahrhundert. Vgl. dazu JÜTTE (2005).

57 Siehe dazu BERGDOLT (1999), 249, und LABISCH (1989), 19. Labisch weist in diesem Zusammenhang darauf hin, dass die vermehrte Verbreitung der Gesundheitsanweisungen allerdings nicht uneingeschränkt begrüßt, sondern auch als „Despotismus" kritisiert wurde.

Quellen- und Literaturverzeichnis

Alber (1986)
Alber, Wolfgang: Leib – Seele – Kultur. Diätetik als Modell sozialer Wirklichkeit. Skizzen zur Ideen- und Wirkungsgeschichte. In: Tübinger Beiträge zur Volkskultur 69 (1986), 29–49.

Beisswanger (2003)
Beisswanger, Gabriele: Der Arzneimittelmarkt um 1800: Arzneimittel zwischen Gesundheits-, Berufs- und Gewerbepolitik. In: Wahrig, Bettina; Sohn, Werner (Hrsg.): Zwischen Aufklärung, Policey und Verwaltung. Zur Genese der Medizinalwesens 1750–1850. Wiesbaden: Harrassowitz, 2003, 147–161.

Bergdolt (1999)
Bergdolt, Klaus: Leib und Seele. Eine Kulturgeschichte des gesunden Lebens. München: Beck, 1999.

Emch-Dériaz (2007)
Emch-Dériaz, Antoinette: Artikel „Tissot, Samuel Auguste Andre David“. In: Bynum, W.F. und Helen (Hrsg): Dictionary of Medical Biography. Vol. 5. Westport: Greenwood Press, 2007, 1229.

von Engelhardt (1996)
von Engelhardt, Dietrich: Gesunde Lebensführung als Präventivmedizin. Antike Diätetik im Ausgang von Galen. In: Schott, Heinz (Hrsg.): Meilensteine der Medizin. Dortmund: Harenberg, 1996, 107–113.

Frevert (1984)
Frevert, Ute: Krankheit als politisches Problem 1770–1880 (Kritische Studien zur Geschichtswissenschaft 62). Göttingen: Vandenhoeck & Ruprecht 1984.

Helm & Stukenbrock (2007)
Helm, Jürgen; Stukenbrock, Karin: Artikel „Friedrich Hoffmann“. In: Bynum, W.F. und Helen (Hrsg): Dictionary of Medical Biography. Westport: Greenwood Press, 2007, 657–658.

Hoffmann (1695)
Hoffmann, Friedrich: Fundamenta medicinae ex principiis naturae mechanicis et practicis. Halle: Hübner, 1695.

Hoffmann (1715)
Hoffmann, Friedrich: Gründliche Anweisung, wie ein Mensch vor dem frühzeitigen Tod und allerhand Arten Kranckheiten durch ordentliche Lebens-Art sich verwahren könne. Halle: Renger, 1715.

Hoffmann (1722)
Hoffmann, Friedrich: Gründlicher Unterricht, wie ein Mensch nach den Gesundheits-Regeln der Heil. Schrifft und durch vorsichtigen Gebrauch weniger außerlesener Artzneyen, [...] sein Leben und Gesundheit lang conserviren könne: Deme noch beygefüget ein [...] Bericht von der Natur, [...] deß Ungarischen Weins, und von dem [...] Nutzen der Wasserbäder [...], wie auch von dem Gebrauch und Missbrauch deß Schnupff-Tobacks. Ulm: Bartholomaei, 1722.

Hoffmann (1744)
Hoffmann, Friedrich: Kurzgefaßte Diätetic, oder hinlänglicher Unterricht, wie ein Mensch durch ordentliche Lebensart, auch wenige und wohlfeile Mittel sich lange Zeit gesund und beim Leben erhalten könne. 2. Aufl. Jena, Leipzig: Gollner, 1744.

Jütte (1997)
Jütte, Robert: Therapie im Wandel. Krankheit und Gesundheit im interkulturellen Kontext. In: Neue Rundschau 108 (1997), Heft 2, 37–50.

Jütte (2005)
Jütte, Robert: Krankheit und Gesundheit im Spiegel von Hermann Weinsbergs Aufzeichnungen. In: Groten, Manfred (Hrsg.): Hermann Weinsberg (1518–1597). Kölner Bürger und Ratsherr. Studien zu Leben und Werk. Köln: SH-Verl., 2005, 231–251.

Kümmel (1984)
Kümmel, Werner Friedrich: Der Homo litteratus und die Kunst, gesund zu leben. Zur Entfaltung eines Zweiges der Diätetik im Humanismus. In: Schmitz, Rudolf; Keil, Gundolf (Hrsg.): Humanismus und Medizin. Weinheim: Acta Humaniorum, 1984, 67–85.

Labisch (1989)
Labisch, Alfons: Gesundheitskonzepte und Medizin im Prozeß der Zivilisation. In: Labisch, Alfons und Spree, Reinhard (Hrsg.): Medizinische Deutungsmacht im sozialen Wandel des 19. und frühen 20. Jahrhundert. Bonn: Psychiatrie-Verlag, 1989, 15–36.

Lanz (1995)
Lanz, Almut: Arzneimittel in der Therapie Friedrich Hoffmanns (1660–1742) unter besonderer Berücksichtigung der Medicina consultatoria (1721–1723). Braunschweig: Dt. Apotheker-Verlag, 1995 (Braunschweiger Veröffentlichungen zur Geschichte der Pharmazie und der Naturwissenschaften 35).

Lempa (2007)
Lempa, Heikki: Beyond the Gymnasium. Educating the Middle-Class Bodies in Classical Germany. Lanham, MD: Lexington Books, 2007.

Mai (1793)
Mai, Franz Anton: Medicinische Fastenpredigten oder Vorlesungen über Körper- und Seelen-Diätetik, zur Verbesserung der Gesundheit und Sitten. 1. Teil, Mannheim: Schwan & Götz, 1793.

Mai (1794)
Mai, Franz Anton: Medicinische Fastenpredigten oder Vorlesungen über Körper- und Seelen-Diätetik, zur Verbesserung der Gesundheit und Sitten. 2. Teil, Mannheim: Schwan & Götz, 1794.

Müller (1991)
Müller, Ingo Wilhelm: Iatromechanische Theorie und ärztliche Praxis im Vergleich zur galenistischen Medizin (Friedrich Hoffmann – Pieter van Foreest, Jan van Heurne). Stuttgart: Steiner, 1991 (Historische Forschungen 17).

Müller (1996)
Müller, Ingo Wilhelm: Das mechanistische Körpermodell in der Praxis. Die „Fundamenta“ des Friedrich Hoffmann. In: Schott, Heinz (Hrsg.): Meilensteine der Medizin. Dortmund: Harenberg, 1996, 227–233.

Pieper (1998)
Pieper, Markus: Der Körper des Volkes und der gesunde Volkskörper. Johann Peter Franks „System einer vollstaendigen medicinischen Polizey“. In: Zeitschrift für Geschichtswissenschaft 46 (1998), 97–119.

Reiber (1999)
Reiber, Matthias: Anatomie eines Bestsellers: Johann August Unzers Wochenschrift „Der Arzt” (1759–1764). Göttingen: Wallstein 1999.

Riha (2001)
Riha, Ortrun: Diät für die Seele. Das Erfolgsrezept von Hufelands Makrobiotik. In: Internationale Zeitschrift für Geschichte und Ethik der Naturwissenschaften, Technik und Medizin 9 (2001), 80–89.

Rosen (1993)
Rosen, George: A history of Public Health. Baltimore, London: Johns Hopkins University Press 1993.

Seidler (1975)
Seidler, Eduard: Lebensplan und Gesundheitsführung. Franz Anton Mai und die medizinische Aufklärung in Mannheim. Mannheim: Boehringer, 1975.

Steger (2004)
Steger, Florian: Antike Diätetik – Lebensweise und Medizin. In: Internationale Zeitschrift für Geschichte und Ethik der Naturwissenschaften, Technik und Medizin 12 (2004), 146–160.

Wahrig (2003)
Wahrig, Bettina: „Alle Aerzte sollten also zu redlichen Männern gemacht werden.“ Der Zeitschriftendiskurs zur medicinischen Policey 1770–1810. In: Wahrig, Bettina; Sohn, Werner (Hrsg.): Zwischen Aufklärung, Policey und Verwaltung. Zur Genese der Medizinalwesens 1750–1850. Wiesbaden: Harrassowitz, 2003, 39–69.

Zedler (1734)
Zedlers Universallexikon: Artikel „Diätetica“. Bd. 7, Halle/Leipzig: Zedler, 1734.

Part II:
Therapeutic Uncertainties

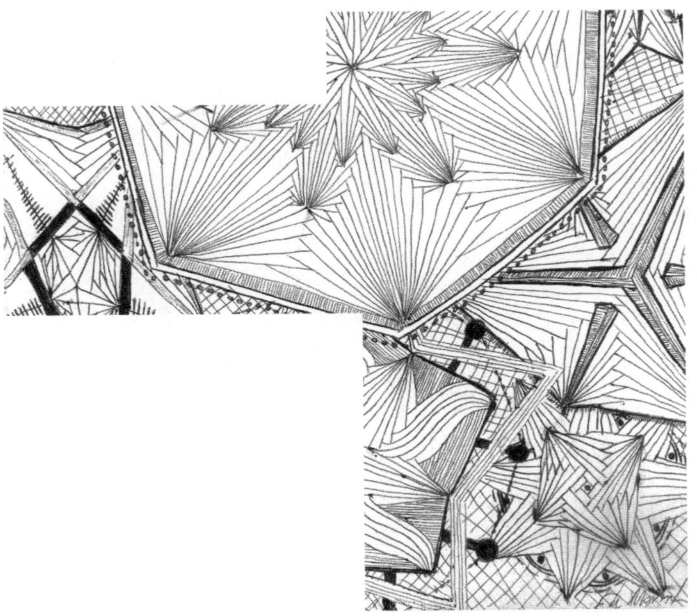

THERAPEUTIC PLURALISM AND CONFLICTING MEDICAL OPINIONS IN THE EIGHTEENTH CENTURY: THE PATIENT'S VIEW

Michael Stolberg

When patients seek medical treatment today, they frequently make a disconcerting experience. The physician seems to arrive at a clear diagnosis and prescribes the necessary medication. But if they then consult another doctor, perhaps because they have not seen the improvement they were hoping for, or simply to get a second opinion, they are given quite different advice or indeed a different diagnosis. In extreme cases, one practitioner may recommend a serious operation, while another advises against it. Getting a third or even a fourth opinion is usually not of much help either. On the contrary, the patients may find themselves confronted with an ever wider range of diagnoses or therapeutic options – even more so if they decide to consult practitioners of alternative medicine, who may have a completely different view of how illnesses arise and should be treated. Their health and even life may be at stake – yet the patients have nothing on which they might base a reliable judgment. The result can be deepening dismay.

The frequent encounters with conflicting medical judgments contribute substantially to an ambivalent perception of professional medical practice among the general public and in the media. The numerous advances and discoveries of modern medicine arouse fascination and admiration. However, they also generate high expectations, which only too often remain unfulfilled when it comes to the individual patient. That is especially true for the chronic-degenerative diseases which loom so large in the daily practice of many physicians. On top of that, doubts and disappointment in the face of limited therapeutic results often combine with a pervasive sense of powerlessness, of being at the mercy of the experts. The concepts and theories of modern medicine, their explanations for the genesis of diseases and for the ways in which they can successfully be treated, remain largely incomprehensible even to highly educated patients.

Faced with this complexity and lack of comprehensibility, many a patient today may harbor nostalgia for the good old days of earlier centuries, when physicians and patients still largely used the same language and operated within a shared world of humoral medicine. However, as this essay seeks to show for the eighteenth century, everyday medical practice in the pre-modern era was in many respects marked to an even greater degree by the patient's experience of contradictory medical opinions. Educated patients were at least able to comprehend the general medical theories and to discuss their diagnosis and therapy on a par with their physicians. But that did not save them from the frequent experience of doctors arriving at widely diverging diagnostic and therapeutic conclusions in the same case.

I will explore this experience of medical disagreement principally from the patient's perspective.[1] My findings will be based primarily on a large number of early modern letters in which the sick or their relatives contacted a physician and asked for his advice.[2] They are the product of the practice of long-distance treatment, which was then quite widespread among the upper classes. Patients with chronic diseases in particular liked to seek additional advice from a distant physician, often a prominent figure in the field. Since this physician was expected to arrive at an exact diagnosis solely on the basis of a written description of the complaint, these letters were often quite detailed. They recounted previous therapeutic efforts and, of special interest for the present research, described previous experiences with other physicians.

My analysis will be based in particular on the correspondence of three physicians: Étienne-François Geoffroy (1672–1731) in Paris, Christoph Jakob Trew (1695–1769) in Erlangen, and Samuel Auguste Tissot (1728–1797) in Lausanne.[3] For comparative purposes, I will also include the extensive correspondence which the famous Paracelsian Leonhard Thurneisser (1531–1596) conducted with his patients a good two centuries earlier.[4] In geographic terms, most letters therefore come from Germany, France, and Switzerland. In addition to these manuscript sources, I have also used patient letters inserted into contemporary collections of medical case histories as well as published private correspondence and autobiographies. In these contexts, criticism of the physicians involved and of their contradictory judgments is sometimes expressed far more clearly and sharply than in the direct epistolary exchanges between patients and physicians.

A major limitation of all these sources is, of course, that they largely reflect the views and experiences of educated patients. The experiences and practices of the lower orders are accessible only in exceptional cases, for example through records of proceedings against irregular healers.[5] For the purpose of this study this is not a serious drawback, however, because in the eighteenth century, upper-class patients predominated in many doctors' offices. Poorer and less educated patients in turn may well have had quite similar experiences with the contradictory diagnoses and advice of barber-surgeons and village healers. Indeed in these milieus, patients often found themselves confronted with an even broader range of possible interpretations and treatment options, including supernatural forces and corresponding magical, sympathetic, and religious healing practices.

1 Since the mid-1980s, medical history from the patient's view has developed into a fruitful subfield; see PORTER (1985a and 1985b); DUDEN (1987); PORTER & PORTER (1989a and 1989b); JÜTTE (1991); STOLBERG (2003).

2 On the genre of *Patientenbriefe*, see STOLBERG (1996).

3 For the sources, see Bibliothèque Interuniversitaire de Médecine (BIM), Paris, Mss. 5241–5245; Bibliothèque Cantonale et Universitaire, Lausanne-Dorigny, Fonds Tissot (hereafter: FT); Universitätsbibliothek Erlangen, Trew-Korrespondenz (hereafter: TREW).

4 Staatsbibliothek Berlin, Ms. germ. fol. 99 and 420a–426 (hereafter: SBB).

5 POMATA (1994).

Medical Disagreement in Everyday Life

Eighteenth-century letters of consultations provide ample evidence that patients and their families often found that their physicians arrived at very different conclusions. One reason for this was that patients with prolonged disorders or diseases were seldom satisfied with a single medical opinion. Many of them had a personal doctor, a *medicus ordinarius,* whom they usually consulted first. But when their health did not seem to improve, they frequently asked for a second opinion from another doctor. The chronically ill in particular, who had consulted various medical practitioners simultaneously or one after the other, talked bitterly and indeed desperately about how they had been confronted time and again with new and conflicting diagnoses and prescriptions. For example, a Mme Konauw reported how she had consulted more than 10 doctors, and how each had started all over again from the beginning. Now she set her hopes on Tissot's advice.[6] Many patients like her spent large amounts of money on physicians and medicines, only to find that they were growing ever weaker from the medication or that their intestines were "clogged" or "overheated" by laxatives, or that their whole body was wrecked by the medication which they had been administered in all too copious amounts.

To be sure, complaints about mutually exclusive medical opinions can be found even earlier, in the heyday of Galenic medicine. Thus, in 1614, P. D. Steelant lamented that he no longer knew whom to believe and what to do, since his doctors' advice was so contradictory.[7] "One says this, another that," the Augsburg merchant Lucas Rem summed up his experience in 1520. His doctors could not agree whether his disease was due to excessive humoral flows, as he himself thought, or to other natural causes, or if it stemmed from poison, or was the work of the spell caused by a woman.[8] Some thought he had intestinal colic, others suspected a diseased gall bladder, reported the exasperated Guido von Boetzelaar in 1591. In his view, the location of his acute pain and the perceptible hardening over his navel spoke against both diagnoses. He believed his stomach was to blame.[9]

For the eighteenth century, such accounts are legion. Sometimes the physicians disagreed about simple practical questions. Thus, in the early eighteenth century, a young woman turned in despair to her female friend. She had been suffering for a number of days from a terrible shortness of breath. She could hardly take two steps and was immediately overcome by an intolerable feeling of constriction in her chest. Her breathing was accompanied by a rattling sound, as she wrote, as though she were in agony, on the brink of death. In addition she

6 FT, letter from Mme de Konauw, 26 January 1773.

7 Rijksarchief Arnhem, Archive of the Counts of Coulembourg, Ms. 403, letter from P. D. Steelants: September 17, 1614.

8 Rem (1861), 23: "[...] ainer diz, ander jens."

9 Universiteitsbibliotheek Leiden, Ms. Marchand 3, letters to Johannes and Otto Heurne, here letter from G. von Boetzelaar, 14 December 1591.

had intense pains in her shoulders, legs and head, and sometimes also around the heart. One of her doctors had recommended urgent phlebotomy. Perhaps he thought the cause of the malady was a "plethoric" congestion of the tissues and the heart. But another doctor had been just as adamant in dissuading her from blood-letting. She was dismayed: what should she do? It was a quite simple question: phlebotomy, yes or no? But for her it was literally a matter of life and death. Whichever way she decided, she risked making a fatal mistake. She was without a clue.[10]

Some patients found themselves facing a whole array of differing opinions and plans for treatment. Giuseppe Barbaroux from Turin had long felt morose and was plagued by melancholy. He complained of constant pains in his back and loins and a feeling of heaviness in his buttocks. He was also suffering from a urethral discharge and nocturnal seminal pollutions, which were at the time dreaded as a cause of emaciation and other maladies. In Tissot's famous work on onanism[11] he had, according to his own words, found his malady "described at length" and attributed his disease especially to his earlier habitual masturbation. But the success of the treatment left much to be desired. The first doctor gave him an elixir of sulphuric acid, which caused him to vomit profusely. The doctor insisted on his therapy, but Barbaroux did not want to continue and consulted a second physician who chose a quite different approach. He recommended whey in which a glowing iron had been dipped, and alcohol with dulcamara as a remedy. The complaints improved temporarily, but then returned. So Barbaroux went to a third physician, who harshly took issue with the two previous colleagues and their choice of remedy. In the end, the patient was left bewildered and had no idea whom he should trust. So he decided to put his hope in the famous Docteur Tissot.[12]

In other cases not only the right treatment but the very nature of the disease was a matter of dispute. A 44-year-old army captain complained in 1773 that

> I see that each and every one I have consulted about the causes of my illness gives an elusive answer, and for that reason are very uncertain as to what remedies they should give me.[13]

He suffered from a stubborn rash and had tried a whole series of remedies. But instead of helping him, they had given him a colic or "set his body on fire."[14] For the patients and their loved ones, this was a very disconcerting experience. Like the medical profession, patients believed that an effective therapy required a

10 BIM, Ms. 5241, fol. 79r–v undated letter from a patient with "asthma."

11 TISSOT (1760).

12 FT, letter from Giuseppe Barbaroux (Turin), 21 August 1793: "[...] a lungo trattato del mio male."

13 FT, letter from M. Herbelot (Antibes), 9 June 1773: "[…] je vois tous ceux que j'ai consulté tergiverser sur les causes de mon mal et par conséquent très incertains sur les remèdes qu'ils doivent me donner."

14 FT, letter from M. Herbelot (Antibes), 9 June 1773: "[...] m'a mis le feu dans le corps."

clear diagnosis. For only if the malady and its effect on the body had been deciphered was it possible to treat it specifically, by addressing its roots or causes.

As often, the individual doctor decided on a specific diagnosis but was soon contradicted by another. M. de Walmoden, for example, consulted Tissot, asking him to help him regain his trust in the medical profession. Among other complaints, he suffered from pain in the chest, a foul-smelling expectoration, stomach pains and cramps, along with a cloudy urine. His physicians had led him down a confusing path from one speculation or presumption to the next.

> First they thought everything was a disease of the chest, then a weakness of digestion, then an expectoration of pus, after that poisonous morbid matter, then hemorrhoids.

In the end he feared that instead of getting any nearer to the truth about his condition, they were getting ever further away from it. But his own arguments were insufficient to confront and refute the contradictory judgments of his physicians.[15]

The Limits of Medical Diagnosis

The range of contradictory diagnoses described by Walmoden was exceptional. Yet a profound sense of insecurity among patients due to contradictory and conflicting medical opinions can be found in numerous other letters from patients and families. As the examples suggest, the reasons for such contradictions were many and diverse.

Viewed from today's vantage point, a first important cause was the limited reach of contemporary diagnosis. Physicians had to base their judgment principally on the patient's narrative. Indeed, as the popularity of consulting by letter shows, a mere written account could seem sufficient. At the patient's bedside, the physicians might also note visible external changes, swollen limbs for example, or a dry tongue or a rash. Contrary to what is widely believed, patients in the eighteenth century were also quite often given a direct physical examination when a tumor or a local accumulation of morbid matter was suspected. Within the various, mostly humoral medical theories of the day, however, the patient's narrative, even when it was supported by a physical examination, often offered only very limited and ambiguous diagnostic clues. Especially in the case of chronic or more complicated diseases, the physician frequently could only put forward the most likely among various possible explanations to account for the patient's complaints. The physicians at the time were quite aware of this and

15 FT, letter from M. de Walmoden, n.d.: "[...] un moment tout a été reputé maux de poitrine, un autre tout foiblesse de digestion, un autre tout crachemant de pus, tubercule, ensuite tout virus, ensuite tout hemorrhoides, enfin vous scavez, Monsieur, qu'en me faisant aller de supposition en supposition et toujours éloigner de la veritable, je ne pourrois jamais couper court a ces jugemens par mes propres argumens; je dois les trouver dans la bonté que vous aurez de me donner."

sometimes openly communicated their uncertainty to their patients. Expressions such as "the most probable explanation as I see it" were widespread. They clearly indicated to patients and relatives that the physician was not completely confident about his diagnosis and could therefore not assume full responsibility should either diagnosis or prognosis turn out to be mistaken.

This sense of diagnostic uncertainty was further heightened by the fact that learned physicians usually wanted to offer a causal explanation of the complaint or disease in question. The claim that they alone, thanks to their learning, could explain the underlying pathological processes within the body and could target their treatment accordingly was a major aspect of their professional self-fashioning. It served as a mark of distinction in their fierce battle against the unlearned "empirics." And their educated patients had come to expect such an explanation of the causes of their problem and the way the proposed therapy was going to act against it. For example, a physician might attribute a patient's visible physical deterioration, weakness, and lack of appetite to the effect of phlegm which had accumulated in the upper abdomen due to a weak stomach and insufficient digestion. Based on this assessment he might suggest medicine to empty out the phlegm and strengthen the stomach. Yet another physician might explain the disease in a rather different but similarly plausible manner, arguing it was the consequence of acrid or "scorbutic" blood, which called for blood-letting and medicines which would soften the "sharpness" of the blood.

The Pluralism of Theories

In addition to the limited and often ambiguous diagnostic value of subjective complaints and physical signs, medical disagreement at the bedside was further intensified by conflicting medical theories. Depending on the theoretical framework, symptoms and diagnostic signs could assume widely divergent meanings.[16] It goes without saying that physicians who did not even agree on the most basic premises of physiology and pathology were bound to arrive also at a different diagnosis and therapeutic recommendations when they put their theories into practice at the bedside.

The various medical schools of the eighteenth century and their leading representatives have been studied extensively. Some physicians walked in the footsteps of Johann Baptist van Helmont (1579–1644) and iatrochemistry; they based their diagnoses on acidities and alkalis, fermentations and effervescences. Others resorted to mechanistic-hydraulic theories. For example, they attributed paramount importance to the "plethora," that is to the effects of excessive amounts of blood in the body, which led to local or general blood congestion and slowed down the circulation. Georg Ernst Stahl (1660–1734) and his followers,

16 For overviews of European medicine in the 18th century see KING (1958); PORTER (1995); LINDEMANN (1996 and 1999).

in turn, attributed illness primarily to a disturbance of the governance of the soul. Over the course of the eighteenth century, the Montpellier school of medical vitalism gained ground. Sensibility and irritability as specific capacities of living tissue came to play a major role and there was a massive upsurge of interest in the nerves and in "nervous diseases," which rapidly gained popularity among the general public. In the late eighteenth century, the theories of William Cullen (1710–1790) and John Brown (1735–1788) spread throughout Europe, which classified diseases into "sthenic" and "asthenic" depending on whether they were characterized by an excessive degree or lack of irritation or stimulation. Mesmerism came into vogue, and around 1800, Samuel Hahnemann (1755–1843) presented his new homeopathic principle of "similia similibus curentur" for determining the healing powers of medicinal drugs by observing the symptoms they produced in healthy subjects.[17]

Contemporary physicians deplored this multitude of theories and therapeutic approaches:

> Unfortunately, it has nearly gotten to the point where, like every school principal wanting to formulate his own logic and every superintendent his own catechism, so almost every famous professor will come up with his own theory [...],

Friedrich Hoffmann (1660–1742) noted. Young people did not know which way to turn, "because there are so many principles and hypotheses floating around these days."[18] This diversity was not just disorienting for medical students, who might encounter a completely new perspective on medicine when they moved from one university to another. The dissent between different medical currents also threatened to compromise the very authority of learned medicine as a whole. It undercut the physicians' vociferous claims that they were the exclusive representatives of a truly reliable and scientific medicine.

It remains uncertain, however, to what extent the patients themselves viewed the contradictory judgments by physicians at their bedside as a consequence of conflicting medical theories. Patients' letters and other sources permit only limited generalizations on this point. They do suggest another conclusion, however, which may seem paradoxical at first glance. They indicate that educated laypeople were more acutely aware of theoretical differences in the sixteenth and early seventeenth centuries, when medicine was comparatively homogeneous, than later on in the eighteenth century. In the sixteenth and early seventeenth centuries, the patients and their relatives could still clearly distinguish between two fundamentally different medical schools of thought and practice, the Galenists and the Paracelsians. In 1571, Georg Stange from Magdeburg complained,

17 SCHOTT (1985); HAHNEMANN (1810).

18 HOFFMANN (1721–1739), Vol. 3, Foreword: "Es ist ja leider fast so weit gekommen, dass fast wie ein jeglicher Schuhl-Rector seine eigne Logic, ein Superintendens einen Catechismum, also auch fast ieglicher berühmter Professor eine sonderliche Theorie formiren und schreiben will, [....] da denn so vielerley principia und hypotheses vorkommen, daß die Jugend nicht weiß, wohin sie sich wenden soll."

for example, about of the Galenist physicians he had consulted about the brown spots which had appeared all over his body. They claimed that his condition came from excessive consumption of alcohol and a heated liver, and that the spots were "liver spots." According to Stange, the advice and the medicines of the Galenists were of little value, however, and had achieved less than nothing, because they did not use quintessences and did not know how to prepare them. This is why he had decided to write to the famous Paracelsian physician Leonhard Thurneisser in Berlin.[19] In a similar manner, an unnamed 42-year old patient who sought Thurneisser's advice had initially consulted Galenist physicians but found their advice unhelpful. One doctor had said that he had overheated his stomach with too much wine, and injured his brain with sharp, acrid phlegm. By contrast, another doctor asserted that his stomach was not overheated and that his illness stemmed from cold moisture in the stomach, but his medicines had brought him close to the graveyard. Also, one said there was a kidney stone, the other claimed there was none. Because these humoralist doctors disagreed in their judgments and came to contradictory therapeutic conclusions, he no longer wanted to submit himself "to their uncertain art."[20] He believed he had a violent "tartar" in his body, a Paracelsian term for morbid matter which tended to form deposits in the joints, the kidneys, and elsewhere.

Although medicine had grown much more pluralistic by the eighteenth century and far more patient letters have survived, we rarely find patients who expressed explicit awareness of distinct medical schools. While the frontline between the warring camps of Galenists and Paracelsians was easily visible to ordinary laypersons, the multitude of different medical currents and schools in the eighteenth century and the theoretical eclecticism of many physicians seem to have made it very difficult for patients and their relatives to assign their medical providers to one particular school. At most, we find a certain distrust of medical systems in general. Some letter writers feared that a physician who adhered to a specific medical system might reach prejudiced, one-sided conclusions. Thus a high-ranking court official in Montpellier preferred to describe his spouse's malady to Tissot in his own words. Doctors undoubtedly understood better how to write a medical history, he explained, but they might "present their own views rather than report to you on the malady in question."[21] But even that was unusual.

19 SBB Ms. 420a, fol. 293r–294r, letter from G. Stange (ca. 1580).

20 SBB Ms. 422a, fol. 101r–102r, letter, n. d., presumably presented during a personal visit (ca. 1578): "[...] weitter ihrer vngewissen Kunst nicht vnterwerffen."

21 FT, letter from M. Serres, September 30, 1785: "[…] mais peut-etre en donneroit ils leur idées au lieu de vous rendre compte de la maladie."

The Distinguished Physician

From the vantage point of the patients and their family members, the contradictory medical opinions they frequently encountered were not caused by the multiplicity of competing medical theories. They saw them above all as resulting from differences in the individual physician's ability, experience, power of judgment and skill. If doctors came to opposite conclusions in a given case, that was mainly due to the fact that some of them were better than others and that some were more likely to arrive at the truth – or the most effective therapy – than others.

Yet that left patients and their families with a difficult question. How could they determine which physician best to trust? A key criterion for judging medical competence was how plausibly the physician could explain the disease in question, and educated patients and their relatives did not hesitate to pass judgment on that. They confidently weighed differing medical opinions one against the other and expressed their own views.[22] Trew's council, wrote the Baron von Schlammersdorff about the sick wife of his prince, the Margrave of Brandenburg-Ansbach, had pleased Her Highness greatly and she almost agreed with Trew's opinion.[23] Often patients openly contradicted their physician and offered their own interpretation. A lady suffering from a tightening of the chest and severe upper abdominal pain wrote, for example: "A famous medical doctor and physician here claims it comes from bad digestion in the stomach." But she believed she had an "acrid salty flux in the stomach."[24] When, on top of that, new complaints arose, which the patients suspected to be side effects of the treatment, the therapy was almost bound to be discontinued. "My much devastated body now will not permit me to continue with the internal medicines," declared the ailing pastor Streubel.[25]

A second and indeed frequently decisive criterion for judging a physician's competence was his reputation. The more experienced the practitioner and the better known he was for his successful cures, the greater the confidence in his judgment. Therefore patients considered it indispensable to learn as much as possible about the skills and therapeutic successes of the authorities they might want to consult. People avidly exchanged information about their respective experiences, recommended one physician and advised against another or reported about his failures in treating other patients. Whoever could afford to do so seemed of course best advised to consult eminent physicians of international renown, such as Samuel Tissot, Albrecht von Haller (1708–1777) or Friedrich

22 For a general discussion, see STOLBERG (1999).

23 TREW, letter, September 21, 1760.

24 Letter from the sick "A. R.", October 15, 1704, reproduced in FISCHER (1712), 161–165: "Ein berühmter Medicus und Physicus allhier giebet vor, es käme von der üblen Verdauung des Magens; [...] scharffen Saltz-Fluß in dem Magen."

25 TREW, letter, December 14, 1754: "Mein sehr ruinirter Leib will jetzo nicht gestatten, mit den Internis fort zu fahren."

Hoffmann, who were praised for their outstanding diagnostic and therapeutic genius. If the local doctors disagreed, then the medical genius offered a final resort. Thanks to his acumen and experience, he appeared most likely to grasp the nature of the disease or disorder and propose the right therapy, provided he accorded their case sufficient attention despite the large number of his patients.

Though the patients were not aware of this, the great importance they and their families attributed to the personal reputation of a physician indirectly promoted medical pluralism, however, and further increased the likelihood of medical disagreement at the patient's bedside. Physicians who sought to acquire a good reputation and a lucrative, affluent clientele were well advised to distinguish themselves in some way from their colleagues and their numerous less learned competitors. If a doctor was asked for his opinion on a case where other doctors had also been consulted, there were definite advantages if his diagnostic findings and therapeutic recommendations differed somewhat from those of his colleagues. Provided his advice was accepted and the patient improved at least temporarily under his treatment – which is often the case in many diseases, no matter what the therapy – then he had put his diagnostic and therapeutic skills to a successful test in the eyes of the public. He had enhanced his reputation and could count on attracting new patients.[26] Furthermore, when physicians considered their specific treatment successful in a certain case, they were of course well advised to use a similar approach when treating other patients with more or less the same kind of disease. As a result, many physicians over time developed preferences for certain medications or mixtures that they believed to be especially effective. Some even had their names associated in public with a particular approach. Théodore Tronchin (1709–1781), for example, praised the therapeutic virtues of a good stroll, and "tronchiner" became a popular term. Tissot in turn was known to treat numerous ailments with whey and donkey's milk and Pierre Pomme (1735–1812) became famous for the lengthy therapeutic baths he prescribed to his many "nervous" patients, in order to soften up their hardened and contracted nerves. Other physicians, including even renowned practitioners such as Hoffmann, created and marketed their own pharmaceutical compounds. In extreme cases, physicians relied almost exclusively on a single therapeutic method, like Mesmer's "animal magnetism."[27]

If a physician managed to become associated with a particular therapeutic approach or to be praised as a specialist for certain forms of disease, then he could present himself as a genuine alternative, as someone whose skills might still be worth a try when others had failed. Medical disagreement at the bedside damaged the reputation and image of the medical profession as a whole and left patients and relatives with a disconcerting feeling of insecurity. But for the individual doctor it held out the chance to prove his special worth and enhance his

26 An analysis of the drama which the doctor sometimes had to stage is found in LACHMUND & STOLLBERG (1992).

27 POMME (1763); KLEIJ (2003); SCHOTT (1985).

own reputation by demonstrating the value of his personal experience and his particular, if often idiosyncratic approach – provided his treatment was followed by a favorable outcome.

Blaming Medical Colleagues

Some physicians were not content with merely emphasizing their own skills and special abilities. They also strove to undermine confidence in their competitors. Barely embellished by a thin veil of politeness, they talked badly about fellow physicians, doubting their choice of treatment or even their medical competence. Johann Andreas Fischer (1667–1729), for example, told a patient who was suffering from excruciating pain that it was no great surprise that in these circumstances the acidulous mineral waters and Carlsbad spa cures recommended by other doctors not only had not achieved their intended effect, but had made the malady worse.[28] Even physicians of great renown could become the targets of criticism from colleagues who sought to undermine their authority. For example, a little known physician by the name of Jullien rejected, one after the other, all instructions which the famous doctor Geoffroy had given to a common patient of theirs. He conceded that the milk prescribed by Geoffroy was an effective means to eliminate the acrimony, but the patient in question, alas, could not tolerate milk. The phlebotomy recommended was basically a good idea, Jullien noted, but the patient's swollen legs indicated the danger of an imminent dropsy. Blood-letting would make the watery, serous parts predominate even more and was therefore dangerous. Geoffroy's suggestions that the patient's urinary incontinence was caused by a kidney stone was, in Jullien's view, utter nonsense. A large kidney stone would cause marked pain, he argued, and a small stone would simply be excreted.[29]

The degree to which such a critique could serve primarily as a means to enhance one's own standing becomes especially clear in cases in which the differences of opinion were, at closer analysis, extremely subtle or had no practical relevance. He had to confess, wrote Dr. Antoine Louis (1723–1792) in Metz, commenting on the case of a man who had suddenly turned deaf, that he was not satisfied at all with the measures which had been taken against the humming in the ears, which then provoked the subsequent deafness. The means themselves were good, he explained, but they had been applied empirically, without paying sufficient attention to the relation between their effect and the causes of the problem. Even the best remedies had to be utilized with a clear aim in mind, however, otherwise they would prove useless or even detrimental.[30]

28 Responsum, October 19, 1704, in FISCHER (1712), 168–170: "[...] wann bey diesen Zufällen die von denen Medicis vorgeschlagene und auch von deroselben gebrauchte Sauer-Brunnen und Carls-Bad-Cur nicht allein ihren abgerichten Effect nicht erreichet."

29 BIM Ms. 5241 fol. 102r–103r, letter, July 31, 1728.

30 Médiathèque de la Ville de Metz, Ms. 1317, consultation for the deaf patient M. Danneville.

When the competitor came from a lower rung of the social and medical hierarchy, a more or less condescending condemnation of his approach could almost be taken for granted. Academic physicians often spoke with disdain about barber-surgeons and even more so about the numerous empirics who enjoyed great popularity among the lay public. When Mme Serres in Montpellier was suffering from loss of appetite, a feeling of disgust for meat, nausea, vomiting and fainting spells, the local surgeon provided a well-reasoned explanation for her ailment. The affliction, he argued, had originated from a local deposit of milk after the patient had suffered a miscarriage. Eventually the milk had accumulated in the lower abdomen. In addition, her portal vein was excessively filled, which explained her irritable stomach and irregular menstrual periods. He advised her to drain off the milk using foot baths, steam sitz baths, and leeches. These diagnostic and therapeutic conclusions were perfectly in line with contemporary standards and could easily have come from a learned physician. But the university-trained physicians who were consulted on the same case brushed aside his explanation as "mere theory," disdaining even to deal with it.[31]

Individualization

A final important cause of contradictory judgments at the bed-side was the great value which contemporary physicians placed on tailoring diagnosis and therapy to the individual patient. The choice of medication and other therapeutic measures always had to take the nature of the patient into account, his or her manner of living, age, physical disposition, etc. Like the learned causal explanation of the patient's disease, this was an important and much publicized asset of academic medicine as a whole. By tailoring diagnosis and therapy to the individual patient, university-trained physicians sought to distinguish themselves from the empirics who were considered unable to perform the complex act of balancing so many and different factors in arriving at diagnosis and treatment decisions. For their part, many educated patients insisted on such an individualizing approach. They shared the belief that therapy could only be truly efficacious if the physician were familiar with their temperament, living circumstances, eating habits, and so forth and knew how they reacted to various types of medicine. They expected a treatment and regimen specifically suited to their body and their lifestyle. Closer analysis of the prescriptions which doctors like Tissot and Geoffroy wrote for their patients[32] reveals that they dealt with most patients much more schematically than the patients themselves believed or hoped. Nevertheless, in view of the numerous factors which had to be taken into account in each case and which could be weighed differently against each other, physicians could

31 FT, letter from M. Serres: September 30, 1785.

32 Tissot's answers have not been preserved, but, presumably as a mnemonic aid, he often wrote a brief diagnosis on the patients' letters along with the medicines he had prescribed.

hardly avoid arriving at different conclusions in the same case. Again, that was detrimental to the authority of learned medicine as a whole. However, the individual physician who thus underscored his ability to tailor his therapy to the body and life-style of his patients improved his chances to build himself a faithful clientele. For obviously the longer he had known and treated a patient, the better he presumably knew his or her characteristic responses to illness and to various types of regimen and medicines. "Since my complexion, nature and illness are quite familiar to you," wrote Caspar von Hobergk to Leonhard Thurneisser, he wished once more to obtain some advice.[33] A 44-year-old woman did not want to confide in any other doctor at all after her ordinary physician had passed away, who had "known my nature," as she wrote. Only later did she consult the famous Friedrich Hoffmann.[34]

In retrospect, this ideal of a decidedly individualizing approach was also a major reason why a statistical comparison of different therapeutic approaches to the same type of sickness was virtually unthinkable. That changed only in the 19th century, when the hospital became a principal site of medical research. The numerous, mostly lower-class patients in the large hospitals could not command the same respect from the physicians as affluent, upper-class patients; their sheer number would have made a detailed exploration of their individual physical characteristics, like life-style and related factors, very difficult anyway. Physicians were now free to use a more or less standardized approach and to compare groups treated with different therapeutic regimes or indeed not treated at all, something very few upper-class patients would have tolerated.[35] Over the longer term, the increasing use of standardized clinical trials led, in turn, to a standardization of medical treatment and a marked reduction in therapeutic pluralism.

Conclusion

Medical disagreement at the bedside was a common experience in the eighteenth century. Even if the doctors agreed on the diagnosis, they often differed considerably in their choice of regimen and medication. A uniform treatment *lege artis* did not exist for most maladies. As we have seen, a number of factors contributed to this situation, in particular the plurality of medical theories, limited diagnostic means and the often almost exclusive reliance on the patient narrative, the emphasis placed on tailoring diagnosis and therapy to the individual patient, and the physician's pursuit of individual distinction.

In no small measure, medical disagreement thus resulted from the expectations and wishes which patients and their families communicated to their physi-

33 SBB Ms. germ. fol. 421b, foll. 118r–119r, letter from Caspar von Hobergk, March 9, 1577: "Die weill euch mein Complecktion, Natur vnnd Kranckheit sunderlichen woll bekhant."

34 HOFFMANN (1721–1739), Vol. 10, 279–282, letter from a 44-year-old patient, "der meine Natur gekant."

35 LESKY (1965).

cians. It was a consequence of the way patients viewed the trustworthiness and reputation of physicians, and thus their social status and professional advancement. In this sense, the much-cited power of the patient in early modern medicine[36] had ambivalent effects. For the patients and their families, contradictory medical opinions could be deeply unsettling and burdensome. They consulted one doctor after the other and spent large amounts of money. Yet their condition often worsened. But from the individual patient's point of view, there were also positive sides to this therapeutic pluralism. For one thing, medical pluralism and the contradictory medical opinions on the same case could be a source of hope. As long as physicians offered quite different explanations and opted for different kinds of therapy, the prospect remained that one of them might be right after all, that he would, thanks to his great experience or brilliant intuition, finally fathom the true nature of the patient's illness and find a successful treatment. Furthermore, diagnostic and therapeutic disagreement among the physicians gave more decision-making power to the patients. Many of them had quite specific ideas about their sickness and the way it should be treated. When the physicians consulted unanimously proposed a diagnosis and therapy, the patient was under considerable pressure to follow their advice, even more so when the family supported the medical verdict. But when physicians contradicted one another, patients were basically free to choose whatever explanation suited them best and whatever therapy they were willing to put up with. If a physician wanted the patient to accept their judgment and submit to their treatment rather than someone else's, he therefore had to make an effort to convince the patient. He had to explain his diagnosis and his plan of treatment in the most plausible way possible and he had to be prepared to deal with the questions and doubts of the patients. In other words, he had to take the patient seriously as a competent partner in a joint decision-making process. In certain respects patient autonomy and informed consent were thus, among the upper classes, not an abstract idea but, much more than today, lived reality. Though admittedly, just as today, many patients would probably have preferred an incontrovertible and infallible verdict to freedom of choice.

36 JEWSON (1974) and JEWSON (1976).

Unpublished Sources and References

BIM
Bibliothèque Interuniversitaire de Médecine, Paris, Mss. 5241–5245 (2 undated letters 5241 fol. 79r–v; 102r–103r.)

FT
Bibliothèque Cantonale et Universitaire, Lausanne-Dorigny, Fonds Tissot (letters from Konauw, Barbaroux, Herbelot, v. Walmoden, Serres).

Médiathèque de la Ville de Metz, Ms. 1317 (consultation Danneville).

Rijksarchief Arnhem, Archive of the Counts of Coulembourg, Ms. 403 (letter from Steelants).

SBB
Staatsbibliothek Berlin, Ms. germ. fol. 99 and 420a–426 (letters from Stange: Ms. 420a, fol. 293r–2946; n. d.: Ms. 422a, fol. 101r–102r; v. Hobergk: 421b, fol. 118r–119r).

Trew
Universitätsbibliothek Erlangen, Trew-Korrespondenz (letters from v. Schlammersdorff, Streubel).

Universiteitsbibliotheek Leiden, Ms. Marchand 3 (letter from v. Boetzelaar).

Duden (1987)
Duden, Barbara: Geschichte unter der Haut. Ein Eisenacher Arzt und seine Patientinnen um 1730. Stuttgart: Klett-Cotta, 1987.

Fischer (1712)
Fischer, Johann Andreas: Consilia medica iterum continuata, quae in usum practicum et forensem pro scopo curandi et renunciandi adornata atque singularibus experimentis, inter arcana domestica hactenus reservatis, illustrata sunt. Frankfurt: Apud Joh. Maximil. a Sande, 1712.

Helmont (1683)
Helmont, Johann Baptist van: Aufgang der Artzney-Kunst. Sulzbach: Endters, 1683.

Hahnemann (1810)
Hahnemann, Samuel: Organon der rationellen Heilkunde. Dresden: Arnold, 1810.

Hoffmann (1721–1739)
Hoffmann, Friedrich: Medicina consultatoria. 12 Vols. Halle: Renger, 1721–1739.

Jewson (1974)
Jewson, N. D.: Medical Knowledge and the Patronage System in 18th Century England. In: Sociology 8 (1974), 369–385

Jewson (1976)
Jewson, N. D.: The Disappearance of the Sick Man from Medical Cosmology, 1770–1870. In: Sociology 10 (1976), 225–244.

Jütte (1991)
Jütte, Robert: Ärzte, Heiler und Patienten. Medizinischer Alltag in der frühen Neuzeit. München, Zürich: Artemis & Winkler, 1991.

King (1958)
King, Lester S.: The Medical World of the Eighteenth Century. Chicago: University of Chicago Press, 1958.

Kleij (2003)
Kleij, Thomas: Zur Entwicklungs- und Herstellungsgeschichte der „Hoffmannstropfen“ und ihrer Darstellung und Interpretation in den medizinischen Werken des 19. und 20. Jahrhunderts. Dresden 2003 (MD thesis).

Lachmund & Stollberg (1992)
Lachmund, Jens; Stollberg, Gunnar: The Doctor, his Audience, and the Meaning of Illness. The Drama of Medical Practice in the Late 18th and Early 19th Centuries. In: Lachmund, Jens; Stollberg, Gunnar (Eds.): The Social Construction of Illness. Stuttgart: Franz Steiner, 1992 (Medizin, Gesellschaft und Geschichte, Beiheft 1), 53–66.

Lachmund & Stollberg (1995)
Lachmund, Jens; Stollberg, Gunnar: Patientenwelten. Krankheit und Medizin vom späten 18. bis zum frühen 20. Jahrhundert im Spiegel von Autobiographien. Opladen: Leske & Budrich, 1995.

Lesky (1965)
Lesky, Erna: Die Wiener medizinische Schule im 19. Jahrhundert. Graz: Böhlau, 1965

Lindemann (1996)
Lindemann, Mary: Health and Healing in Eighteenth-Century Germany. Baltimore, London: Johns Hopkins University Press, 1996.

Lindemann (1999)
Lindemann, Mary: Medicine and Society in Early Modern Europe. Cambridge: Cambridge University Press, 1999.

Pomata (1994)
Pomata, Gianna: La promessa di guarigione. Malati e curatori in antico regime. Bologna XVI–XVIII secolo. Bari: Laterza, 1994.

Pomme (1763)
Pomme, Pierre: Traité des affections vaporeuses des deux sexes. Lyons: Duplain, 1763.

Porter (1985a)
Porter, Roy: The Patient's View. Doing Medical History from Below. In: Theory and Society 14 (1985), 175–198.

Porter (1985b)
Porter, Roy (Ed.): Patients and Practitioners. Lay Perceptions of Medicine in Pre-Industrial Society. London: Cambridge University Press, 1985.

Porter (1995)
Porter, Roy: Medicine in the Enlightenment. Amsterdam, Atlanta: Rodopi, 1995.

Porter & Porter (1989a)
Porter, Roy and Dorothy: In Sickness and in Health. The British Experience, 1650–1850. New York: Blackwell, 1989.

Porter & Porter (1989b)
Porter, Dorothy and Roy: Patient's Progress. Doctors and Doctoring in Eighteenth-Century England. Cambridge, Oxford: Polity Press, 1989.

Rem (1861)
Rem, Lucas: Tagebuch des Lucas Rem aus den Jahren 1494–1541. Ein Beitrag zur Handelsgeschichte der Stadt Augsburg. Edited by B. Greiff. In: 26. Jahresbericht des Historischen Kreis-Vereins im Regierungsbezirke Schwaben und Neuburg für das Jahr 1860. Augsburg, 1861.

Schott (1985)
Schott, Heinz (Ed.): Franz Anton Mesmer und die Geschichte des Mesmerismus. Stuttgart: Franz Steiner, 1985.

Stolberg (1996)
Stolberg, Michael: „Mein äskulapisches Orakel!" Patientenbriefe als Quelle einer Kulturgeschichte der Krankheitserfahrung im 18. Jahrhundert. In: Österreichische Zeitschrift für Geschichtswissenschaften 7 (1996), 385–404.

Stolberg (1999)
Stolberg, Michael: La négociation de la thérapie dans la pratique médicale du XVIIIe siècle. In: Faure, Olivier (Ed.): Les thérapeutiques. Savoirs et usages. Lyons: Fondation Mérieux, 1999, 357–368.

Stolberg (2003)
Stolberg, Michael: Homo patiens. Krankheits- und Körpererfahrung in der Frühen Neuzeit. Weimar: Böhlau, 2003.

Tissot (1760)
Tissot, Samuel Auguste: L'onanisme ou dissertation physique sur les maladies produites par la masturbation. Lausanne: Chapuis, 1760.

Vila (1998)
Vila, Anne C.: Enlightenment and Pathology. Sensibility in the Literature and Medicine of Eighteenth-Century France. Baltimore, London: Johns Hopkins University Press, 1998.

DIE MEDIKAMENTE DES WAISENHAUSES. EIN BEISPIEL FÜR DIE ETABLIERUNG UND VERBREITUNG THERAPEUTISCHER PRAKTIKEN IM 18. JAHRHUNDERT

Jürgen Helm

Am 5. September 1748 wandten sich die beiden Halleschen Apotheker Christian Friedrich Zepernick und Carl Christian Schultze an den Magistrat der Stadt Halle. Weil sie die Kosten für die angekündigten Visitationen der von ihnen geleiteten Stadtapotheken kaum tragen konnten, baten sie um einen Aufschub des Verfahrens. Die schlechte wirtschaftliche Lage ihrer Apotheken hing nach Aussage der beiden Apotheker vor allem mit dem Erfolg der Apotheke des Waisenhauses zusammen. Kein „Medicus" verschreibe mehr „ein Recept in unsere Officinen", denn jedermann „suchet die Waysenhäußer Apotheque". Dies geschehe entweder aus „Superstition" oder aus Unbedachtheit, vielleicht aber auch deswegen, weil „alle Leuthe ihr Artzney von der Waysenhäußer Apotheque hohleten".[1]

Offensichtlich hatte der Erfolg der Apotheke der Franckeschen Anstalten die Stadtapotheken in Bedrängnis gebracht. Im Gefüge des städtischen Gesundheitsmarktes gaben die beiden Apotheker, wie sie schrieben, „bloß Zuschauer" ab; eine Teilhabe am Markt war ihnen versagt.[2] Insofern hatte sich August Hermann Franckes (1663–1727) Versprechen, das er am 10. November 1711 dem preußischen Kronprinzen und späteren Friedrich Wilhelm I. gegeben hatte, als nicht tragfähig herausgestellt. Francke hatte damals behauptet, dass die Halleschen Apotheken keine Verluste durch die Anstalten erleiden würden, „weil die Medici in Halle nicht aus der Apothecke des Waysenhauses verschreiben, sondern bey denen in Halle bißher bleiben".[3]

Nicht nur in Halle, sondern auch in anderen Teilen Preußens sorgte der Erfolg der Medikamente des Waisenhauses für Unruhe. Am 4. April 1744 hatten sich die Apotheker im pommerschen Stargard beim *Obercollegium medicum* in Berlin über „eindringende" Medikamente beschwert, die ihnen die Nahrung raubten. Das *Obercollegium medicum*, die oberste preußische Gesundheitsbehörde, erstattete knapp drei Wochen später dem König Friedrich II. pflichtgemäß Bericht. Darin heißt es, dass nicht nur aus Stargard, sondern auch aus anderen Provinzen Beschwerden über den „alzustarcken Vertrieb der Hallischen Medi-

1 Stadtarchiv Halle XIV, A, 4, Schreiben vom 5. September 1748.

2 Nach Aussage der beiden Apotheker hing die Ertragslage der Apotheken in erster Linie vom Verschreibungsverhalten der Ärzte ab: „Der meiste profit, welchen unsere Stadt-Apothequen der Medicinal-Ordnung und Billigkeit nach haben sollten, bestehet in Verschreibung derer Recepte; [...]." Diese Behauptung wird durch Beisswangers Untersuchungen zu den Apotheken Braunschweigs bestätigt, denen zufolge im 18. Jahrhundert bis zu zwei Drittel der Gesamteinnahmen der Apotheken auf ärztliche Rezepte zurückzuführen waren; vgl. BEISSWANGER (2003), 149.

3 AFSt/W II/-/11, fol. 2v.

camenten eingegangen" seien. Insbesondere werde beklagt, „daß selbige von Buchhändlern, alten Weibern, Predigern und Personen von allerley Stande debitiret und verkauffet" würden. Der Verkauf der Halleschen Medikamente führe dazu, dass in den Apotheken „die nach dem Dispensatorio dem Publico zum besten im Überschuß [...] vorhandene praeparata zum Verderben und ihrem größesten Schaden stehen" blieben.[4]

Die beiden Beispiele zeigen die Kehrseite einer Erfolgsgeschichte, die in den vergangenen Jahrzehnten mehrfach dokumentiert wurde. Die Apotheke und der Medikamentenversand (die so genannte Medikamentenexpedition) hatten sich in der ersten Hälfte des 18. Jahrhunderts zu einem überaus wichtigen wirtschaftlichen Standbein der Franckeschen Anstalten entwickelt. Die Medikamente wurden im In- und Ausland verkauft und erzielten (wie Renate Wilson in ihrer Monographie zum Einfluss der Halleschen Medikamente auf den kolonialamerikanischen Gesundheitsmarkt aufgezeigt hat) vielfach Reingewinne von mehr als 20.000 Reichstalern jährlich.[5] Man kann mit Recht behaupten, dass sich die Franckeschen Anstalten auf der rechtlichen Grundlage des kurfürstlichen Privilegs vom Jahr 1698, das die Führung einer Apotheke zuließ,[6] zu einem pharmazeutischen Großunternehmen mit internationalen Geschäftsbeziehungen entwickelt hatten.[7]

In den bisherigen Arbeiten[8] zum großen Erfolg der Halleschen Medikamente werden auch die Faktoren angesprochen, die diesen Erfolg bedingten: Auf der Anbieterseite waren dies in erster Linie marktgängige Verkaufsformate – man denke nur an die Haus-, Feld- und Reiseapotheke, in der die wichtigsten Medikamente handlich verpackt waren – und eine auch nach heutigen Maßstäben fast professionell zu nennende Werbekampagne, die der Internationalität der Absatzmärkte Rechnung trug.[9] Auf der Seite der Nachfragenden trug zum einen die unkomplizierte Therapie mit den Medikamenten, die mit den vielfach gedruckten Anleitungen auch ohne Konsultation eines Arztes möglich war, zum Erfolg bei.[10]

4 GStA PK, I. HA, Rep. 52 Magdeburg, Nr. 131 b2, fol. 72–76 (Zitate fol. 75r). Beisswanger führt aus, dass im Herzogtum Braunschweig-Wolfenbüttel die Halleschen Medikamente in größerem Umfang auch über die Apotheken vertrieben wurden; vgl. BEISSWANGER (1996), 152–158.

5 Vgl. WILSON (2000), 91. Zu Beginn der Sechzigerjahre des 18. Jahrhunderts wurden jährliche Gewinne in Höhe von 35.000 Reichstalern erzielt.

6 Vgl. GITTNER (1948), 5–7; POECKERN (1984), 10.

7 Die Formulierung ist angelehnt an WELSCH (1956).

8 Zu nennen wären neben Renate Wilsons Monographie: GITTNER (1948), KAISER & PIECHOCKI (1969), POECKERN (1984), POECKERN (2004).

9 Vgl. WILSON (2000), 69–71. Die gedruckten Werbeschriften für die Arzneien erschienen u.a. in englischer, französischer, niederländischer und neugriechischer Sprache. Vgl. dazu auch die Faksimiles der Titelblätter in GITTNER (1948).

10 Der vollständige Titel des 1705 erschienenen *Kurtzen und deutlichen Unterrichts* von Christian Friedrich Richter bringt klar zum Ausdruck, dass das Buch und die Medikamente der – durchaus zeitüblichen – Selbstbehandlung dienen sollten; vgl. RICHTER (1705).

Zum anderen war natürlich auch die Herkunft der Arzneien von Bedeutung: In dem Pietismus nahe stehenden Milieus genossen die Medikamente sicherlich allein deshalb einen guten Ruf, weil sie aus den Franckeschen Anstalten stammten.[11] Dies werden die beiden Halleschen Apotheker auch gemeint haben, als sie im Zusammenhang mit dem wirtschaftlichen Erfolg der Waisenhausapotheke von „Superstition“ auf Seiten der Patienten und Ärzte sprachen.

Diese Sicht auf den Erfolg der Medikamentenherstellung und des Medikamentenverkaufs durch die Franckeschen Anstalten beruht weitgehend auf einer Außenwahrnehmung der Vorgänge um die Waisenhausmedikamente. Im Folgenden soll diese Außensicht um eine Innenperspektive der Anbieter erweitert werden. Konkret sollen grundlegende Argumentationsstrategien der zwischen 1700 und 1710 in den Anstalten für die Entwicklung und den Vertrieb der Medikamente verantwortlichen Ärzte untersucht und dargestellt werden. Wie begründete man den Gebrauch und den Nutzen der von ihnen vertriebenen Medikamente? Inwiefern evaluierte man deren Wirkung? Und wie ging man mit Kritik um, die auch in dieser frühen Zeit schon an den Medikamenten geübt wurde? Damit soll gewissermaßen die Vorgeschichte zu der bekannten Erfolgsgeschichte erzählt werden, denn es wird sich zeigen, dass sich die genannten Faktoren, die zur erfolgreichen Etablierung einer bestimmten therapeutischen Praxis führten, zumindest zum Teil aus den Argumenten der Ärzte ableiten lassen. Und daher wird erst durch die Berücksichtigung der Argumentation der Mediziner der Erfolg der Medikamente nachvollziehbar und verständlich.

Grundlage der Analyse ist eine Sammlung von mehr als 160 Briefen, die zwischen 1701 und 1711 von den beiden Waisenhausärzten Christian Friedrich Richter (1676–1711) und Christian Sigismund Richter (1672/73–1739) an Carl Hildebrand Baron von Canstein (1667–1719) in Berlin gesandt wurden.[12] Canstein war ein enger Vertrauter Franckes am Berliner Hof.[13] Er hatte Zugang zu den entsprechenden Hofkreisen und versorgte – das wird aus den Briefen deutlich – sein Umfeld mit den neuen Medikamenten des Waisenhauses. Die beiden Mediziner waren für die Ausarbeitung der Medikamente zuständig.[14] Sie sandten alte und neue Präparate an Canstein, der sie weitergab, um anschließend nach Halle über den Zustand der Patienten und den Erfolg der Therapie zu be-

11 Zur Verteilung der Medikamente in „pietistischen Netzwerken“ vgl. den Beitrag von Elisabeth Quast in diesem Band.

12 AFSt/H C 285:15. Da einige Briefe nur als Fragmente vorliegen, ist die genaue Gesamtzahl der Schreiben noch nicht exakt zu bestimmen. Eine kritische Edition der Briefe, herausgegeben von Elisabeth Quast und Jürgen Helm, ist in Vorbereitung.

13 Zu Canstein vgl. SCHICKETANZ (1972), IX–XI; SCHICKETANZ (2002).

14 Die Frage, ob die Brüder Richter tatsächlich neue Medikamente „erfunden“ oder lediglich in die Anstalten gelangende Rezepte „nachgekocht“ haben, war bereits im 18. Jahrhundert Ursache schwerwiegender Streitigkeiten; vgl. dazu POECKERN (1984), 15–25, 32–35. Weil es in der hier untersuchten Argumentation der beiden Ärzte nicht um das Urheberrecht, sondern in erster Linie um die Legitimation der Therapieverfahren geht, ist diese Frage für die vorliegende Untersuchung nachrangig.

richten. Die Ärzte reagierten darauf ihrerseits mit Anweisungen, ob die Therapie beizubehalten oder zu ändern war. Leider sind nur die Briefe der Halleschen Ärzte erhalten, Cansteins Schreiben liegen nicht mehr vor. Ein weiteres kleineres Quellenkorpus der Analyse sind gedruckte Schriften über die Medikamente, die zwischen 1701 und 1708 erschienen sind und die zu unterschiedlichen Genres gehören.[15]

In den folgenden Ausführungen wird zunächst aufgezeigt, wie die Ärzte eine positive Wirkung der von ihnen vertriebenen Medikamente plausibel machten. Im zweiten Schritt soll die Frage beantwortet werden, ob und wie die Mediziner Beobachtungen und Erfahrungen über die Medikamentenwirkung in ihre Argumentation einfließen ließen. Im dritten Abschnitt wird dargestellt, wie Kritik an den Waisenhausmedikamenten aufgenommen und wie mit ihr umgegangen wurde. Abschließend werde ich die Ergebnisse zusammenfassen und vor diesem Hintergrund nochmals auf den eingangs dargestellten Erfolg der Medikamente eingehen.

Plausibilität des therapeutischen Konzepts

In den Briefen der Brüder Richter finden sich zahlreiche therapeutische Anweisungen für Patienten im Umfeld Cansteins, die in den allermeisten Fällen namentlich benannt werden. Neben den eigenen Medikamenten empfehlen die Ärzte gelegentlich auch Drogen aus der traditionellen *materia medica* sowie konventionelle therapeutische und prophylaktische Maßnahmen wie den Aderlass. Zum weit überwiegenden Teil aber sollten die Patienten mit den in Halle hergestellten Medikamenten behandelt werden.

In ihren therapeutischen Anweisungen bewegten sich die Ärzte weitgehend im Rahmen sehr allgemeiner Überlegungen und Deutungsmuster, von denen sowohl das ärztliche als auch das laienmedizinische Denken in der Frühen Neuzeit geprägt war. Michael Stolberg hat vor kurzem derartige Überlegungen und Denkmuster aus Patientenbriefen rekonstruiert.[16] In den Briefen der Gebrüder Richter über die Patienten imponieren als wichtigste Krankheitsursache Verstopfungen (*obstructiones*) der verschiedenen Organsysteme – je nach Symptomatik etwa der Lunge[17], des Darms[18] oder des Unterleibs[19]. *Obstructiones* führen dazu,

15 BERICHT (1701), SELECTUS (1702), BERICHT (1703), RICHTER & RICHTER (1703), RICHTER (1705), RICHTER (1708).

16 Vgl. STOLBERG (2003).

17 Vgl. z.B. AFSt/H C 285:15, Nr. 23 (2. Mai 1702): „Daß die Lunge schon solte angegangen seyn, halte wol nicht, weil sichs sonst in mehrern Umständen zeigen würde: sonderl. würde sich auch ein Auswurff einer purulenten materie dabey finden: es scheinet aber mehr eine Stagnatio materiae acris biliosae in pulmonibus zu seyn, aus welcher endlich eine erosio und laesio in der Lunge, und also vera phthysis leicht entstehen könte; [...].“

dass schädliche Materien nicht ausgeschieden werden können. Der Abfluss dieser schädlichen Substanzen ist gehemmt, sodass es – so die Vorstellung – zum Stau, zur *stagnatio*, dieser Materien kommt. Nahezu alle Beschwerden werden in den Briefen letztlich auf diese Überschwemmung der Organe mit nicht ausgeschiedenen „Unreinigkeiten", wie es meist heißt, erklärt.[20]

Die Wirkung, die man den verordneten Halleschen Medikamenten zuschrieb, entsprach dieser Krankheitsvorstellung. Die Medikamente öffnen den Leib,[21] und sie reinigen die Organe, etwa den Darm[22], die Lunge[23] oder den Uterus[24]. Dies tun sie, indem sie die Unreinigkeiten zerteilen und „die Materie zum Auswurff bequem"[25] machen. Die Ausscheidung erfolgt dann über verschiedene Wege. Als den Patienten zu sehr belastend und eher nicht erwünscht wurde das Erbrechen angesehen.[26] Besser (und so sollte ein Teil der verordneten Arzneien wirken) sei die Ausscheidung als Husten über die Lunge oder als Durchfall über

18 Vgl. z. B. AFSt/H C 285:15, Nr. 65 (20. März 1703): „Daß sich beym Hn. Ober Jäger Meister ein pallor im Gesichte und Alvi et haemorrhoidum Obstructio ereügnet, sind nicht gutte indicia."

19 Vgl. z. B. AFSt/H C 285:15, Nr. 39 (31. Oktober 1703): „Die benennten Umstände von der Fräul. von Friedeborn deuten gar offenbarl. auf einen affectum hystericum, oder Mutter=Kranckheit, zu welchem doch leichtlich eine Suffocatio uterina oder Catharrhus Suffocativus, Starck=Fluß schlagen könte. Die auf der Brust sich ereignende Beschwerungen, und Beklemmung, wie auch die Kopf=Schmertzen rühren von der bekandten communication dieser Theile des Leibes mit dem Utero her. Dannenhero vermuthlich einige Unreinigkeit der Mutter vorhanden seyn wird, ob gleich die monatliche Reinigung zu gehörigen Zeiten sich einfindet: [...]."

20 Zum Konzept der „Verstopfungen und gestörten Ausscheidungen" vgl. STOLBERG (2003), 172–182.

21 Vgl. z. B. AFSt/H C 285:15, Nr. 58 (20. Januar 1703): „Ich halte dafür, mann würde sehr wohl thun, wenn man den Hn Ober Jäger=Meister vom Elixir Polychr. in Gottes Nahmen brauchen ließe. Dadurch würde die Hitze gedämpfet, der Leib geöffnet und die Haemorrhoides befördert werden."

22 Vgl. z. B. AFSt/H C 285:15, Nr. 8 (28. Januar 1702): „Sind obstructiones alvi dabey, so wäre das Elixir Polychr freilich gut, wil er es aber nicht brauchen, so müßen doch dieselbe auf andere und in Fiebern dienliche Weise gehoben werden, wenigstens durch Clystire, sonst schlagen die Medicamente nicht recht durch."

23 Vgl. z. B. AFSt/H C 285:15, Nr. 10 (27. Februar 1702): „Daß der Phthysicus nach dem Gebrauch des Bezoard. solaris mehr ausgeworffen, hat nichts zu bedeuten gehabt, denn die Pulmones sind durch solche Evacuation gereinigt worden, [...]."

24 Vgl. nochmals AFSt/H C 285:15, Nr. 8 (28. Januar 1702): „Es könnten zur Reinigung des Uteri erstl. die Pilul. polychr. hernach pulvis antispasmodicus, oder beydes mit einander gebraucht werden." Vgl. auch AFSt/H C 285:15, Nr. 39 (31. Oktober 1703): „Außer dem aber ist auf einige gebräuchliche Reinigung und Stärckung der Mutter vornehmlich zu dencken, welches durch die essentiam dulcem, und durch das Bezoardicum solare mercklich geschiehet, [...]."

25 AFSt/H C 285:15, Nr. 21 (17. April 1702).

26 Vgl. ebenfalls AFSt/H C 285:15, Nr. 21 (17. April 1702): „Daß man kein Vomitiv in die Reise=Apothecken genommen, rühret daher, weil sie mit mehrerer Behutsamkeit müßen gebraucht werden, als andere Medicamenta, [...]."

den Darm. Auch so genannte *haemorrhoides*, Blutflüsse, dienten neben der Therapie der Blutfülle der Ausscheidung schädlicher Materien und wurden von den Präparaten reguliert.[27] Diese Blutflüsse konnten als Nasenbluten, als Monatsblutung bei Frauen oder auch als Fluss der so genannten Goldenen Ader auftreten. Als ideale Ausscheidungsform der Unreinigkeiten galt jedoch der Schweiß.[28] Die Patienten wurden dabei nicht durch Erbrechen, Durchfälle oder Blutungen gestört und dennoch von den krankmachenden Materien befreit. Gerade diese Wirkung, die bei den Ärzten in „größtem aestim“ stehe, schrieb man einigen der Arzneien zu.[29]

Weitere Krankheits- und Therapiekonzepte, die in den konkreten Anweisungen der Halleschen Ärzte zutage treten, waren die so genannten „Schärfen“, die durch die Medikamente gedämpft werden sollten.[30] Außerdem ist mehrfach von der bereits erwähnten Blutfülle, der „Plethora“, die Rede, die in der Regel durch den Aderlass behandelt wurde.[31] Auch mit diesen Begrifflichkeiten bewegten sich die Halleschen Ärzte im Rahmen des allgemeinen frühneuzeitlichen Diskurses[32] – ein Bezug zu einer der zeitgenössischen medizinischen Theorien, etwa zu

27 Vgl. AFSt/H C 285:15, Nr. 27 (24. Juni 1702): „Das (*sic!*) pulvis antispasmodic. ist sehr dienl. bey dem fluxu haemorrhoidali, ihn zu temperiren.“

28 Zur heilsamen Wirkung des Schweißes vgl. STOLBERG (2003), 175–178. Vgl. dazu auch die Ausführungen Christian Sigismund Richters zu einem Patienten, der u.a. von Schmerzen und Zittern der Arme gequält wurde, in AFSt/H C 285:15, Nr. 57 (16. Januar 1703): „Ich vermuthe, die arme werden weiter mit fettigkeiten und Salben geschmieret worden seyn, wodurch die Poren verstopffet und die transpiration verhindert wird. Man kann dabey nicht viel thun, als daß man das Fett aus denen poris mit Spiritu vini camphorato fleißig wieder auswaschen, und zugleich den spasmum damit discutiren.“

29 Vgl. AFSt/H C 285:15, Nr. 14 (14. März 1702): „Alle diese Medicamenta würcken per Diaphoresin, wird von den Medicis für ein gutes Zeichen gehalten, wenigstens daß sie sicher zu gebrauchen seyn. Diaphoretica sind bey den Medicis in größten aestim, [...].“

30 Vgl. AFSt/H C 285:15, Nr. 4 (25. Oktober 1701): „Wenn die Frau von Bülow von den pulvere antispasmodico fleißig brauchen wird, so hoffe, daß sie auch wegen der Schärffe große Erleichterung spüren werden. Wolten sie einen Versuch thun, und die Essentiam dulcem mit der Essentia amara zu Dämpfung der Schärffe vermischen, möchte villeicht der Effect desto beßer erfolgen: [...]. “ Vgl. auch AFSt/H C 285:15, Nr. 119 (16. November 1706): „Für die Frau von Löben, welcher mich gehorsamst empfehle, übersende eine Tinctur, [...]: sie pfleget die Schärffe, von welcher sie incommodiret wird, [...] zu dämpfen, und sie guten theils auch durch den Urin abzuführen.“

31 Vgl. z. B. AFSt/H C 285:15, Nr. 22 (25. April 1702): „Wenn die Engbrüstigkeit von der Vollblütigkeit herrühret, so wird derselben durch Medicamenta allein nicht recht abgeholffen, weil sie Plethoram nicht heben können: drum ist dabey Venaesectio und mäßige aber eine Zeitlang anhaltende Bewegung des Leibes dabey nöthig.“

32 Zu den „Schärfen“ vgl. STOLBERG (2003), 139–144 und 155–157; zur „Plethora“ vgl. STOLBERG (2003), 121–125.

den Theorien Georg Ernst Stahls (1659–1734) oder Friedrich Hoffmanns (1660–1742), ist in den konkreten Therapievorschlägen der Briefe kaum greifbar.[33]

Die gedruckten Schriften zu den Arzneien, die vornehmlich dem Verkaufsschlager *Essentia dulcis* gewidmet sind, entwerfen hingegen ein anderes Bild und lassen eine bemerkenswerte Entwicklung erkennen. Im 1701 erschienenen *Bericht von der Artzney / Essentia Dulcis genannt [...]* wird die Wirkung dieses „trinkbaren Goldes" folgendermaßen beschrieben:

> „Die Essentia dulcis ist ein sehr subtiles durchdringendes / doch anbey gelindes und unschädliches Medicament, so in grosser Geschwindigkeit den Leib durchgehet / alle Unreinigkeit / so es findet / es sey in welchem Gliede es wolle / corrigiret / zertheilet und ausführet / die Natur erfreuet und stärcket / und ordinair mit augenscheinlicher Erleichterung der Patienten seine Würckung thut."

Die Essenz wirke – so der Text weiter – bei jedem Patienten so, wie es für ihn und seine Konstitution am besten sei. Bei den meisten führe sie die „Unreinigkeit des Leibes" durch Schweiß aus, bei anderen aber auch durch den Speichel, durch den Urin, durch den Stuhlgang oder durch Schnupfen.[34]

Im 1703 gedruckten *Ausführlichen Bericht* über die *Essentia Dulcis* wird die Wirkung des Medikaments in modifizierter Weise beschrieben. Zwar heißt es immer noch, dass es „subtil, auffgeschlossen und spirituös" sei. „Ohne sich im Magen zu verweilen", durchdringe es schnell den Leib und beweise seine Kraft. Die der Essenz zugeschriebene primäre Wirkung besteht nun allerdings nicht mehr in der Korrektur, Zerteilung und Ausführung der Unreinigkeiten, sondern in einer unmittelbaren Stärkung der Natur. Das Medikament – so heißt es – „erfreuet die Natur und machet sie vigoreus". In diesem Sinn sei es eine „allgemeine Artzney", die bei allen Krankheiten sicher anzuwenden sei. Der Begriff „Natur", der im Text von 1701 in allgemeiner und untergeordneter Bedeutung auftauchte, wird nun zum zentralen Punkt der Argumentation. In diesem Zusammenhang verweisen die Autoren der Schrift – die beiden Briefeschreiber Christian Friedrich und Christian Sigismund Richter – ausdrücklich auf Georg Ernst Stahl: Er habe in seiner Dissertation *De Autocratia Naturae* ausgeführt,[35] dass die Natur des Menschen „das meiste in denen Kranckheiten / unter dem Beystande und direction GOttes / zu Wiederbringung der Gesundheit thun muß", und daher sei die *Essentia dulcis* ein so wertvolles Medikament, weil sie diese Natur aufmuntere und stärke sowie die Lebenskraft unterhalte und vermehre. Und erst durch diese Wirkung auf die Natur führe die *Essentia dulcis* zur Ausscheidung der Unreinigkeiten über Schweiß, Speichel, Urin, Stuhlgang oder Schnupfen.[36]

33 Vereinzelt lassen sich Anklänge an Stahls Überlegungen zur „Natur" des Menschen (s. u.) erkennen, wenn etwa der „motus der wirre gemachten natur" durch den Leib öffnende Präparate besänftigt wird; vgl. AFSt/H C 285:15, Nr. 28 (11. Juli 1702).

34 BERICHT (1701).

35 Vgl. STAHL (1696).

36 BERICHT (1703), 7–8.

Damit hat sich in den gedruckten Schriften zur *Essentia dulcis* die Begründung für deren Wirkung gewandelt: Im *Bericht* von 1701 galt das Medikament als ein besonders schonendes und wirksames Mittel zur Ausführung von schädlicher Materie, im *Bericht* von 1703 hingegen wurde die Essenz als ein Medikament dargestellt, das die Natur in ihrer Tätigkeit im Organismus unterstützt. Natur wurde dabei im Sinne Georg Ernst Stahls verstanden. Bekanntlich war die Bewegung der Seele oder Natur – Stahl gebrauchte diese Begriffe synonym – der Kernpunkt von Stahls medizinischer Theorie: Die Seele verhindere den zwangsläufigen Verfall eines Organismus durch zweckmäßige und gezielte Bewegungen. Die Bewegungen der Seele wirkten auf die Gewebe und Organe des Körpers und steuerten den Kreislauf des Blutes sowie die Sekretion und Exkretion schädlicher Materien.[37] Stahls Fakultätskollege Friedrich Hoffmann hatte im Gegensatz dazu ein „technomorphes" Modell des Organismus vertreten, dessen Bewegungen nicht einer übergeordneten Instanz wie der Seele, sondern den Gesetzen der Mechanik folgten.[38] Mit ihren Theorien versuchten beide, die bei gesunden und kranken Menschen zu beobachtenden Phänomene kausal zu erklären.[39]

Um kurz zusammenzufassen: In den konkreten therapeutischen Anweisungen der Briefe wird weitgehend auf der Grundlage allgemeiner Begrifflichkeiten frühneuzeitlichen medizinischen Denkens argumentiert. Im Vordergrund stehen hier so genannte „Unreinigkeiten des Leibes", deren Ausscheidung durch die Arzneien befördert wird. Der gedruckte *Bericht* von der *Essentia dulcis* folgt in seiner ersten Auflage von 1701 denselben Vorstellungen. Im Unterschied dazu

37 Zu Stahls Theorie vgl. HELM (2006), 29–34; GEYER-KORDESCH (2000), 140–220; BAUER (2000); HARTMANN (2000); MÜLLER (1995); MÜLLER (1994); BAUER (1991); GOTTLIEB (1943); PAGEL (1931); KOCH (1926).

38 Zu Hoffmann vgl. HELM & STUKENBROCK (2007); LANZ (1995), 30–70; MÜLLER (1991).

39 Hoffmann entwarf in den Vorreden seiner *Medicina consultatoria* ein aus „observationes" und „theoria" bestehendes Programm zur Entwicklung der Medizin zur Wissenschaft. Vgl. z.B. HOFFMANN (1721), Vorrede: „Damit man aber sich die observationes recht zu Nutz machen könne / so ist dazu nöthig eine theoria physico-medica, und zwar eine gründliche Erkänntniß des menschlichen Cörpers und dessen Leben und Gesundheit. [...] Denn gleichwie es mit Untersuchung und Erfindung der Wahrheiten insgemein so beschaffen ist / daß keine unbekante könne anders entdecket und erfunden werden / es sey denn / daß solches aus schon bekanten entstehe / und man diese mit jenen vergleiche; also kann man auch ex observationibus keine neuen Wahrheiten oder Ursachen derjenigen factorum, eventuum & effectuum, welche in denen observationibus enthalten / entdecken / es sey denn / daß man zuvor eine theoriam physico-mechanicam & anatomicam habe / [...] Wenn man nun dergleichen theoriam physicam zuerst auf die observationes appliciret / u. dadurch einige Wahrheiten erfindet / so können aus deren vielen hernachmals regulae und axiomata gemacht werden / und hieraus wird alsdenn gebohren die rechte und wahrhafftige theoria medica, die absonderlich dem Medico zu seinem Zweck dienet / und eine universal scienz ist / woraus er hernach alles leicht beurtheilen kann / was er thun und lassen soll."– Zur Ausweitung und Relativierung des Theorie-Begriffs im 18. Jahrhundert vgl. KÖNIG (1998), 1135–1136.

stellt die Nachfolgeschrift aus dem Jahr 1703 das Medikament in einen engen Zusammenhang mit der medizinischen Theorie Georg Ernst Stahls. Die *Essentia dulcis* erscheint nun als das Therapeutikum zur Unterstützung der im Sinne Stahls verstandenen Natur oder Seele des Menschen. Einen Höhepunkt erreichte die Adaptation von Stahls Theorie in Christian Friedrich Richters 1705 erschienenem *Kurtzen und deutlichen Unterricht von dem Leibe und natürlichen Leben des Menschen*: Die Anleitung zum Gebrauch der Medikamente ist hier zu einem medizinischen Handbuch angewachsen, das in seinen allgemeinen Teilen die erste deutschsprachige und populäre Darstellung von Stahls medizinischer Theorie enthält.[40] Bei der Präsentation der *Essentia dulcis* wird wie im *Bericht* aus dem Jahr 1703 ausdrücklich auf Stahls Theorie hingewiesen,[41] und auch bei der Darstellung des *Elixir polychrestum*, der *Pilulae contra obstructiones*, des *Magisterium diaphoreticum*, das *Magisterium solare*, des *Mercurius diaphoreticus* und des *schwarzen Pulvers* wird die Wirkung der Substanz auf die „Natur“ des Menschen erwähnt.[42]

Dieser Befund legt die Vermutung nahe, dass die Halleschen Ärzte zweigleisig argumentierten: In ihrer therapeutischen Praxis stützten sie sich in erster Linie auf allgemein anerkannte Begriffe und Überlegungen. In den im Druck veröffentlichten Darstellungen hingegen versuchten sie, die Wirkung der Medikamente mit der medizinischen Theorie eines anerkannten Universitätsmediziners zu erklären. Offensichtlich wollten die beiden Autoren mit der Übernahme von Stahls Theorie eine Art akademischer Rückendeckung für ihre veröffentlichten Aussagen über die *Essentia dulcis* und die anderen Arzneien erreichen. Für das Verhältnis von medizinischer Theorie und therapeutischer Praxis bedeutet dies, dass die Theorie auf eine bestehende und unverändert beibehaltene medizinische Praxis übertragen und zu deren Legitimation herangezogen wurde.[43]

Beobachtung und Erfahrung

Die moderne Vorstellung von der „Wirksamkeit“ einer Therapiemethode war im 18. Jahrhundert kein verbreiteter Gedanke. Heutzutage wird die Wirksamkeit eines Medikaments durch klinische Prüfungen belegt. In einer solchen Studie werden Patienten, die an einer bestimmten Krankheit leiden, in verschiedene

40 Zu Richters *Unterricht* von 1705 vgl. HELM (2006), 34–42; HELM (2004); POECKERN (1984).

41 Vgl. RICHTER (1705), 399–400.

42 Vgl. RICHTER (1705), 428, 438, 442, 446, 447 und 449.

43 Ein ähnliches Theorie-Praxis-Verhältnis hat Risse für die schottische Medizin des 18. Jahrhunderts festgestellt. Vgl. RISSE (2005), 11: „While Edinburgh physicians such as William Cullen and James Gregory readily accepted a new view of the human body governed by the nervous system in constant contact with environmental stimuli, their therapeutic efforts remained steeped in traditional humoralism.“

Behandlungsgruppen aufgeteilt und entweder mit dem zu testenden Präparat oder mit einem bereits bekannten Medikament oder manchmal auch mit einem Scheinpräparat (Placebo) behandelt. Im Anschluss an die Therapie werden die Ergebnisse mit statistischen Methoden verglichen. Das geprüfte Medikament gilt dann als wirksam, wenn in der Gruppe der mit ihm behandelten Patienten eine größere Zahl von Patienten von der Therapie profitiert als in den Vergleichsgruppen.[44]

Diese Methode des Wirksamkeitsnachweises war im 18. Jahrhundert als allgemein anerkannte Methode medizinischen Wissenserwerbs kaum denkbar.[45] Zum einen ging man davon aus, dass jeder Mensch seine eigenen Krankheiten entwickelte. Denn im Gegensatz zum heutigen Konzept verstand man Krankheiten als allgemeine Veränderungen des individuellen Körpergeschehens, nicht als spezifische organische Störungen, die man bei nahezu allen Individuen in ähnlicher Form erkennen und behandeln kann. Und weil man Krankheit als ein ganz individuelles Geschehen deutete, ließen sich – zum anderen – die beobachteten Wirkungen eines Medikaments auch nicht ohne weiteres von einem Individuum auf ein anderes übertragen.[46] Insofern konnten systematische Untersuchungen, in denen Therapieergebnisse an Patientenkollektiven mit gleichen Krankheitsbildern ausgewertet und verglichen werden, keinen Sinn ergeben und wurden kaum in Erwägung gezogen.[47] Man versuchte stattdessen, die Wirkung der Therapie in Einzelfällen zu beobachten und im Zusammenhang mit der individuellen Krankengeschichte zu verstehen. Aus dieser kausalen Deutung der Wirkungsweise wollte man Schlüsse ziehen, welche Wirkungen das Medikament bei einem anderen Patienten entfalten würde.[48]

44 Das bedeutet nicht, dass jeder Patient zwangsläufig von der Therapie mit dem als „wirksam" bezeichneten Präparat profitieren wird. Die so genannte *evidence based medicine*, die diese Art des Wirksamkeitsnachweises propagiert, kommt ausschließlich zu probabilistischen Aussagen, die die Erfolgswahrscheinlichkeit für den einzelnen Patienten betreffen; ob ein individueller Patient tatsächlich durch die Behandlung geheilt wird, lässt sich dennoch nicht mit Gewissheit voraussagen. Zur *evidence based medicine* vgl. RASPE (1998) und ROGLER & SCHÖLMERICH (2000).

45 Die von TRÖHLER (2000) gefundenen Belege für eine auf empirisch-statistischer Basis beruhende medizinische Praxis betreffen England und die zweite Hälfte des 18. Jahrhunderts.

46 Vgl. HOFFMANN (1721), Vorrede: „Es ist hierbey diese regula physico-mechanica wohl zu mercken / daß die vires corporum und also auch medicamentorum / so weit sie eine Wirckung und effect thun sollen / nicht absolutae, sondern relativae et conditionatae seyn / das ist so viel gesagt: es haben die medicamenta an und vor sich selbst allein keinen nothwendigen und gewissen effect zu schaden oder zu helffen / sonder es muß jederzeit das corpus humanum auf gewisse Art dazu disponiret seyn / und zugleich mitwircken. Derowegen geschiehet es / daß /was einen zur conservation der Gesundheit oder bey einer Kranckheit dienet / dem andern öffters undienlich und gar schädlich sey […]."

47 Zur Situation in England vgl. MAEHLE (1999), 22: „Only exceptionally, simple arithmetics (‚protostatistics') were applied to evaluate treatment in a number of similar cases […]."

48 Vgl. dazu die in Anm. 39 zitierten Ausführungen Hoffmanns, der aus „observationes" und „theoria" die „wahrhafftige theoria medica", die eine „universal scienz sey", entwickeln

In den Briefen an Canstein wird deutlich, dass auch die Ärzte in den Franckeschen Anstalten in dieser Weise vorgingen. Aufgrund der Zusammensetzung der Arznei und ihrer Herstellungsweise vermutete man einen positiven Effekt bei den Kranken, nur genau wusste man das nicht. Canstein wurde daher oft beauftragt, über die Wirkung der Heilmittel zu berichten. Eine typische Formulierung findet sich etwa im Juni 1702: „Daß es ein gut Medicament sey, ist kein Zweifel. Ob es aber das praestiren werde, was man davon bezeuget, verlanget mich aus der Erfahrung zu vernehmen.“[49] An anderer Stelle, am 7. März 1702, heißt es, man habe ein neues Mittel „selber noch nicht experimentiret“. Es könne jedoch „sicher in allen vorfallenden Kranckheiten gebraucht werden, und wenn man fleißig observiret, wie sich die Patienten darauf befinden, so kan man leicht hinter seine Kräffte kommen“.[50] Canstein wurde gelegentlich auch zu vergleichenden Beobachtungen angehalten. Christian Friedrich Richter schrieb beispielsweise im Januar 1702:

> Inzwischen stelle es in Dero Belieben, ob Sie erst die Essentiam dulcem, und so diese nicht effectuiren wollte beygehendes Pulver, so unser neues Medicament ist, brauchen wollen, so würde sich bey diesem casu zeigen, welches unter diesen beyden das kräfftigste.[51]

Die Briefe zeigen, wie man über Fallgeschichten, *case histories*, zu einem Verständnis der Wirkungsweise der Medikamente kommen wollte.[52] Dabei war man nicht unkritisch, sondern versuchte durchaus, die Berichte über Heilungen in ihrer Glaubwürdigkeit und Zuverlässigkeit zu werten. So äußerte sich Christian Friedrich Richter im März 1702 über die Nachricht aus Wien, dass ein fünfzehnjähriger Knabe innerhalb einer Stunde durch die Einnahme von sechs Tropfen der *Essentia dulcis* von einer Kontraktur befreit wurde: „Ist mehr eine miraculöse, als ordinaire operation des medicaments.“[53]

Die Rolle Baron von Cansteins beschränkte sich nicht nur auf die Mithilfe bei der Beobachtung der Medikamentenwirkungen. Er war darüber hinaus maßgeblich daran beteiligt, dass die Fallgeschichten gesammelt und nach und nach gedruckt wurden. Begünstigend wirkte sich hier zweifellos aus, dass gleichzeitig

wollte. Zu diesem Zweck veröffentlichte Hoffmann in den zwölf Bänden seiner *Medicina consultatoria* fast 600 Krankengeschichten.

49 AFSt/H C 285:15, Nr. 27 (24. Juni 1702).

50 AFSt/H C 285:15, Nr. 13 (7. März 1702). Gerade dieses Zitat zeigt, dass es bei der Beobachtung der Medikamentenwirkung nicht um eine allgemeine Wirksamkeit bei definierten Krankheitsbildern, sondern um die Erschließung der Wirkungsweise der Arznei, seiner „Kräffte“, ging. Vgl. zum Humanexperiment im 18. Jahrhundert auch SCHIEBINGER (2004), die meines Erachtens jedoch das den Versuchen zugrunde liegende Erkenntnisinteresse nicht ausreichend differenziert darstellt.

51 AFSt/H C 285:15, Nr. 5 (18. Januar 1702).

52 Vgl. auch AFSt/H C 285:15, Nr. 40 (6. November 1702): „Den effect, den die Tinctura Antimonii gethan, möchte wol gerne wißen. Es ist zwar freyl. auf eine observation nicht gleich zu bauen, inzwischen lernt man doch immer was draus.“ – Zum „case history approach“ in der Medizin des 18. Jahrhunderts vgl. MAEHLE (1999), 21–23.

53 AFSt/H C 285:15, Nr. 12 (4. März 1702).

mit dem Aufbau der Apotheke und der Medikamentenexpedition die Buchhandlung und der Verlag des Waisenhauses als zweites bedeutendes wirtschaftliches Standbein der Franckeschen Anstalten entwickelt wurden.[54] Eine erste größere Sammlung solcher Heilungsberichte erschien im Jahr 1702 unter dem Titel *Merckwürdige Exempel der unter dem Seegen Gottes durch die Essentiam dulcem geschehenen Curen.*[55] Canstein redigierte die von den Brüdern Richter formulierten Berichte und steuerte seinerseits Exempel aus seinem Berliner Umfeld bei. Eine Durchsicht dieser gedruckten Berichte lässt erkennen, dass der kritische Ansatz, der sich in den Briefen gelegentlich findet, keinen Eingang in die Exempel gefunden hat. Ein Beispiel dafür ist der Fall eines Herrn Klein, der in den Briefen gewissermaßen als „Therapieversager" thematisiert wird.[56] Christian Friedrich Richter regte am 28. Oktober 1702 an, diesen Fall auch in die Exempel aufzunehmen, „damit die leute sehen möchten, man handele aufrichtig". Canstein möge sich zu dieser Idee äußern.[57] Cansteins Antwort liegt nicht vor, aber der Fall ist in den gedruckten Berichten nicht zu verifizieren. Zu vermuten ist, dass Canstein aus Werbegründen von einer Publikation abgeraten hatte. Im Übrigen wuchs die Zahl der Heilungsberichte im Laufe der Jahre. In der letzten Auflage der *Merckwürdigen Exempel* von 1708 wurden fast 200 erfolgreiche Therapien mit den Medikamenten der Franckeschen Anstalten aus den Jahren 1701 bis 1708 beschrieben.[58]

Um wiederum kurz zusammenzufassen: Um die Wirkung der Halleschen Medikamente zu begreifen, wurden – wie in der damaligen Zeit nicht ungewöhnlich – Krankengeschichten gesammelt und ausgewertet. Diese Berichte wurden im anstaltseigenen Verlag gedruckt und einem breiten Publikum zugänglich gemacht. Mit dieser Verbindung von medizinischer Beobachtung und pietistischem Publikationseifer begann die in der Forschungsliteratur beschriebene Werbekampagne für die Medikamente des Waisenhauses.

54 Vgl. OBST & RAABE (2000), 72.

55 EXEMPEL (1702).

56 Vgl. AFSt/H C 285:15, Nr. 9 (14. Februar 1702).

57 Vgl. AFSt/H C 285:15, Nr. 36 (28. Oktober 1702). Vgl. auch AFSt/H C 285:15, Nr. 40 (6. November 1702): „Die observation, so sie bey H. Klein gemacht, habe auch schon, in praesentia, gemerckt. Inzwischen praejudicirt es doch der Sache nichts, man läßt das überflüßige weg. Wenn sein Zustand mit gedruckt würde, könte es meinem Bedüncken nach diesen Nutzen haben 1) daß man dadurch bezeuge, man gehe auffrichtig heraus 2) Man halte es nicht pro necessitate, daß alle Gesund würden 3) Man könte dabey am beqvemsten diejenige effecte anzeigen, so das medicament auch bey denen thut, so nicht völlig gesund werden, und wie sich die dem Medicament im Bericht beygelegte Eigenschafften doch dabey exseriren, kurtz, wie das medicament das seine gethan. Sind nur meine zufällige Gedancken."

58 Vgl. RICHTER (1708).

Der Umgang mit Kritik an den Medikamenten

An den Halleschen Medikamenten (und besonders an der *Essentia dulcis*) wurde schon früh massive Kritik seitens anderer Therapeuten geübt.[59] Diese Kritik bewegte sich auf unterschiedlichen Ebenen: Vielfach wurde bezweifelt, dass die Essenz tatsächlich Gold enthielt, oft wurde aber auch die Wirksamkeit der Medikamente in Frage gestellt.

Am 24. Juni 1702 berichtete Christian Friedrich Richter von einer Reise, die er gemeinsam mit August Hermann Francke unternommen hatte.[60] Man hatte Philipp Jakob Spener (1635–1705), Franckes pietistischen Mentor, in Lichtenburg besucht und ihn krank vorgefunden. Richter beobachtete u.a. eine „Abnahme der Kräffte", eine „Trockenheit des Mundes", „Husten" und vor allem eine Kälte der Gliedmaßen. Weiter schrieb Richter:

> Der H. Profess. hat ihm zwar den Gebrauch der Essentiae Dulcis concentratae vorgeschlagen, und selbige ohne Entgeld zu überlaßen versprochen, weil an dem Mann so viel gelegen, und die Essentz gar offenbarlich calorem vitalem foviret und augmentiret.

Aber zur Überraschung der Besucher lehnte Spener die Anwendung des Medikaments ab. Spener verwies auf den Fall des Kindes eines Herrn Troschel, bei dem die Essenz nicht geholfen habe, und außerdem darauf, „daß die Medici zweiffelten, ob in Metallen Kräffte zur Gesundheit des Menschen enthalten wären". Nach Richters Aussage habe man darauf verzichtet, Spener zu überreden, denn es „scheinet nicht dienl. zu seyn", die „Artzney durch persuasiones zu abtrudiren, da keine confidentz vorhanden".

Auf derselben Reise traf Richter in Torgau einen Dr. Zapf, den (wie er schreibt) „Leibmedicus" der Königin, um mit ihm über die *Essentia dulcis* zu sprechen. Dieser habe „alle virtutem des Medicaments schlechterdings" geleugnet, wobei er sich auf seine Erfahrungen mit der Substanz berufen habe. Richter äußert dann im Folgenden die Überzeugung, dass die Essenz nicht richtig angewandt worden sei, und schließt seinen Bericht mit den Worten: „Ich muß bekennen, ich sehe nicht gern, wenn Medici unsere Artzney probiren, denn es ist gar leicht, sie so zu probiren, daß sie nichts hilfft."[61]

59 Vgl. etwa AFSt/H C 285:15, Nr. 4 (25. Oktober 1701): „Es war vor etlichen Tagen ein Medicus von Berlin, D. Abel in unserer Apothecke, und ließ sich die Essentiam dulcem weisen, verachtete sie, sagende, daß er nicht glaube, daß etwas vom Golde drinnen sey, es sey nur spiritus vini, mit spiritu rosarum tingiret, man hätte es an der Fr. Astmannin in Berlin gesehen was es sey, welche bald darüber gestorben wäre etc. Die Medici werden sich sehr widersetzen, sonderl. wenn der Bericht von den Hauß- und Reise-Apothecken publiciret würde." Ähnlich und ausführlich in AFSt/H C 285:15, Nr. 15 (11. März 1702). – Zur Kritik an der *Essentia dulcis* vgl. auch MEYER-HABRICH (1981), 251–258, und POECKERN (1984), 91.

60 Der Bericht zum Treffen mit Spener findet sich in AFSt/H C 285:15, Nr. 27 (24. Juni 1702). Daraus auch die folgenden Zitate.

61 Ebenfalls AFSt/H C 285:15, Nr. 27 (24. Juni 1702).

Die beiden Episoden zeigen, wie mit begründeten Zweifeln an der Wirksamkeit der *Essentia dulcis* umgegangen werden konnte. Kurzerhand bezweifelte man, dass das Medikament in der richtigen Weise angewandt wurde. Im Falle Speners wird dieser Gedanke indirekt deutlich: Als man erkannte, dass er kein Vertrauen in die Therapie hatte, sah man von Überredungsversuchen ab, weil man sich der Wirkung der Arznei in einem solchen Fall nicht sicher war. Offensichtlich nahm man als Voraussetzung einer erfolgreichen Therapie eine positive Einstellung des Patienten an. Weitergedacht bedeutet dies, dass bei einem Therapieversagen die Patienten selbst und ihr mangelndes Zutrauen verantwortlich gemacht werden konnten. Der Kritik des zweifelnden Arztes begegnete Richter mit dem Hinweis darauf, dass Ärzte immer die Möglichkeit hätten, ein Therapieverfahren durch bewusst oder unbewusst falsche Anwendung zu diskreditieren.

Ganz empfindlich reagierte man, als man den Eindruck hatte, Georg Ernst Stahl stelle die Wirksamkeit der *Essentia dulcis* öffentlich in Frage. In Anbetracht der Funktion der Theorie und Autorität Stahls für die Legitimation der Medikamente überrascht die Aufregung nicht. Stahl scheint dem Goldpräparat gegenüber kritisch eingestellt gewesen zu sein, obwohl er es 1702 in seinem *Collegium practicum* empfohlen hatte[62] und obwohl eines seiner Kinder (wie Christian Sigismund Richter im Januar 1703 berichtete) durch die Behandlung mit der *Essentia dulcis* von einer schweren akuten Krankheit genesen war.[63] Allerdings musste Christian Friedrich Richter in einem Brief an Canstein auch berichten, dass Stahl (wie in dem eben geschilderten Beispiel des Dr. Zapf) ausdrücklich auf Patienten hingewiesen habe, bei denen er keine Wirkung habe feststellen können. Und darüber hinaus habe Stahl vermutet, dass die vorgeblich durch die *Essentia dulcis* genesenen Patienten nicht durch die Substanz selbst, sondern lediglich durch ihr Vertrauen in deren Wirksamkeit gesund geworden seien.[64] Dass Stahl hier einen Placebo-Effekt annahm, verwundert – wenn überhaupt – nur auf den ersten Blick: In Stahls Theorie übten die Affekte einen starken Einfluss auf die Seele und deren Bewegungen aus, sodass dieser Gedanke durchaus nahe lag.[65]

62 Vgl. AFSt/H C 285:15, Nr. 40 (6. November 1702): „So viel habe gehöret, er habe denen Studiosis, im Collegio practico unter andern Medicamentis auch essentiam dulcem recommendirt, et in calamum dictirt, davon ich aber auch noch Gewißheit erwarte." Vgl. auch AFSt/H C 285:15, Nr. 44 (25. November 1702). Richter gibt hier den lateinischen Text des *Collegium* wieder.

63 Vgl. AFSt/H C 285:15, Nr. 56 (13. Januar 1703).

64 AFSt/H C 285:15, Nr. 36 (28. Oktober 1702): „Inzwischen objicirte er doch, sagende, es sey gleich wol eine wichtige objection, wenn man unterschiedene nennen könte, denen es gar nichts geholffen, wie er es denn selbst bey unterschiedenen gebraucht, an welchen er nicht den geringsten effect gemercket, da er ihnen hernach nur ein gemein Pulver gegeben, welches seinen effect gleich bewiesen. In übrigen wären die Patienten so dadurch gesund worden […] gute Leute, […] die eine gute Meynung davon hätten und […] durch das gute Vertrauen gesund worden."

65 Vgl. HELM (2006), 31.

Stahls Kritik rief aufgeregte Reaktionen in den Franckeschen Anstalten hervor, die sich in den Briefen der beiden Ärzte widerspiegeln. Stahl hatte sich Ende 1702 und im Jahr 1708 abschätzig geäußert.[66] In beiden Fällen verwies man als Beleg für die Wirkung der Medikamente auf die zahlreichen Berichte von gelungenen „Curen".[67] Damit konnte man die Kritik Stahls, der seinerseits Beispiele von nicht erfolgreichen Anwendungen vorbringen konnte, vielleicht nicht grundsätzlich entkräften. Auf der anderen Seite aber – und dies war für die weitere Geschichte der Halleschen Medikamente bedeutsam – musste man sich auch nicht beirren lassen. Die große Zahl der positiven Berichte konnte als eindrucksvoller Beleg dafür gelten, dass die Medikamente (und insbesondere die *Essentia dulcis*) tatsächlich wirkten. Denn vielen kranken Menschen war offensichtlich durch die Arzneien geholfen worden. In der damaligen Zeit, als man durch Überlegung, Beobachtung und erneutes Nachdenken die jeweils individuell wirksamen „Kräffte" einer Substanz erschloss, galten glaubhafte Berichte über erfolgreiche Therapien so viel, dass Einzelfälle, in denen die Behandlung versagt hatte, keine grundsätzlichen Zweifel an den positiven Eigenschaften eines Medikaments wecken konnten.[68]

Schluss

Die Medikamente des Halleschen Waisenhauses etablierten sich im Verlauf des 18. Jahrhunderts auf den deutschsprachigen und überregionalen Gesundheitsmärkten. Etliche Bedingungen dieses Erfolgs wurden in der Literatur beschrieben. Nach der Analyse der hier vorgestellten internen Quellen sollen noch drei Voraussetzungen hinzugefügt werden:

66 Vgl. AFSt/H C 285:15, Nr. 163 (vermutlich 13. Oktober 1702); AFSt/H C 285:15, Nr. 36 (28. Oktober 1702); AFSt/H C 285:15, Nr. 167 (Oktober/November 1702); AFSt/H C 285:15, Nr. 140 (ohne Datum, 1708): „Herr D. Stahl disputiret heute De multitudinis Remediorum abusu, in welcher er virtutem Auri in Morbis negiret, und an statt des Beweises refutiret er die Effectus von einer Gold=Tinctur, und die davon edirten Exempel, daß niemand, der es lieset, anders gedencken kan, als daß er von der Essentia dulcis handele, [...]." Vgl. STAHL (1708), 28–31; dazu auch ALTMANN (1972), 82–83.

67 Vgl. AFSt/H C 285:15, Nr. 167 (Oktober/November 1702): „Inzwischen eröfnete er unterschiedene dubia so er gegen das Medicament hatte, und bekante, daß, da er offt schrifft= und mündl. deswegen sey befraget worden er frigide geantwortet. Ich producirte ihm darauf unterschiedene Briefe einiger Patienten, so an die Frl. Kroßig geschrieben waren, und benahm ihm seine dubia, so gut ich konte, so schien es doch, als wenn er sich faßte, [...]". AFSt/H C 285:15, Nr. 140 (ohne Datum, 1708): „Inzwischen habe ich doch dem H. D. Stahl die lezt edirten Exempel communiciret."

68 Auch in der modernen Medizin wird die Aussage über die mit statistischen Methoden ermittelte ‚Wirksamkeit' einer Therapiemethode durch Einzelfälle nicht wesentlich beeinflusst.

(1) Mit der gezielten Übernahme von Stahls Theorie in die gedruckten Texte zu den Medikamenten lieferte man eine zumindest die Stahl-Anhänger überzeugende Erklärung für deren Wirkungsprinzip.

(2) Zwischen der im 18. Jahrhundert durchaus üblichen Sammlung von Fallberichten zum besseren Verständnis von Arzneimittelwirkungen und den missionarischen und verlegerischen Aktivitäten der Franckeschen Anstalten kam es zu einer Synergie, deren Resultat eine für die damalige Zeit erstaunliche Werbekampagne war.

(3) Der individualisierende Ansatz der Medizin in der ersten Hälfte des 18. Jahrhunderts und die umfangreiche Sammlung von Heilungsberichten ermöglichten es, Berichte über erfolglose Therapieversuche zu entkräften.

Aber dennoch: Betrachtet man die Halleschen Arzneien als Beispiel für eine erfolgreiche Etablierung spezifischer therapeutischer Praktiken in der Frühen Neuzeit, bleibt deren rasche Verbreitung auf den regionalen, nationalen und überregionalen Gesundheitsmärkten auch nach der Analyse dieser Voraussetzungen ein bemerkenswertes Phänomen.

Quellen- und Literaturverzeichnis

Archiv der Franckeschen Stiftungen zu Halle / Wirtschafts- und Verwaltungsarchiv (AFSt/W)
AFSt/W II/-/11: Verschiedene Nachrichten besonders was bey Antritt Sr. Kgl. Majt. von Preußen Friedrich Wilhelms Regierung und besonders deroselben hohen persönlichen Besuchung des Waisenhauses ergangen betr.

Archiv der Franckeschen Stiftungen zu Halle / Hauptarchiv (AFSt/H)
AFSt/H C 285:15: Corresp. mit denen Herrn Christian Friedrich u. Christian Sigismund Richtern als denen Medicis des Waisenhauses. 1699 seqq.

Geheimes Staatsarchiv Preußischer Kulturbesitz Berlin-Dahlem (GStA PK)
GStA PK, I. HA, Rep. 52 Magdeburg, Nr. 131 b2: Waysenhauß, Päedagogium etc. 1698–1755.

Stadtarchiv Halle, Kap. XIV, Abt. A, Nr. 4: Apotheken-Visitation und Taxe u.a. 1711–1754.

Altmann (1972)
Altmann, Eckhard: Christian Friedrich Richter (1676 – 1711). Arzt, Apotheker und Liederdichter des Halleschen Pietismus. Witten: Luther-Verlag, 1972 (Arbeiten zur Geschichte des Pietismus 7).

Bauer (2000)
Bauer, Axel: Der Körper als Marionette? Georg Ernst Stahl und das Wagnis einer psychosomatischen Medizin. In: Engelhardt, Dietrich von; Gierer, Alfred (Hrsg.): Georg Ernst Stahl (1659–1734) in wissenschaftshistorischer Sicht. Leopoldina-Meeting am 29. und 30. Oktober 1998 in Halle (S.). Halle: Deutsche Akademie der Naturforscher Leopoldina, 2000 (Acta Historica Leopoldina 30), 81–95.

Beisswanger (1996)
Beisswanger, Gabriele: Arzneimittelversorgung im 18. Jahrhundert. Die Stadt Braunschweig und die ländlichen Distrikte im Herzogtum Braunschweig-Wolfenbüttel. Braunschweig: Deutscher Apotheker-Verlag, 1996 (Braunschweiger Veröffentlichungen zur Geschichte der Pharmazie und der Naturwissenschaften 36).

Beisswanger (2003)
Beisswanger, Gabriele: Der Arzneimittelmarkt um 1800. Arzneimittel zwischen Gesundheits-, Berufs und Gewerbepolitik. In: Wahrig, Bettina; Sohn, Werner (Hrsg.): Zwischen Aufklärung, Policey und Verwaltung. Zur Genese des Medizinalwesens 1750–1850. Wiesbaden: Harrassowitz, 2003 (Wolfenbütteler Forschungen 102), 147–161.

Bericht (1701)
Bericht von der Artzney, Essentia Dulcis genannt, durch welche unter dem Seegen Gottes allerley schwere Kranckheiten [...] curiret werden. Halle: Krebs, 1701.

Bericht (1703)
Ausführlicher Bericht von der Artzney Essentia Dulcis genannt. Durch welche unter dem Seegen Gottes allerley schwere Kranckheiten [...] bißher curiret worden. Zum drittenmahl und verbessert in Druck gegeben aus der Apothecke des Wäysen-Hauses zu Glaucha an Halle. Halle: Waisenhaus, 1703.

Exempel (1702)
Merckwürdige Exempel der unter dem Seegen Gottes durch die Essentiam dulcem geschehenen Curen, zum klaren Beweiß desjenigen, was von dieser Artzney in dem davon edirten Bericht angezeigt worden. Halle: Waisenhaus, 1702.

Geyer-Kordesch (2000)
Geyer-Kordesch, Johanna: Pietismus, Medizin und Aufklärung in Preußen im 18. Jahrhundert. Das Leben und Werk Georg Ernst Stahls. Tübingen: Niemeyer, 2000 (Hallesche Beiträge zur Europäischen Aufklärung 13).

Gittner (1948)
Gittner, Hermann: 250 Jahre Waisenhaus-Apotheke und Medikamenten-Expedition der Franckeschen Stiftungen zu Halle an der Saale. Halle: Niemeyer, 1948.

Hartmann (2000)
Hartmann, Fritz: Die Leibniz-Stahl-Korrespondenz als Dialog zwischen monadischer und dualistisch-„psycho-somatischer" Anthropologie. In: Engelhardt, Dietrich von; Gierer, Alfred (Hrsg.): Georg Ernst Stahl (1659–1734) in wissenschaftshistorischer Sicht. Leopoldina-Meeting am 29. und 30. Oktober 1998 in Halle (S.). Halle: Deutsche Akademie der Naturforscher Leopoldina, 2000 (Acta Historica Leopoldina 30), 97–124.

Helm (2004)
Helm, Jürgen: Christian Friedrich Richters ‚Kurtzer und deutlicher Unterricht' (1705) – Medizinische Programmschrift des Halleschen Pietismus? In: Toellner, Richard (Hrsg.): Die Geburt einer sanften Medizin. Die Franckeschen Stiftungen zu Halle als Begegnungsstätte von Medizin und Pietismus im frühen 18. Jahrhundert. Halle: Verlag der Franckeschen Stiftungen zu Halle, 2004, 25–37.

Helm (2006)
Helm, Jürgen: Krankheit, Bekehrung und Reform. Medizin und Krankenfürsorge im Halleschen Pietismus. Tübingen: Verlag der Franckeschen Stiftungen Halle im Max Niemeyer Verlag, 2006 (Hallesche Forschungen 21).

Helm & Stukenbrock (2007)
Helm, Jürgen; Stukenbrock, Karin: Artikel „Friedrich Hoffmann". In: Bynum, W.F. und Helen (Hrsg): Dictionary of Medical Biography. Westport: Greenwood Press, 2007, 657–658.

Kaiser & Piechocki (1969)
Kaiser, Wolfram; Piechocki, Werner: Die Familie Richter – ein Beitrag zur Geschichte der Medikamenten-Expedition des halleschen Waisenhauses. In: Kaiser, Wolfram; Beierlein, Christine (Hrsg.): In memoriam Hermann Boerhaave (1668–1738). Halle: Martin-Luther-Universität, 1969 (Wissenschaftliche Beiträge der Martin-Luther-Universität Halle-Wittenberg 1969/2 [R 103]), 139–151.

Hoffmann (1721)
Hoffmann, Friedrich: Medicina Consultatoria. Worinnen Unterschiedliche über einige schwehre Casus ausgearbeitete Consilia, auch Responsa Facultatis Medicæ enthalten, Und in Fünf Decurien eingetheilet, Dem Publico zum besten herausgegeben. Erster Theil. Halle: Rengerische Buchhandlung, 1721.

Koch (1926)
Koch, Richard: War Georg Ernst Stahl ein selbständiger Denker? In: Sudhoffs Archiv für Geschichte der Medizin 18 (1926), 20–50.

König (1998)
König, Gert: Artikel „Theorie I". In: Ritter, Joachim; Gründer, Karlfried (Hrsg. in Verbindung mit Günther Bien): Historisches Wörterbuch der Philosophie, Bd. 10. Basel: Schwabe, 1998, 1128–1146.

Lanz (1995)
Lanz, Almut: Arzneimittel in der Therapie Friedrich Hoffmanns (1660–1742). Unter besonderer Berücksichtigung der Medicina consultatoria (1721–1723). Braunschweig: Dt. Apotheker-Verl., 1995 (Braunschweiger Veröffentlichungen zur Geschichte der Pharmazie und der Naturwissenschaften 35).

Maehle (1999)
Maehle, Andreas-Holger: Drugs on trial. Experimental pharmacology and therapeutic innovation in the eighteenth century. Amsterdam: Rodopi, 1999 (Clio Medica 53).

Meyer-Habrich (1981)
Meyer-Habrich, Christa: Untersuchungen zur pietistischen Medizin und ihrer Ausprägung bei Johann Samuel Carl (1677–1757) und seinem Kreis. Habilitationsschrift LMU München, 1981.

Müller (1991)
Müller, Ingo Wilhelm: Iatromechanische Theorie und ärztliche Praxis im Vergleich zur galenistischen Medizin (Friedrich Hoffmann – Pieter van Foreest, Jan van Heurne). Stuttgart: Steiner, 1991 (Historische Forschungen 17).

Müller (1995)
Müller, Ingo W.: Seele statt Mechanismus. Medizinische Theorie und Praxis bei Ernst Georg Stahl (1659–1734). In: Hartwich, Hans-Hermann; Berg, Gunnar (Hrsg.): Bedeutende Gelehrte der Universität Halle seit ihrer Gründung im Jahr 1694. Opladen: Leske & Budrich, 1995 (Montagsvorträge zur Geschichte der Universität Halle 2), 37–57.

Obst & Raabe (2000)
Obst, Helmut; Raabe, Paul: Die Franckeschen Stiftungen zu Halle (Saale). Geschichte und Gegenwart. Halle: Fliegenkopf, 2000.

Pagel (1931)
Pagel, Walter: Helmont, Leibniz, Stahl. In: Sudhoffs Archiv für Geschichte der Medizin 24 (1931), 19–59.

Poeckern (1984)
Poeckern, Hans-Joachim: Die Hallischen Waisenhaus-Arzeneyen. Kommentar, Glossar und Transkription. Leipzig: Edition Leipzig, 1984.

Poeckern (2004)
Poeckern, Hans-Joachim: Waisenhaus-Apotheke und Medikamenten-Expedition der Franckeschen Stiftungen zu Halle a. d. Saale. In: Toellner, Richard (Hrsg.): Die Geburt einer sanften Medizin. Die Franckeschen Stiftungen zu Halle als Begegnungsstätte von Medizin und Pietismus im frühen 18. Jahrhundert. Halle: Verlag der Franckeschen Stiftungen zu Halle, 2004, 73–86.

Raspe (1998)
Raspe, Hans Heinrich: Evidence based medicine. Modischer Unsinn, alter Wein in neuen Schläuchen oder aktuelle Notwendigkeit?. In: Meyer zum Büschenfelde, Karl-Hermann; Gethmann, Carl F.; Raspe, Hans H.; Schott, Heinz: Fragen an die moderne Medizin. Stuttgart: Steiner, 1998 (Akademie der Wissenschaften und der Literatur, Mainz; Abhandlungen der Mathematisch-Naturwissenschaftlichen Klasse 1998, 1), 21–41.

Richter & Richter (1703)
Richter, Christian Friedrich; Richter, Christian Sigismund: Fernerer Bericht von der Gesegneten Würckung der Essentiae Dulcis, in welchem zugleich von einigen andern Medicamenten Erwehnung geschiehet. Halle: Waisenhaus, 1703.

Richter (1705)
Richter, Christian Friedrich: Kurtzer und deutlicher Unterricht von dem Leibe und natürlichen Leben des Menschen: Woraus ein jeglicher / auch Ungelehrter erkennen kan / Was die Gesundheit ist / und wie sie zu erhalten: auch welches die menschlichen Kranckheiten / deren Ursachen und Kennzeichen sind / Und wie sie Von einem jeden zu verhüten / oder auch bey Ermangelung eines Medici, ohne Gefahr und mit gutem Success zu curiren: Nebst einem Selectu Medicamentorum, oder XIII. der sichersten und besten Artzneyen / zu einer kleinen / auff alle gewöhnliche Kranckheiten eingerichteten Haus- Reise- und Feld-Apothecken / Mit gnugsamen Bericht von deren Eigenschafften und rechtem Gebrauch. Halle: Waisenhaus, 1705.

Richter (1708)
Richter, Christian Friedrich: Merckwürdige Exempel sonderbahrer durch die Essentiam dulcem von 1701 bis 1708 geschehenen Curen, nebst einer Vorrede in welcher auf die in den [...] unschuldigen Nachrichten unbillig gefällte Censur über Franckens gedruckte Nachrichten vom Waysen-Hause [...] geantwortet wird. Halle: Waisenhaus, 1708.

Risse (2005)
Risse, Guenter B: New medical challenges during the Scottish enlightenment. Amsterdam: Rodopi, 2005 (Clio medica 78).

Rogler & Schölmerich (2000)
Rogler, Gerhard; Schölmerich, Paul: „Evidence-Biased Medicine“ – oder: Die trügerische Sicherheit der Evidenz. In: Deutsche Medizinische Wochenschrift 125 (2000), 1122–1128.

Schicketanz (1972)
Schicketanz, Peter (Hrsg.): Der Briefwechsel Carl Hildebrand von Cansteins mit August Hermann Francke. Berlin: De Gruyter, 1972 (Texte zur Geschichte des Pietismus Abt. III, Band 1).

Schicketanz (2002)
Schicketanz, Peter: Carl Hildebrand Freiherr von Canstein. Leben und Denken in Quellendarstellungen. Tübingen: Verlag der Franckeschen Stiftungen im Max Niemeyer-Verlag, 2002 (Hallesche Forschungen 8).

Schiebinger (2004)
Schiebinger, Londa: Human Experimentation in the Eighteenth Century. Natural Boundaries and Valid Testing. In: Daston, Lorraine; Vidal, Fernando (Hrsg.): The moral authority of nature. Chicago, IL: Univ. of Chicago Press, 2004, 384–408.

Selectus (1702)
Selectus Medicamentorum zu einer compendieusen Hauß- , Reise- Und Feld-Apothecke. Aus eilff Stücken derer erlesensten Medicamentorum Arcanorum und Specificorum zusammen getragen, und auff alle Kranckheiten und Fälle eingerichtet, nebst gegenwärtigen ausführlichen deutlichen Bericht von derselben rechten Gebrauch [...] / publiciret aus der Apothecke des Waisen-Hauses zu Glaucha an Halle. Halle: Waisenhaus, 1702.

Stahl (1696)
Stahl, Georg Ernst: Dissertatio medico-practica de autokratia naturae, sive spontanae morborum excussime et convalescentia. Halle, Med. Diss., vermutlich 1696 (Resp. Johannes Albertus Lasius).

Stahl (1708)
Stahl, Georg Ernst: Dissertatio medica inauguralis de multitudinis remediorum abusu. Halle: Henckel, 1708 (Resp. Barthold Wichers).

Stolberg (2003)
Stolberg, Michael: Homo patiens. Krankheits- und Körpererfahrung in der Frühen Neuzeit. Köln: Böhlau, 2003.

Tröhler (2000)
Tröhler, Ulrich: „To improve the evidence of medicine“. The 18th century British origins of a critical approach. Edinburgh: Royal College of Physicians of Edinburgh, 2000.

Welsch (1955)
Welsch, Heinz: Die Franckeschen Stiftungen als wirtschaftliches Großunternehmen. Untersucht aufgrund der Rechnungsbücher der Franckeschen Stiftungen. Phil. Diss. Halle, 1955.

Wilson (2000)
Wilson, Renate: Pious traders in medicine. A German pharmaceutical network in eighteenth-century North America. University Park, Pennsylvania, PA: Pennsylvania State University Press, 2000.

Part III: Materia Medica and Their Uses

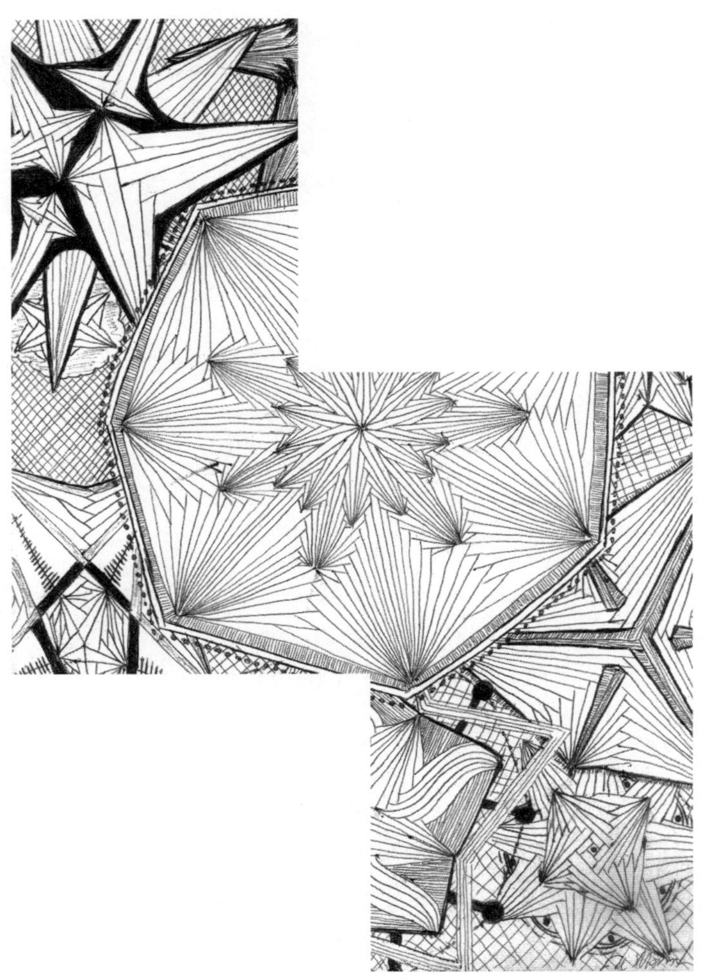

MENSCHLICHE GEWEBE UND ORGANE ALS BESTANDTEIL EINER RATIONALEN MEDIZIN IM 18. JAHRHUNDERT

Robert Jütte

1995 verurteilte das Amtsgericht Tiergarten in Berlin zwei frühere Sektionsassistenten des Zehlendorfer Behring-Krankenhauses, die Hirnhäute Verstorbener verkauft hatten, wegen Störung der Totenruhe zu Geldstrafen von 6.000 und 3.500 D-Mark. Zwei Jahre lang hatten die langjährigen Krankenhausmitarbeiter Hirnhäute, die bei den Obduktionen zur Feststellung der Todesursache den Leichnamen entnommen worden waren, verschwinden lassen. Die Leichenteile wurden in Kochsalzbehälter gepackt und an eine auf Medizinprodukte spezialisierte Firma in Hessen geschickt. 30 D-Mark pro Hirnhaut zahlte damals das Unternehmen, an jeden rund 3.000 D-Mark. Harte Hirnhäute werden für die Heilung von Schädelverletzungen dringend benötigt. Hätte der Institutsleiter die Entnahme gebilligt, hätten sich die Angeklagten nicht strafbar gemacht, denn damals, kurz vor der Verabschiedung des Transplantationsgesetzes (26. September 1997), bewegte man sich noch in einer rechtlichen Grauzone.[1]

Mehr Glück hatten der Münchner Scharfrichter und sein Sohn, denen man 1640 das „hochsträffliche Verhalten“ der Leichenschändung vorwarf. Die gerichtliche Untersuchung brachte folgendes an den Tag. Eine Kindsmörderin war nach der Hinrichtung von einem Knecht des Scharfrichters fachgerecht enthäutet worden. Der Scharfrichtersohn entnahm anschließend noch der Leiche das Herz, das bei der vom Gericht angeordneten Hausdurchsuchung in der Stube „hinder dem Ofen an einem bändtl hangen“[2] gefunden wurde. Auf Nachfrage kam heraus, dass das entnommene Herz an diesem Ort zum Trocknen aufgehängt worden war und später zu Arznei verarbeitet werden sollte. Der Scharfrichter und sein Sohn gingen schließlich straffrei aus, weil sie nachweisen konnten, dass der zuständige Richter die Leiche, für welche die Angehörigen eine christliche Beerdigung erwirkt hatten, versehentlich zur üblichen Verwertung durch den Scharfrichter freigegeben hatte.

In beiden Fällen geht es also auf den ersten Blick um den Handel mit Leichenteilen, der an sich als legal angesehen wurde, aber sich durch die angebliche oder tatsächliche Nichteinhaltung der entsprechenden Rechtsvorschriften als problematisch erwies. In beiden Fällen geht es um die medizinische Nutzung dieser Leichenteile. Der Unterschied liegt lediglich in der Bewertung dieser Praktiken. Während wir es in dem zeitnahen Fall mit einem Beispiel für den angeblichen Fortschritt in der Medizin (Stichwort Transplantationsmedizin) zu tun haben, sieht man in der Geschichte, die sich vor über 350 Jahren zugetragen hat, üblicherweise eine Manifestation volksmedizinischen Aberglaubens. Dass die Dinge

1 Berliner Zeitung vom 1. Juni 1995.

2 Zitiert nach NOWOSADTKO (1993), 50.

komplizierter liegen und es mehr Gemeinsamkeiten zwischen den beiden Fällen gibt, als man zunächst vermutet, das ist das Thema dieses Beitrags, dessen zeitlicher Schwerpunkt auf dem 18. Jahrhundert liegt – also einer Zeit, in der sich nach landläufiger Sicht die medizinische Aufklärung allmählich Bahn brach.

Im Folgenden wird gezeigt, dass uns heute als „irrational" erscheinende Therapieverfahren aus der Zeit vor 1800 nach damaliger Auffassung durchaus „rational" und damit Bestandteil des offiziellen Arzneischatzes waren. So wurden beispielsweise auch die Scharfrichter-Kuren mit Leichenfett und Menschenhaut als rational im Sinne der damals herrschenden humoralpathologischen Medizin angesehen.

In einem ersten Schritt werden die betreffenden Bestandteile der Materia medica des 17. und 18. Jahrhunderts kurz in ihrem zeitgenössischen Kontext vorgestellt und dann im Einzelnen abgehandelt, von der Haut über einzelne Organe bis hin zu Körpergeweben und dem Blut.

Das Warenlager

„Ausserhalb der Mumie, die sich in unseren Läden befindet, verkauffen wir auch Menschenfett, das wir von unterschiedlichen Orten bringen lassen. [...] Auch verkauffen wir, ohne das Menschenfett, annoch das flüchtige und fixe Saltz vom Menschenblute und dem Hirschedel, dem Haar und Urin, samt vielen andern auf Chymische Weise bereiteten Artzneyen mehr",[3] so preist 1717 der Pariser „Spezerey-Händler" Pierre Pomet (1658–1699) sein einschlägiges Warenangebot an Arzneiprodukten aus menschlichen Geweben und Körpersubstanzen an. Es fehlt zudem nicht der Hinweis, dass man beim Kauf auf die Qualität der Produkte achten solle und nicht so sehr auf den Preis. Deshalb sei es besser, diese Arzneisubstanzen nicht beim Scharfrichter zu kaufen, sondern beim Apotheker, da jene nur den Rohstoff lieferten, die Apotheker diesen aber „mit aromatischen Kräutern" zurichteten, was die Wirksamkeit erhöhe.

Was uns heute wie ein Greuelmärchen anmutet, war noch im 18. Jahrhundert gängige Praxis. Meist waren es zum Tode verurteilte Verbrecher, deren Leichen zur Herstellung von Arzneistoffen dienten. Aber auch auf den Schlachtfeldern der Frühen Neuzeit gehörte das Menschenfett zum Beutegut.[4] Begehrt waren neben Schädel, Daumen (Diebesdaumen) und Fett (Menschenschmalz, lat. *axungia hominis*) auch Haut und Knochen eines Menschen, der nicht eines natürlichen Todes gestorben war. Aus diesen Körperteilen wurden damals relativ kostbare und als hochwirksam eingeschätzte Arzneien hergestellt, die gegen eine Vielzahl von Krankheiten helfen sollten. Christoph Hellwigs *Lexicon pharmaceuticum* von 1709 enthält Artikel über die unterschiedlichsten Arzneimittel, die damals im Gebrauch waren. Die meisten der dort beschriebenen Medikamente

3 POMET (1717), 470.
4 Vgl. GROEBNER (2003), 22.

entstammen dem Pflanzenreich (370). An zweiter Stelle stehen die Animalia (109), gefolgt von den Mineralia (61) und den Composita (10), das heißt den aus mehreren Ingredienzien zusammengesetzten Arzneimitteln, von denen der Theriak das bekannteste ist.[5] Zu den Animalia gehören auch die Arzneien, die vom Menschen stammen. Der entsprechende Abschnitt ist überschrieben: „Vom Menschen / so wohl vom lebenden / als vom ertödeten / wird viel gebrauchet / auch unterschiedliche Präparata von ihm in Officinis gefunden."[6] Er folgt in seiner Aufzählung der üblichen Unterteilung, wie sie sich beispielsweise in Johann Schröders bekanntem Arzneibuch von 1685 findet. Vom lebenden Menschen werden danach folgende Stoffe verwendet: Haare, Nägel, Speichel, Ohrenschmalz, Schweiß, Milch, Menstrualblut, Nachgeburt, Urin, Kot, der Samen, Blut, Blasen- oder Nierensteine sowie die Haut, die den Kopf des Foetus umgibt (*membrana caput foetus cingens*, vermutlich sind damit Reste des Amnions gemeint). Es folgen die Stoffe, die dem toten Körper zu medizinischen Zwecken entnommen werden: „der gantze todte Körper" (Mumien), die Haut, das Fett, die Knochen (*ossa*), die Hirnschale, das Gehirn, die Galle und das Herz.[7] Es fehlt in dieser Aufzählung das Blut frisch verstorbener Menschen, das bei Hinrichtungen reißenden Absatz fand. In unserem Zusammenhang sollen uns nur diejenigen Substanzen interessieren, die aus Leichen gewonnen wurden, und zwar in einer Zeit, die noch kein Transplantationsgesetz kannte und auch keine Richtlinien oder Vorschriften für die Entnahme oder Aufbewahrung von menschlichem Gewebe.

Mumia

Der Pharmaziehistoriker Hermann Schelenz berichtet in einem Zeitungsartikel aus dem Jahre 1907, dass noch im 19. Jahrhundert eine kleine Kindermumie, die in einem Glasschränkchen aufbewahrt wurde, zu den Schätzen in der Materialkammer der Engelapotheke in Halle gehörte.[8] Um 1757 kostete *Mumia vera* in der Leipziger Materialienhandlung von David Heinrich Brückner 9 Groschen das Lot.[9] In der Straßburger Apothekertaxe von 1760 wird Mumie als Heilmittel für unterschiedliche Indikationen aufgeführt, ebenfalls in der Württembergischen Pharmakopoe von 1750.[10] Erst gegen Ende des 18. Jahrhunderts verschwindet die Mumie aus den offiziellen Arzneibüchern. Hahnemann bemerkt in seinem *Apothekerlexikon* von 1793, dass Mumien von den „Voreltern" zum Kurieren

5 BRACHMANN (1956), 21–30.
6 HELLWIG (1709).
7 SCHRÖDER (1686), 1286.
8 Zitiert bei HOVORKA & KRONFELD (1908), 315.
9 Vgl. HOVORKA & KRONFELD (1908), 315.
10 PHARMACOPEA WIRTENBERGICA (1750), 132–133.

von allerhand Krankheiten gebraucht worden seien.[11] Im 19. Jahrhundert findet die Mumie gelegentlich noch in der Veterinärmedizin Verwendung.[12]

Doch was verstand man in der Frühen Neuzeit eigentlich unter einer Mumie? In Zedlers *Universal-Lexicon* wird der schillernde Begriff der Mumie wie folgt definiert: „ein schwartzes, hartes, hartziges Wesen von balsamirten Menschen-Cörpern herrührend."[13] Es handelte sich bei diesem kostbaren Arzneimittel ursprünglich um paraffinische Erdölprodukte (Bitumen), die bereits im Alten Ägypten neben Harzen zum Einbalsamieren benutzt wurden. Solche Leichenfüllungen, auch Totenpech genannt, wurden bereits im frühen Mittelalter durch arabische und jüdische Händler in den Westen exportiert, bis der Nachschub versiegte. Dann kam man auf die naheliegende Idee, „solche künstlicher Weise aus dem Menschenfleisch nachzumachen [...] ohne Unterscheid, ob sie von ansteckenden Seuchen oder anderen Kranckheiten gestorben, also zubereitet und angeschmieret, vor die rechte Mumien verkauffet [...]".[14] Fortan wurden die echten Mumien als „mumia vera" bezeichnet und waren entsprechend teuer, wenngleich man weiterhin nicht vor Fälschungen sicher sein konnte, wie sich bei Apothekenvisitationen immer wieder herausstellte. Auch gab es in der Frühen Neuzeit einen Gelehrtenstreit darüber, was eigentlich als echte Mumie anzusehen ist, das „balsamirte Menschfleisch", oder, wie es Zedler ausdrückte, „dasjenige Hartz oder Erdpech, so mit dem Geblüt sich vereinigt", also die bitumenhaltigen Bestandteile der Mumie. Ob Haut- oder Knochenreste an dem „Totenpech" kleben mussten, blieb ebenfalls weiterhin umstritten. Wichtig war, beim Einkauf auf die folgenden Qualitätsmerkmale zu achten. Man solle, so der Materialienhändler Pierre Pomet, solche Mumien nehmen, „welche fein sauber, gläntzend, hübsch, schwartz, ohne Bein und Staub sind, gut riechen, und nicht wie Pech stincken, wenn sie angezündet werden".[15]

Ein weiteres Problem der Bezeichnungsvielfalt ist, dass die Anhänger von Paracelsus unter Mumie etwas völlig anderes verstanden. Sie sei ein „subtiler geistiger Theil, der einem jeden Menschen angebohren, und in und nach seinem Tode, ja sogar auch in denen Excrementen eine zeitlang verharret".[16] Die Rede ist von der sogenannten *virtus mumialis*, die sich angeblich übrigens auch in Reliquien findet.[17] Paracelsus unterscheidet unterschiedliche Arten von Mumien, je nachdem, mit welchem Element (Luft, Wasser oder Feuer) der Leichnam in Berührung gekommen ist. Hier soll uns nur die zuerst genannte Mumienart interessieren: „[...] mumia des Lufts, das ist der leib der an dem luft oder im luft zu einem mumia ist worden, der mensch, der erhenkt, gespießet oder geradbrecht ist

11 HAHNEMANN (1793-1799), Bd. 1, 84.
12 SCHNEIDER (1985), 185.
13 ZEDLER (1732-1754), Bd. 22, Sp. 735.
14 ZEDLER (1732-1754), Bd. 22, Sp. 741.
15 POMET (1717), Sp. 468.
16 ZEDLER (1732-1754), Bd. 22, Sp. 745.
17 Vgl. HERZOG (1994), 330.

worden […].“[18] Ihre Heilkraft wird von Paracelsus besonders hoch eingeschätzt, insbesondere, wenn der Rohstoff vom Scharfrichter stammt, denn dieser eignet sich die Lebenskraft des Delinquenten durch die Exekution gleichsam an. Daneben gibt es noch die Mumien, „die von einem lebendigen leib separirt und praeparirt wird“, denn „ein ieglicher mensch kann seinen leib in mumiam transmutiren“.[19] Ein Rezept für ein auf diese Weise gewonnenes Arzneimittel liefert uns beispielsweise *Zedlers Universal-Lexicon*.[20] Danach wird Aderlassblut in ausgehöhlte Hühnereier gefüllt, über die Hennen eine Zeit lang brüten sollen. Die bereits weitgehend eingetrocknete Blutmasse sollte dann aus dem Ei entfernt und im Backofen weiter „ausgebacken“ werden. Angeblich lässt sich mit der fertigen Arznei jede Krankheit kurieren.

Doch zurück zu den Mumien, die aus Leichenbestandteilen hergestellt wurden.[21] Zu den Ärzten, die schon früh den Vorschlag machten, statt der teuren ägyptischen Mumien in jüngster Zeit verstorbene Personen zu verwenden, gehört unter anderem der Italiener Petrus Andreas Matthiolus (1501–1577).[22] In seinem immer wieder aufgelegten Kräuterbuch aus dem Jahre 1563 denkt er dabei in erster Linie an Menschen, die im Spital verstorben sind. Paracelsus, wie gesagt, hatte dagegen eine andere Personengruppe im Auge: die zum Tode durch den Strang oder das Feuer verurteilten Verbrecher. Jedenfalls besteht kein Zweifel daran, dass auch Scharfrichter in der Frühen Neuzeit mit Mumienteilen Geschäfte machten. In den Aufzeichnungen des Nürnberger Scharfrichters Meister Franz lesen wir unter dem Datum vom 3. September 1588: „Georg Solen von Nürnberg […] Ist allhie mit den Strang gericht worden, ward nur 8 tag gehangen, da hatt man Ihme den halben Leib mit den Geseß herab geschnitten, und das ander also hangen blieben […].“[23]

Das Anwendungsspektrum der Mumie fasste 1663 der Leibarzt des Kurfürsten von Mainz, Johann Joachim Becher (1635–1682), in seinem Werk *Parnassus medicinalis* wie folgt in Reimen zusammen:

> Die Mumi resolvirt geronnenes Geblüt / Vor Milzes stechen und vor Husten es behüt / Blähung und Wind dess Leibs / verhaltne Weiberzeit / Zwey Quintlein öffnen die / zum Pulver seynd bereit.[24]

Daran hat sich auch im 18. Jahrhundert wenig geändert, wie ein Blick in die einschlägigen Arzneibücher jener Zeit zeigt.

18 PARACELSUS (1931), 345.
19 PARACELSUS (1931), 346.
20 ZEDLER (1732-1754), Bd. 22, Sp. 745.
21 Vgl. vor allem WIEDEMANN (1998), 248–249.
22 MATTHIOLUS (1565), 117–118.
23 TAGEBUCH DES MEISTER FRANZ (1980), 39.
24 Zitiert nach BARGHEER (1931), 235.

Haut

Doch nicht nur in Form von Mumienteilen kam Menschenhaut in der Frühen Neuzeit in den Apotheken zum Verkauf, wie ein Blick in eines der populärsten und einflussreichsten Arzneibücher des späten 17. Jahrhunderts belegt. Unter dem Stichwort Menschenhaut findet sich dort der Hinweis, wozu diese gut ist:

> Die Haut wird gebraucht in der schweren Geburt / und Mutter Beschwerden / (wann man den Bauch damit bindet) in Dörre und Contractur der Gelencke / (wann man die Handschuch davon anziehet.) Sie tauget auch in *suffocatione hypochondriaca*, und bereitet man auch ein edles Wundpflaster daraus.[25]

Dass gegerbte Menschenhaut tatsächlich bei den hier genannten Indikationen Verwendung fand, belegen nicht nur damals weit verbreitete Arzneibücher, sondern auch frühneuzeitliche Gerichtsakten. Anfang des 17. Jahrhunderts gebrauchte der Münchner Scharfrichter Hans Stadler Menschenhaut „für den Kramphff und für dez Zittern".[26] Unter Krampf verstand man damals nicht nur die unwillkürliche Kontraktion der Glieder (Spasmus), auch das Podagra (Gicht) konnte darunter begriffen werden. Mit Zittern sind wohl ganz allgemein diskontinuierliche Zuckbewegungen bestimmter Muskeln gemeint. Noch 1747 benutzte der Augsburger Scharfrichter Johann Georg Tränkler Menschenhaut bei ähnlichen Krankheitszuständen, nämlich „Krampf, Kröpf und Schwinden der Glider und anderen leibs Schmerzen".[27] Wer sich Menschenhaut nicht leisten konnte, der konnte es auch mit der Haut eines frisch geschlachteten Hundes versuchen, die noch warm über die vom „Schwund" betroffenen Körperteile des Kranken gestülpt werden sollte.[28]

Vor allem aber fand Menschenhaut Anwendung in der frühneuzeitlichen Geburtshilfe, und zwar meist in Form einer Leibbinde. Was dieses Mittel bewirken sollte, geht aus der zeitgenössischen Literatur nicht eindeutig hervor. Der bereits erwähnte Scharfrichter Hans Stadler, der einer Münchner Hebamme, die bei den Geburten seiner Ehefrau half, „claine Stuckhl Menschenheuttl"[29] kostenlos überließ, hätte es eigentlich wissen müssen. Doch auch er beschränkte sich darauf, die Vermutung zu äußern, dass dieses Mittel bei schwangeren Frauen wohl ebenfalls krampflindernd wirke. Dass sogar gelehrte Mediziner sich dieses Mittels bedienten, um Beschwerden vor oder nach der Geburt zu lindern, belegt das Zeugnis des Arztes Christoph Hellwig (1663–1721), dessen Frau nach der Entbindung einen lahmen Fuß bekam und durch das Tragen von Pantoffeln aus Menschenhaut nach einigen Tagen angeblich wieder unbeschwert gehen konn-

25 SCHRÖDER (1686), 1305.

26 Stadtarchiv München, Stadtgericht Nr. 866/8, fol. 249–250, zitiert nach NOWOSADTKO (1994), 171.

27 Stadtarchiv Augsburg, Reichsstadt, Akten Nr. 1081, zitiert nach NOWOSADTKO (1994), 171.

28 Vgl. Höfler (1888), 161.

29 Stadtarchiv München, Stadtgericht Nr. 866/8, fol. 249–250, zitiert nach NOWOSADTKO (1994), 171.

te.[30] Ähnlich positiv äußerte sich 1747 der bereits erwähnte Augsburger Scharfrichter Johann Georg Tränckler, der behauptete, dass den „gebehrenden frauen durch die applicirung der menschen haut sehr gut hilfe gelaistet“[31] werden könne.

Auch der Gebrauch von Menschenhaut zu nicht-therapeutischen Zwecken ist quellenmäßig belegt. Ein „Gauner“, der 1769 im Vogtland verhaftet wurde, trug als Amulett „einen aus einem armen Sünder geschnittenen Riemen“[32] bei sich. Außerdem wird die Geschichte eines Hussiten-Oberst kolportiert, der verfügt haben soll, dass man ihm nach dem Tod die Haut abzieht und damit die Feldtrommeln seines Regiments bespannt, damit die Feinde auch nach seinem Tod „von solchem Trummelschlag so bald flüchtig und siegloß werden“.[33] Dabei spielte ebenfalls die Vorstellung eine Rolle, dass die ursprünglich vorhandene Lebenskraft über den Tod hinaus im Leichnam erhalten blieb und sogar auf andere Menschen übertragen werden konnte.

In ländlichen Gegenden Österreichs traf man bis ins 20. Jahrhundert gelegentlich auf die Vorstellung, dass jede Apotheke das Recht habe, jährlich einen, zwei, drei oder vier Menschen zu Arzneimitteln zu verarbeiten.[34] Angesichts der Tatsache, dass Menschenhaut und andere Teile des menschlichen Körpers erst im späten 18. und frühen 19. Jahrhundert endgültig aus dem offiziellen Arzneischatz verschwanden, überrascht es nicht, dass sich dieser „Aberglaube“ so lange halten konnte. Doch die Apotheker waren lediglich für die Weiterbearbeitung zuständig, das Liefermonopol hatten die Scharfrichter, die daraus reichlich Gewinn zogen. Von dem Nürnberger Scharfrichter Franz Schmidt, der ein Tagebuch hinterlassen hat, wissen wir beispielsweise, dass ihm der Magistrat bereits 1580 erlaubt hatte, „den enthaupteten cörper zu schneiden, und, was ime zu seiner arznei dienstlich, davon zu nehmen“.[35]

Wie man sich dieses uns heute schaurig anmutende Ausweiden des menschlichen Körpers vorzustellen hat, zeigt der Fall der 1640 hingerichteten Kindsmörderin Barbara Schmidt, deren Leiche der Scharfrichtergeselle enthäutete, indem er einen Längsschnitt am Rücken entlang führte und dann mit Hilfe einer weiteren Person die Haut „vornen her von den brüsten an biß auf die khnie und als hinterwerts“[36] ablöste. Anschließend musste die Haut – ähnlich wie eine Tierhaut – gegerbt werden. Das unternahm der Henker selbst, denn ein Gerber wäre durch diese schandbare Arbeit unehrlich geworden, wie ein Vorfall in Augsburg im Jahre 1562 dokumentiert.[37] Das Tragen der Menschenhaut wirkte

30 Vgl. HELLWIG (1709).
31 Stadtarchiv München, Stadtgericht Nr. 866/8, fol. 249–250, zitiert nach NOWOSADTKO (1994), 171.
32 Zitiert bei SEYFARTH (1913), 286.
33 Zitiert nach HANDWÖRTERBUCH DES DEUTSCHEN ABERGLAUBENS, Bd. 3, Sp. 1584.
34 Vgl. GRABNER (1985), 196.
35 Zitiert nach NOWOSADTKO (1994), 168.
36 Zitiert nach NOWOSADTKO (1993), 50.
37 STUART (1999), 173.

dagegen für die Kranken – ähnlich wie die Berührung durch die Hand des Henkers – erstaunlicherweise nicht stigmatisierend. Im therapeutischen Kontext war das Tabu, das den Umgang mit dem Scharfrichter betraf, offenbar zeitweilig außer Kraft gesetzt. Da es schwer war, einen Gerber zu finden, der dieses Risiko auf sich nahm, existierten sogar Gebrauchsanweisungen, wie man notfalls dieses Geschäft selbst erledigen konnte – und das in einem vielbändigen Nachschlagewerk, das im Zeitalter der Aufklärung herauskam! Im Band 68 (1785 erschienen) der berühmten ökonomisch-technologischen Enzyklopädie, die von Johann Georg Krünitz herausgegeben wurde, findet sich der Hinweis:

> Es kann sich daher ein Jeder gelegentlich eine solche Haut, oder ein Stück davon, selbst bereiten. Wenn nämlich zuvor, so viel möglich, das Fett davon abgesondert worden ist, darf man nur die Haut mit Alaun und etwas Salz wohl einreiben, in einen Topf thun, und mit einem Gewichte oder Steine beschweren. Nach etlichen Tagen kann man es heraus nehmen, auswaschen, und in der Luft trocknen, hernach über einem hölzernen Stuhle oder einem andern Brete reiben, oder mit einem hölzernen Schlägel klopfen, auch mit Kreide oder Mehl reiben, so wird die Haut zum Aufbewahren ganz geschickt sein.[38]

Allerdings musste man sich zuvor erst Menschenhaut besorgen. Auf legale Weise ging das nur über einen Scharfrichter, der hier eine Art Monopol besaß und sich dieses teuer bezahlen ließ.

Fett

Unter Leichenfett, auch Armesünderfett genannt, versteht man zum einen Leichenwachs (*Adipocire*) oder wachsartiges Fett, das sich bei der Verwesung teils aus vorhandenem Körperfett, teils aus dem Eiweiß der Gewebe, zumal der Muskeln, bei Luftabschluss bilden kann, wodurch der Zerfall des Körpers lange aufgehalten wird. Zum anderen kann es sich auch um Fett handeln, das aus der Leiche herausgeschnitten oder aus fetthaltigen Leichenteilen gewonnen wird. *Axungia hominis*, Menschenfett, erscheint noch um die Mitte des 18. Jahrhunderts in deutschen Pharmakopoen oder Apothekentaxen.[39] Selbst im 19. Jahrhundert war dieses populäre Heilmittel fast in jeder Apotheke zu haben, wenngleich der Käufer getäuscht wurde; denn es handelte sich dabei in der Regel um Schweineschmalz oder andere tierische Fette, die unter dieser Bezeichnung vertrieben wurden. Noch kurz vor dem Ersten Weltkrieg bot ein Totengräber in einer Apotheke in Fischern (Rybáře) bei Karlsbad Leichenfett zum Kauf an. Man zeigte ihn an, und er wurde wegen Störung der Totenruhe verurteilt.[40] Traditionelle Lieferanten des Leichenfetts waren auch im 18. Jahrhundert noch die Scharfrich-

38 KRÜNITZ (1785), 383.

39 Vgl. SEYFARTH (1913), 286. Laut Iburger Apothekertaxe von 1616 kostete ein Lot Menschenfett 4 Gute Groschen, während ein Lot Hühnerfett bereits für einen Pfennig zu haben war, vgl. das Faksimile der Taxe http://www.apohirsch.de/taxe2.htm (Zugriff am 22. August 2007).

40 Vgl. JUNGBAUER (1934), 154.

ter, wie der bereits erwähnte Pariser Spezialitätenhändler Pierre Pomet bezeugt.[41] Doch war dieser Berufsgruppe damals schon eine starke Konkurrenz erwachsen: die Anatomischen Institute an den Universitäten. Im Jahre 1753 beschwerte sich der Münchner Scharfrichter Johann Peter Spann beim Hofrat, dass die Anatomie die begehrte Substanz direkt an die Apotheken liefere und damit sein Monopol verletze.[42] Mit der in vielen Territorien im 18. Jahrhundert durch Gesetz gebotenen regelmäßigen Ablieferung der Leichen von Hingerichteten an das nächstgelegene Anatomische Institut[43] war den Scharfrichtern die Rohstoffquelle abgeschnitten worden. Um dieses zu verhindern, hatte der Augsburger Henker Johann Georg Tränckhler bereits 1747 beim Rat der Stadt den Antrag gestellt, auch „bey anatomirung eines Cörpers" wenigstens die „haut und Schmalz zu hechster nothdurft abnehmen zu dürfen".[44] Mit dem Verweis, dass ihm die medizinische Behandlung untersagt sei, wurde diese Bitte abgeschlagen. Gleichzeitig wies der Magistrat die Ärzte und Wundärzte, die eine anatomische Sektion durchführten, an, die städtischen Apotheken mit Menschenfett nach Bedarf zu versorgen.

Das „Armesünderfett", das von Hingerichteten gewonnen wurde, galt als das beste Menschenschmalz, denn es stammte von einem gesunden Menschen, den ein gewaltsamer Tod meist in der Blüte seiner Jahre ereilt hatte.[45] Verwendung fand dieses Mittel als Beimischung zu Salben für Knochenbrüche, Lähmungen und Verletzungen jeder Art, aber auch gegen Kopfläuse sollte Menschenfett helfen. Über weitere Indikationen weiß Schröders *Arzeney=Schatz* (1685) zu berichten:

> Das Fett stärcket / zertheilet / lindert die Schmertzen / nimmet die Contracturen hinweg / lindert die Hartigkeit der Wunden-Mähler / und füllet die Gruben nach den Kindsblattern aus. Wann mans innerlich frisch gebrauchet / so tauget sie zur Lungensucht / und das Abnehmen des Leibes.[46]

Das Hauptanwendungsgebiet waren und blieben jedoch Lähmungen, wie ein Merkvers besagt: „Zerlassen Menschenfett ist gut vor lahme Glieder, / So man sie damit schmiert, sie werden richtig wieder."[47]

Heute verarbeiten Künstler menschliches Fett, das bei Schönheitsoperationen angefallen ist. Das behauptet jedenfalls der Schweizer Künstler Gianni Motti, der auf der Kunstmesse „Art Basel" ein Stück Seife, hergestellt angeblich aus dem Körperfett des italienischen Ministerpräsidenten Silvio Berlusconi, zum Kauf anbot. Das eher unansehnliche Kunstwerk sollte 15.000 Euro bringen und trägt den Titel „Mani pulite", was auf deutsch „saubere Hände" bedeutet und auf das Schlagwort der Antikorruptions- und Anti-Mafia-Kampagne der italienischen Justiz in den 1990er Jahren anspielt. Das Fett, so behauptet der Künstler, habe er

41 POMET (1717), Sp. 469.
42 Vgl. NOWOSADTKO (1993), 53.
43 Vgl. STUKENBROCK (2001).
44 Zitiert nach NOWOSADTKO (1993), 53.
45 Vgl. GRABNER (1985), 200. Zu anderen Todesarten vgl. GROEBNER (2003).
46 SCHRÖDER (1686), 1305.
47 Zitiert nach HANDWÖRTERBUCH, Bd. 2, Sp. 1384.

von der Klinik in Lugano erhalten, in der Berlusconi sich einer Schönheitsoperation unterzogen hatte. „Es war so eine gallertartige Masse, die schrecklich stank, wie verdorbene Butter oder altes Fritieröl“,[48] so Motti.

Knochen (*ossa*)

Über die Verwendung menschlicher Knochen in der therapeutischen Praxis des 18. Jahrhunderts schreibt *Zedlers Universal-Lexicon*:

> Die Gebeine des Menschen, als eine Artzney innerlich gebrauchet, zertheilen, trocknen, reinigen, daher sie in Bauchflüssen, der rothen Ruhr u. d. g. wie auch zur starcken Monatszeit und anderen Flüssen gut sind. In den Apotheken findet man sie gepulvert, präpariert, ingleichen ein Magisterium und Oel daraus bereitet, welches letztere vornemlich äusserlich zum Podagra dienen soll.[49]

Als medizinische Autoritäten werden Galen, der pulverisierte Menschenknochen gegen Gicht empfiehlt, und Paracelsus mit einem Rezept für ein Gichtpulver aus Menschenknochen, Scammonium, Hermodactyli (Art der Herbstzeitlose) und Turbithwurzel zitiert. Ähnlich lautet die Indikation in Schröders *Arzeney=Schatz* (1685) und in Hellwigs *Lexicon pharmaceuticum* (1714). Gegen Schwindel empfahl die *Dreck-Apotheke* (1714) Späne von getrockneten Menschenknochen mit Honig vermischt.[50] Ein Südtiroler Heiler verarbeitete noch in der zweiten Hälfte des 18. Jahrhunderts Menschenknochen zu einem Pulver gegen Muskelerkrankungen.[51] Zu den Knochen zählte man damals auch die Zähne, die man Toten aus dem Kiefer brach und gegen Karies oder zur Erleichterung des Zahnens gebrauchte. Gegen Zahnschmerz sollte ein in der Tasche bei sich getragener Zahn eines Toten helfen. Der Leipziger Mediziner Carly Seyfarth (1890–1950) berichtet von einem Prozess, der 1907 vor dem Landgericht in Freiberg/Sachsen stattfand.[52] Damals wurden ein Totengräber und ein Arbeiter angeklagt, einer Leiche, die bereits in der Verwesung begriffen war, Zähne ausgebrochen und für volksmedizinische Zwecke missbraucht zu haben. Noch schauriger ist die Geschichte, die in einer Sammlung kurioser Geschichten aus Sachsen von 1699 kolportiert wird:

> Eines [Erz-]Gebirgischen Diaconi Eheliebste hatte eine Befreundin / welche unerträgliche Zahnschmertzen gehabt / und vermeynet sich durch einen Todten-Zahn auch Ruhe zu schaffen. Gehet hin / und beißet einer auffgebahrten Leichen im Grimm der Schmertzen einen Zahn aus / aber mit Verlust aller ihrer Förder-Zähne oben und unten.[53]

48 http://www.n24.de/boulevard/vip/index.php/n2005061313171400002 (Zugriff am 11. August 2005). Die mexikanische Künstlerin Teresa Margolles malt mit bei Schönheitsoperationen abgesaugtem Fett.

49 ZEDLER (1732-1754), Bd. 25, Sp. 2196.

50 DRECK-APOTHEKE (1714), 48.

51 ASCHE & SCHULZE (1996), S. 306; S 5 Nr. 10.

52 SEYFARTH (1913), 289-290.

53 LEHMANN (1699), 824.

Heute wird autolog gewonnenes Mehl aus menschlichen Kieferknochen zur knöchernen Augmentation des atrophischen Oberkiefers vor der Insertion enossaler Implantate benutzt.[54]

Hirnschale

Noch in der Königlich Preußischen Medizinaltaxe von 1749 wird Menschenhirn-Spiritus erwähnt.[55] Über die Verwendung der Hirnschale (*cranium humanum*) als Arznei macht *Zedlers Universal-Lexicon* detaillierte Angaben:

> Man soll sich eine erwählen, von einem jungen Menschen, guten Temperaments, welcher eines gewaltsamen Todes gestorben und nicht begraben worden ist. Oder man soll die Hirn-Schedel von denenjenigen nehmen, so im Kriege umgekommen sind, weswegen im letzten Türken-Kriege gantze Säcke voll Türcken-Köpfe nach Leipzig bracht worden.[56]

Dagegen seien die Schädel von normal verstorbenen Personen, die gelegentlich auch in Apotheken vertrieben würden, ein Betrug am Kunden, denn diese hätten „weder Safft noch Krafft". Als Beleg dient Zedler ein Fall aus dem Jahre 1701. Damals habe der berühmte Gießener Arzt Michael Bernhard Valentini (1657–1729) ein Kleinkind, das an „schwerer Noth" (Fallsucht) litt, zunächst mit „praeparirten Menschen-Hirn-Schedel" aus der Apotheke behandelt, aber keinen Erfolg erzielt. Erst als er dem kleinen Patienten ein Schädelknochenfragment aus eigenem Besitz verabreicht habe, sei eine Besserung eingetreten. Noch besser seien aber Schädelstücke, die von einem noch lebenden Menschen stammten. Nach Paracelsus sei insbesondere das dreieckige Knochenteil (*os triquetrum*) zwischen Hinterhauptbein und den beiden Scheitelbeinen das beste Antiepileptikum.

Nicht nur gegen die Fallsucht sollte die menschliche Gehirnschale helfen. Ein *Wunderbuch* aus dem Jahre 1700 empfiehlt dieses Mittel gegen „den heftigen rothen Fluß der Weiber".[57] Als weitere Indikationen finden sich in der zeitgenössischen Arzneimittellehre: Kopfkrankheiten jeglicher Art, Kropf, Gelbsucht und Vergiftungen. Ein Irrglauben sei es jedoch, so Zedler, darauf zu vertrauen, dass das Trinken aus einer Hirnschale Unverwundbarkeit verleihe, wie manche meinten.[58] Als Gegenbeweis wird der damals offenkundig unter Medizinstudenten übliche Brauch angeführt, nach Abschluss einer anatomischen Sektion gemeinsam aus einer Hirnschale zu trinken. Näheres über die Zubereitung von Arzneien aus *cranium humanum* erfahren wir beispielsweise aus Schröders

54 http://www.zm-online.de/m5a.htm?/zm/8_03/pages2/zmed1.htm (Zugriff am 22. August 2007).

55 Vgl. BARGHEER (1931), 249.

56 ZEDLER (1732-1754), Bd. 13, Sp. 193.

57 GLOREZ (1700), 23.

58 Diese Vorstellung war noch im 18. Jahrhunderts in Italien verbreitet; vgl. CAMPORESI (1990), 51.

Arzney-Schatz (1685). Genannt wird dort unter anderem die Kalzination.[59] Zedler empfiehlt dagegen, die Knochen nicht in den Brennofen zu legen, sondern bloß zu raspeln und dann zu pulverisieren, da sich ansonsten das Salz verflüchtige.[60] Ein weiteres Heilmittel, das in diesem Zusammenhang erwähnt werden muss, ist das Schädelmoos. Die Medizinalordnung von Hessen-Kassel aus dem Jahre 1656 führt unter anderem auch „Moeß von eines Menschen Hirnschal" (*muscus cranio humano innascens*) auf.[61] Wegen der Ähnlichkeit mit einer Moosart, die auf Eichenbäumen wächst, wurde dieses Heilmittel auch *Usnea cranii humani* genannt. Am besten sollte wiederum das Moos von solchen Schädeln gewonnen werden, bei denen ein gewaltsamer Tod zu vermuten war. Schröder spricht von einer „mumialische[n] Krafft",[62] die dem Schädelmoos innewohne und empfiehlt das Mittel vor allem bei Nasenbluten. Hahnemann bezeichnete dagegen in seinem *Apotheker-Lexikon*, das damals als Standardwerk gelobt wurde, sowohl den Gebrauch der menschlichen Hirnschale als auch des Schädelmooses als „Geistesverirrungen" beziehungsweise als „Unsinn",[63] die gleichwohl keiner Kritik bedürften.

Gehirn

Auch der Inhalt der Gehirnschale fand noch bis weit ins 18. Jahrhundert pharmazeutische Verwendung. Ein entsprechendes Rezept lautet:

> Das Gehirn von einem jungen (24. Jahr alten) gesunden Menschen / der gewaltsamer Weise getödtet worden / mit allen Häutlein / Arterien / und Nerven zusammt dem gantzen Rückgrat / zerstoß / und gieß daran Haupt-Wasser [...] laß eine weil stehen / dann destillirs durch etliche Cohobationen. Zieh aus denen calcinirten fecibus das Saltz / und conjungirs mit dem Spir[itus], und behalts.[64]

Johann Joachim Becher dichtete 1663 den folgenden Merkvers: „So aus dem Menschenhirn ein Wasser wird bereit / Ein Scrupel dessen hilft und stillt das böse Leid".[65] In einem anderen Verfahren wurde menschliches Gehirn zu einem ölhaltigen Arzneimittel verarbeitet, das ebenfalls gegen Epilepsie helfen sollte. Die Verwendung von Gehirnen von Kindern zu therapeutischen Zwecken wird übrigens schon bei Plinius beschrieben.[66]

59 SCHRÖDER (1686), 1307.
60 ZEDLER (1732-1754), Bd. 13, Sp. 194.
61 PECHAČEK (2003), 237.
62 SCHRÖDER (1686), 1308.
63 HAHNEMANN (1793-1799), Bd. 2, 84, 120.
64 SCHRÖDER (1686), 1309.
65 BECHER (1663), 12.
66 PLINIUS (1988), 15. Vgl. HÖFLER (1910) 56; BARGHEER (1931), 248; GRASSET (1900), 606.

Galle

Während in den meisten frühneuzeitlichen Arzneitaxen fast nur Ochsengalle als Heilmittel für die unterschiedlichsten Krankheiten aufgeführt wird, empfehlen einige Ärzte auch Menschengalle. Bei Becher heißt es: „Extract von Menschen-Gall getröpffelt in die Ohren / Den Tauben hilffts / ob sie gleich weren so gebohren.“[67] In der Antike war dagegen Menschengalle das Mittel der Wahl bei Augenleiden, wenngleich Plinius gewisse Vorbehalte gegen die Verwendung hatte und deshalb einen Gewährsmann vorschiebt.[68] Nach der Säftelehre sollte die Bitterkeit der Galle die kalten *humores* beseitigen, die als Auslöser von Augenkrankheiten angesehen wurden.[69] Wie man die Menschengalle beschaffte, darüber lassen sich die Arzneibücher nicht näher aus.

Herz

Das Herz galt nicht nur bei den Germanen als Sitz der Seele.[70] Menschenopfer, bei denen anschließend das Herz verspeist wurde, sind Bestandteil der mythologischen Überlieferung aus den unterschiedlichsten Kulturen. Im Arzneischatz des 17. und 18. Jahrhunderts kommt das menschliche Herz ebenfalls vor. Schröder nennt folgende Verwendung: „Das Hertz heilet die schwehre Not / (wann mans tröcknet und giebet).“[71] Ähnlich lautet das Rezept in einem Arzneibuch aus dem Jahre 1714.[72] Dass bei der Herstellung solcher uns heute äußerst merkwürdig anmutenden Arzneien gegen die Epilepsie Menschenherz tatsächlich ein Bestandteil war und nicht durch Tierherzen substituiert wurde, belegt der bereits erwähnte Vorfall in Augsburg im Jahre 1640, als man im Haus des Scharfrichters „hinder dem Ofen an einem bändtl hangen“ ein menschliches Herz fand, das dort getrocknet und anschließend zu einem Medikament weiterverarbeitet werden sollte.

Blut

In der Auflistung der pharmazeutischen Verwertbarkeit der Leiche fehlt sowohl in Schröders *Arzeney=Schatz* (1685) als auch in Hellwigs *Lexicon pharmaceuticum* (1714) das Blut. Dabei spielte gerade dieser „Stoff des Lebens“ in der Scharfrichterpraxis eine große Rolle, wie zahlreiche Berichte über Hinrichtungen bis sogar in das 20. Jahrhundert hinein belegen. Als im Juli 1908 in Freiberg in

67 BECHER (1663), 13.
68 PLINIUS (1988), 17.
69 Vgl. BARGHEER (1931), 288.
70 Vgl. BARGHEER (1931), 230–232; HÖFLER (1910), 258–260.
71 SCHRÖDER (1686), 1309.
72 Vgl. BRACHMANN (1956), 29.

Sachsen eine Frau hingerichtet wurde, bat eine ältere Frau aus einem Dorf in der Umgebung einen Justizbeamten, ob sie nicht eine kleine Menge Blut von der Delinquentin nach der Hinrichtung durch das Fallbeil bekommen könne. Sie habe in ihrer Bekanntschaft ein junges Mädchen, das an Epilepsie leide, und diesem wolle sie mit dem Blut helfen.[73] Die ersten Belege für die Praxis, bei Hinrichtungen das Blut für Heilzwecke „abzuzapfen“, datieren aus dem 17. Jahrhundert. Aus Nürnberg wird 1674 berichtet, dass das aus dem Hals schießende Blut eines hingerichteten Verbrechers in einer Schale aufgefangen worden sei, um es „armen und preßhaften Leuthen, welche mit der schweren Kranckheit oder hinfallenden Sucht beladen gewesen, zu trinken [...] zu geben, wovon sie curirt, gesund und heil worden“.[74] Im Jahr 1731 vermeldete die Vossische Zeitung über eine Hinrichtung in Dresden:

> Bey der am verwichenen Dienstag erfolgten Enthauptung des Unter-Officiers Jacobi hat eine junge Weibes=Person, welche mit der fallenden Sucht behafftet gewesen, nach erlangter Erlaubnis, einen guthen Theil von dessen warmen Blut, um dadurch curiret zu werden, zu sich genommen, welcher dann hierauf Platz gemacht worden, daß sie durch beständiges Lauffen die verhoffte Würckung davon erlangen möchte.[75]

Durch die Bewegung des Laufens sollte offenbar das Blut des Hingerichteten mit dem der Frau besser vermischt werden. Auch bei der Enthauptung des berühmten Räuberhauptmanns Schinderhannes in Mainz im Jahre 1803 gaben Scharfrichterknechte einigen Zuschauern, die an Epilepsie litten, das in einem Becher aufgefangene Blut zu trinken, während gleichzeitig die Ärzte galvanometrische Experimente mit dem abgetrennten Räuberhaupt unternahmen.[76] Und noch 1814 schilderte ein Beobachter einer Hinrichtung in Stralsund die Szenen, die sich vor seinen Augen abspielten, wie folgt:

> Die merkwürdige Erscheinung bei dieser Exekution waren zwei Reiter, anscheinend Fremde. Sie führten einen elenden Kranken, wahrscheinlich einen Epileptischen mit sich, und füllten ein mäßiges Töpflein mit dem Blute des Hingerichteten bis an den Rand. Nachdem der Kranke hilfesuchend und gierig den schauerlichen Inhalt bis auf den Boden geleert hatte, wurde er von den beiden Reitersmännern mit starken Riemen zwischen den Pferden festgebunden und im sausenden Galopp davongeführt.[77]

Über die Glaubwürdigkeit dieses Berichts lassen sich keine Angaben machen, doch dürften die damaligen Leser daran keine Zweifel gehabt haben.

Ähnliche Szenen spielten sich noch um die Mitte des 19. Jahrhunderts bei öffentlichen Hinrichtungen ab. Um 1850 reagierte die Obrigkeit auf ein solches Ansinnen jedoch nicht mehr so bereitwillig wie in den Jahrzehnten zuvor. Als sich 1843 in Groß-Schneen im damaligen Königreich Hannover sechs Epileptiker mit Trinkgefäßen in der Hand zum Schafott begeben wollten, verweigerten

73 Freiberger Anzeiger vom 24. Juli 1908, zitiert bei BARGHEER (1931), 264.

74 Zitiert nach van DÜLMEN (1985), 163.

75 BUCHNER (1922), 35.

76 Vgl. FRANKE (1984), 318.

77 Zitiert nach BARGHEER (1931), 266.

ihnen die Sicherheitskräfte den Zugang mit dem Hinweis, dass medizinische Autoritäten dieses offenbar immer noch populäre Heilmittel für unwirksam hielten. Ein Gerichtsassessor aber hatte Mitleid mit den Kranken und holte ein Gutachten zweier Göttinger Professoren ein, die bescheinigten, dass der Genuss des Blutes eine heilsame seelische Wirkung haben könne.[78] So kamen die Kranken schließlich doch zu ihrem Ziel.

Die früheste Erwähnung, dass frisches Menschenblut gegen Epilepsie helfe, finden wir bei Plinius, der auf die Gladiatorenpraxis verweist.[79] Um 1400 rät Ortolff von Bayrlandt in seinem Arzneibuch, Aderlassblut mit Eidotter vermischt einem Fallsüchtigen zu verabreichen.[80] Der bereits mehrfach zitierte Johann Joachim Becher empfiehlt in seinem Arzneibuch von 1663 ebenfalls die Anwendung, nennt aber nicht die Quelle des Blutes, warnt dafür aber vor den Risiken und Nebenwirkungen: „[...] wiewol in dieser Cur große Gefahr obstehet / gestaltsam Etliche durch solche Cur ohnsinnig worden / auch an statt daß sie die Epilepsia verlassen sollte / dieselbe erstlich recht bekommen haben."[81] In allen Fällen äußert sich die Vorstellung, dass Blut Lebenskraft in sich birgt und durch die unmittelbare Übertragung schwere Krankheiten, wie beispielsweise die Epilepsie, heilen kann. Dass es nicht unbedingt das Blut von Hingerichteten sein musste, zeigt der Brauch, der für das 19. Jahrhundert mehrfach belegt ist, dass Eltern sich in den Finger stachen, um dann die Blutstropfen ihren an Krämpfen oder an Epilepsie leidenden Kindern einzuflößen.[82]

Rationale Medizin

Was wir heute in den Bereich der Zauberei oder des volksmedizinischen Sympathieglaubens verweisen würden (z. B. die Vorstellung, dass Lungenkraut aufgrund seiner Form bei Erkrankungen der Lunge hilft), war bis ins 18. Jahrhundert durchaus Bestandteil der „rationalen" Medizin. Rational hieß, nicht nur die Ursachen einer Krankheit zu kennen, sondern „man muß auch die Mittel kennen, von denen die Erfahrung gelehrt hat, daß sie hierzu geschickt sind [...]".[83] So war Menschenhaut zwar ein ungewöhnliches, aber durchaus „natürliches" Heilmittel, das nichts mit weißer Magie im damaligen Sinne zu tun hatte, denn man kannte seine Wirkung aus Erfahrung und hatte dazu auch die passende medizinische, auf Kausalität abzielende Theorie. Als der Münchner Scharfrichter Hans Stadler 1609 in den Verdacht geriet, magische Praktiken anzuwenden, verteidigte er sich mit dem Hinweis, dass er nur natürliche Mittel, nämlich allerlei Kräuter, Wurzeln und Menschenfett anwende. Und auch die Tatsache, dass Leichen-

78 Vgl. EVANS (2001), 127.
79 PLINIUS (1988), 15.
80 ORTOLFF VON BAYRLANDT (1477), Bl. 19r.
81 BECHER (1663), 12.
82 Vgl. die Beispiele bei BARGHEER (1931), 268.
83 J. G. Krüger, Naturlehre (1765), zitiert nach WITZEL (1990), 35.

bestandteile in der Frühen Neuzeit als Heilmittel in offiziellen Pharmakopoen erwähnt werden, belegt, dass man sich eine „natürliche" Wirkung dieser Arznei vorstellte. Der Kurfürstlich-brandenburgische Hofmedicus Daniel Beckher (1594–1655), der als Professor für Medizin in Königsberg wirkte, legte großen Wert darauf, seinen Lesern zu erklären, dass der Gebrauch menschlicher Körperteile, auch von Toten, nach göttlichem und weltlichem Recht erlaubt sei.[84] Im 17. Jahrhundert rechtfertigten Theologen den Verzehr von Menschenfleisch (Kannibalismus) in extremen Notlagen mit dem Hinweis, dass Menschenfleisch in Arzneimitteln Verwendung finde und damit dem Lebenserhalt diene.[85]

Die Scharfrichter-Kuren mit Leichenfett und Menschenhaut waren also rational im Sinne der damals herrschenden humoralpathologischen Medizin, aber auch der naturphilosophischen Vorstellungen eines Paracelsus, die sich auch im 18. Jahrhundert noch einer großen Beliebtheit erfreuten. So hatte beispielsweise einer der Begründer der modernen Naturwissenschaft, Robert Boyle (1627–1691), keinerlei Probleme, das Bestreichen eines Gichtkranken mit der abgehauenen Hand eines frisch hingerichteten Verbrechers damit zu begründen, dass natürliche Kräfte dabei am Werk seien, die er mit dem Magnetismus verglich.[86]

Nicht immer war die Grenze zwischen Natürlichem und Übernatürlichem leicht zu ziehen. So sah sich der Jesuit Jacob Schmid 1738 zu der Warnung veranlasst:

> Und wann du gleich sagest: Es seynd ja natürliche Sachen / mithin ja auch verlaubt? So gibe ich dir zur Antwort / daß es freylich natürliche Sachen seynd / aber zu solchen Umbständen nicht verlaubt; maßen sie darzu von der Natur die Krafft nicht haben / sondern von dem Höllischen tausend Künstler / und folglich verbotten seynd / aus Ursach / daß sich die Beyhilff des vermaledeyten Seelen-Feindes einmische.[87]

Für die Obrigkeit war dagegen die Trennlinie in der Praxis leichter zu markieren: Wer Zaubersprüche zu Hilfe nahm und sich nicht auf die materielle Wirkung allein verließ, der kam – ob nun Heiler oder Patient – in den Ruf, unerlaubte schwarze Magie zu betreiben, was im schlimmsten Fall sogar den Vorwurf der Hexerei einbringen konnte.

Der seit dem 18. Jahrhundert zu beobachtende Ausschluss der magischen Mittel aus dem Therapieangebot wurde, wie Jutta Nowosadtko nachgewiesen hat, auch von den Scharfrichtern, denen äußerliche und manchmal sogar innere Kuren erlaubt waren, mitgetragen. Als Heiler beschränkten sie sich in der Regel auf die Verwendung natürlicher Mittel, die sie entweder aus den Apotheken bezogen oder an diese sogar verkauften. Ein Problem entstand erst, als sich das medizinische Paradigma zu ändern begann und seit dem ausgehenden 17. Jahrhundert eine neue Weltsicht und auch Körpervorstellung immer mehr an Einfluss gewann: Der von der Seele getrennte Leib (Descartes), das Maschinenmodell des

84 BECKHER (1660), 293–294.
85 MENOCHIO (1699), 212–213. Diesen Hinweis verdanke ich Stefanie Winter (Stuttgart).
86 Vgl. THOMAS (1973), 242.
87 Zitiert nach NOWOSADTKO (1993), 62.

Körpers (LaMettrie) waren Ausdruck einer neuen rationalistischen Weltsicht, die den Weg zu einer naturwissenschaftlichen Medizin freimachte. Fortan verstand man unter Rationalität der Medizin, dass eine rationale Therapie auf den von der Physiologie und anderen medizinischen Grundlagenfächern experimentell gefundenen Erkenntnissen beruhen müsse. Für nicht wenige Ärzte wurde die Newtonsche Physik das paradigmatische Vorbild einer Wissenschaft, die sich auf Vernunftprinzipien gründete. Im ausgehenden 18. Jahrhundert nahmen z. B. die Reiz-Erregungslehre (Brownianismus), aber auch die Homöopathie für sich in Anspruch, eine rationale Heilkunde zu sein.[88] „In Deutschland", so der Berliner Medizinhistoriker Volker Hess, „mündete die Kernfrage, die die Ärzte des 18. Jahrhunderts so beschäftigt hatte, wie nämlich die Medizin nach ‚Vernunft' und ‚Erfahrung' betrieben werden könne, in den Versuch, die Medizin als Wissenschaft zu begründen."[89] In diesem System hatten die Erfahrungsmedizin, aber auch das Analogiedenken, das mehr als zweitausend Jahre die Medizingeschichte prägte, keinen Platz mehr. Oder wie es Friedrich Hoffmann, der bekannte Hallenser Mediziner, bereits 1718 im Vorwort seiner *Medicina rationalis systematica* voraussah, dass nämlich für eine wirksame Therapie die Urteilskraft allein nicht genüge: „Es bedarf darüber hinaus einer fundierten physikalischen, mechanischen, chemischen und medizinischen Theorie, ohne die man beim Beobachten weder eine Wahrheit ans Licht bringen noch die Ursachen irgendwelcher Wirkungen oder Erscheinungen aufdecken kann."[90] Diesem Anspruch genügte offenkundig weder die antike Humoralpathologie noch der Paracelsismus. Und so verschwanden im Zeitalter der Aufklärung die Leichenteile aus der therapeutischen Medizin, um dann im 20. Jahrhundert unter neuen Vorzeichen der Rationalität wieder als medizinischer Fortschritt gepriesen zu werden. Man denke in diesem Zusammenhang nicht nur an die Organtransplantation, bei der Körperteile und Gewebe von Menschen, bei denen der Hirntod festgestellt wurde, übertragen werden. Auch die Plazentatherapie oder die Gewinnung von Wachstumshormon aus Hypophysen von Leichen, wie sie bis vor kurzem noch üblich war, gehören in diesen Kontext. Angesichts des Booms, der heute auf dem Gebiet der Organ- und Gewebetransplantation zu beobachten ist, sprechen einige Kritiker inzwischen vom „Ausdruck eines irrationalen Vertrauens von seiten der Behandelten in die medizinische Rationalität und ihren Fortschritt".[91]

88 Zur Rationalität der Homöopathie vgl. Jütte (1996), 24–25. Zur Bedeutung Newtons für den Brownianismus vgl. Schwanitz (1983), 106.

89 Hess (1993), 155.

90 Hoffmann (1748), 281. Deutsche Übersetzung des ursprünglich lateinischen Texts nach Canguilhem (1989), 45.

91 Canguilhem (1989), 51.

Quellen- und Literaturverzeichnis

Asche & Schulze (1996)
Asche, Roswitha; Schulze, Ernst-Detlef: Die Ragginer. 200 Jahre Volksmedizin in Südtirol. München: Pfeil, 1996.

Bargheer (1931)
Bargheer, Ernst: Eingeweide. Lebens- und Seelenkräfte des Leibesinneren im deutschen Glauben und Gebrauch. Berlin, Leipzig: de Gruyter, 1931.

Becher (1663)
Becher, Johann Joachim: Parnassus medicinalis [...] oder Ein neues Thier-, Kräuter- und Bergbuch. Ulm: Görlin, 1663.

Beckher (1660)
Beckher, Daniel: Medicus microcosmus, seu Spagyria microcosmi exhibens medicinam corpore hominis tum vivo tum extincto docte eruendam, scite praeparandam et dextre propinandam. London: Martin, Allestry & Dicas, 1660.

Brachmann (1956)
Brachmann, Wilhelm: Der Mensch als Arzneimittel in L. Christoph Hellwigs Lexicon pharmaceuticum von 1714. In: Vorträge der Hauptversammlung der Internationalen Gesellschaft für die Geschichte der Pharmazie während des Internationalen Pharmaziegeschichtlichen Kongresses in Rom vom 6. bis zum 10. September 1954. Eutin: Internationale Gesellschaft für die Geschichte der Pharmazie, 1956 (Veröffentlichungen der Internationalen Gesellschaft für die Geschichte der Pharmazie, Neue Folge 8), 21–30.

Buchner (1922)
Buchner, Eberhard: Ärzte und Kurpfuscher. Kulturhistorisch interessante Dokumente aus alten deutschen Zeitungen (17. und 18. Jahrhundert). München: A. Langen, 1922.

Camporesi (1990)
Camporesi, Piero: Das Brot der Träume. Hunger und Halluzinationen im vorindustriellen Europa. Aus dem Italienischen von Karl F. Hauber. Frankfurt a. M., New York: Campus Verlag, 1990.

Canguilhem (1989)
Canguilhem, Georges: Grenzen medizinischer Rationalität. Historisch-epistemologische Untersuchungen. Aus dem Französischen von Monika Noll. Tübingen: Edition diskord, 1989.

Dreck-Apotheke (1714)
Die heylsame Dreck-Apotheke [...]. Frankfurt/Main: Friedrich Knochen und Sohn, 1714 (ND Frankfurt/M.: Govi, 1986).

Dülmen (1985)
Dülmen, Richard van: Theater des Schreckens. Gerichtspraxis und Strafrituale in der Frühen Neuzeit. München: C. H. Beck, 1985.

Evans (2001)
Richard J. Evans: Rituale der Vergeltung. Die Todesstrafe in der deutschen Geschichte 1532–1987. Deutsch von Holger Fliessbach. Berlin: Kindler, 2001.

Franke (1984)
Franke, Manfred: Schinderhannes. Das kurze, bewegte Leben des Johannes Bückler. Nach den alten Dokumenten neu erzählt. Düsseldorf: Claassen, 1984.

Glorez (1700)
Glorez, Andreas: Eröffnetes Wunderbuch [...]. Regensburg, Stadtamhof, 1700 (ND Freiburg i. Breisgau.: Aurum, 1979).

Grabner (1985)
Grabner, Elfriede: Grundzüge einer ostalpinen Volksmedizin. Wien: Verlag der Österreichischen Akademie der Wissenschaften, 1985.

Grasset (1900)
Grasset, Hector: Commentaire scientifique sur l'organothérapie des anciens. In: Janus 5 (1900), 605–610.

Groebner (2003)
Groebner, Valentin: Menschenfett und falsche Zeichen. Identifikation und Schrecken auf den Schlachtfeldern des späten Mittelalters und der Renaissance. In: Martus, Steffen; Münkler, Marina; Röcke, Werner (Hrsg.): Schlachtfelder. Codierung von Gewalt im medialen Wandel. Berlin: Akad.-Verlag, 2003, 21–32.

Hahnemann (1793-1799)
Hahnemann, Samuel: Apothekerlexikon. Bd. 1 und 2. Leipzig: Crusius, 1793–1799.

Handwörterbuch
Bächtold-Stäubli, Hanns (Hrsg.): Handwörterbuch des deutschen Aberglaubens. Berlin: de Gruyter, 2000 (= unveränderter photomechanischer ND der Ausgabe Berlin [u.a.], 1927–1942).

Hellwig (1709)
Hellwig, Christoph: Neu eingerichtetes Lexicon pharmaceuticum Oder: Apothecker-Lexicon: Worinnen teutsch-lateinisch / und lateinisch-teutsch / beyde nach dem. Alphabet, Die Stücke, welche ex triplici Regno, oder dreyfachem Natur-Reiche, als Regno Minerali, Vegetabili, & Animali, in der Medicin, Apothecke und Chirurgie gebräuchlich, zu finden [...]. Frankfurt, Leipzig: Stößl, 1709.

Herzog (1994)
Herzog, Markwart: Scharfrichterliche Medizin. Zu den Beziehungen zwischen Henker und Arzt, Schafott und Medizin. In: Medizinhistorisches Journal 29 (1994), 309–331.

Hess (1993)
Hess, Volker: Von der semiotischen zur diagnostischen Medizin. Zur Entstehung der klinischen Methode zwischen 1750 und 1850. Husum: Matthiesen, 1993.

Hoffmann (1748)
Hoffmann, Friedrich: Opera Omnia. Bd. 1. Genf: Tournes, 1748.

Höfler (1888)
Höfler, Max: Volksmedicin und Aberglaube in Oberbayerns Gegenwart und Vergangenheit. München: Stahl, 1888 (ND Walluf-Nendeln: Sändig, 1976).

Höfler (1910)
Höfler, Max: Die volksmedizinische Organotherapie und ihr Verhältnis zum Kultopfer. Stuttgart: Union Dt. Verl. Ges., 1910.

Hovorka & Kronfeld (1908)
Hovorka, Oskar von; Kronfeld, Adolf: Vergleichende Volksmedizin. Bd. 1. Stuttgart: Strecker & Schröder, 1908.

Jungbauer (1934)
Jungbauer, Gustav: Deutsche Volksmedizin. Ein Grundriß. Berlin, Leipzig: de Gruyter, 1934.

Jütte (1996)
Jütte, Robert: Geschichte der Alternativen Medizin. München: C. H. Beck, 1996.

Krünitz (1785)
Krünitz, Johann Georg: Oekonomisch-technologische Encyklopädie oder allgemeines System der Staats-, Stadt-, Haus- und Landwirthschaft und der Kunst-Geschichte: in alphabetischer Ordnung. Bd. 68. Berlin: Pauli, 1785.

Lehmann (1699)
Lehmann, Christian: Historischer Schauplatz derer natürlichen Merckwürdigkeiten in dem Meissnischen Ober-Erzgebirge: darinnen eine aussführliche Beschreibung dieser ganzen gebirgischen und angräntzenden Gegend. Leipzig: Lankisch, 1699 (ND Stuttgart: v. Elterlein, 1988).

Matthiolus (1565)
Matthiolus, Petrus A.: Commentarii in sex libros Pedacii Dioscoridis Anazarbei de Medica materia [...]. Venedig: Valgrisius, 1565.

Menochio (1699)
Menochio, Joanne Stephano: Nutzliche und sehr gelehrte Zeitvertreibung. Augsburg: Streter, 1699.

Nowosadtko (1993)
Nowosadtko, Jutta: „Wer Leben nimmt, kann auch Leben geben". Scharfrichter und Wasenmeister in der Frühen Neuzeit. In: Medizin, Gesellschaft und Geschichte 12 (1993), 43–74.

Nowosadtko (1994)
Nowosadtko, Jutta: Scharfrichter und Abdecker. Der Alltag zweier „unehrlicher" Berufe in der Frühen Neuzeit. Paderborn: Schöningh, 1994.

Ortolff von Bayrlandt (1477)
Ortolff von Bayrlandt: Artzneipuch. Nürnberg: Anthonius Koburger, 1477.

Paracelsus (1931)
Paracelsus: Sämtliche Werke. Ed. Karl Sudhoff, I. Abt., Bd. XIII. München, Berlin: Oldenbourg, 1931.

Pechaček (2003)
Pechaček, Petra: Scharfrichter und Wasenmeister in der Landgrafschaft Hessen-Kassel in der Frühen Neuzeit. Frankfurt/M.: Lang, 2003.

Pharmacopea Wirtenbergica (1750)
Pharmacopea Wirtenbergica. Stuttgart: Erhard, 1750.

Plinius (1988)
Plinius: Naturkunde, Bd. 28. Herausgegeben und übersetzt von Roderich König in Zusammenarbeit mit Joachim Hopp und Wolfgang Glöckner. München, Zürich: Artemis & Winkler, 1988.

Pomet (1717)
Pomet, Peter: Der aufrichtige Materialist und Specerey-Händler. Leipzig: Gleditsch & Weidmann, 1717 (Nachdruck mit einem Nachwort von Hannsgeorg Löhr. Weinheim: VCH, 1987).

Reitz (1998)
Reitz, Manfred: Mumia – Heilung aus der Mumie. In: Pharmazeutische Industrie 60 (1998), 248–249.

Schneider (1985)
Schneider, Wolfgang: Wörterbuch der Pharmazie. Bd. 4: Geschichte der Pharmazie. Stuttgart, 1985.

Schröder (1686)
Schröder, Johann: Trefflich versehene Medicin=Chymische Apotheke / Oder: Höchstkostbarer Arzeney=Schatz [...]. Nürnberg: Hoffmann, 1686.

Schwanitz (1983)
Schwanitz, Hans Joachim: Homöopathie und Brownianismus 1795–1844. Zwei wissenschaftstheoretische Fallstudien aus der praktischen Medizin. Stuttgart [u.a.]: Fischer 1983.

Seyfarth (1913)
Seyfarth, Carly: Aberglaube und Zauberei in der Volksmedizin Sachsens. Leipzig: Wilhelm Heims, 1913 (ND Hildesheim: Olms, 1979).

Stuart (1999)
Stuart, Kathy: Defiled Trades and Social Outcasts. Honor and Ritual Pollution in Early Modern Germany. Cambridge: Cambridge University Press, 1999.

Stukenbrock (2001)
Stukenbrock, Karin: „Der zerstückte Cörper". Zur Sozialgeschichte der anatomischen Sektion in der frühen Neuzeit (1650–1800). Stuttgart: Steiner, 2001 (Medizin, Gesellschaft und Geschichte, Beiheft 16).

Tagebuch des Meister Franz (1980)
Das Tagebuch des Meister Franz, Scharfrichter zu Nürnberg. Kommentar von Jürgen Carl Jacobs und Heinz Rölleke. Dortmund: Harenberg, 1980.

Thomas (1973)
Thomas, Keith: Religion and the Decline of Magic. Studies in Popular Beliefs in Sixteenth- and Seventeenth-Century England. Harmondsworth: Penguin, 1973.

Witzel (1990)
Witzel, Alexander: Ein Lesebuch zur Unterhaltung & zur Belehrung für Ärzte, zusammengestellt aus einer Arztbibliothek der Goethezeit. Stuttgart: F. Fischer, 1990.

Zedler (1732–1754)
Zedler, Johann Heinrich, Hg. Grosses vollständiges Universal-Lexicon Aller Wissenschaften und Künste [...]. Leipzig und Halle, 1732–1754. [Bd. 13 (1735), Bd. 22 (1739), Bd. 25 (1740)].

FRIEDRICH HOFFMANN: CONCORDANCE BETWEEN MEDICAL THEORY AND PRACTICE

Almut Lanz

This paper[1] describes the relationship between the medical theory and practice of Friedrich Hoffmann (1660–1742), physician and professor of medicine in Halle. It particularly investigates the question to what extent Hoffmann's medical theory influenced his pharmacotherapy and whether it might have led to the prescription of new medicines.

In answering this question I will first of all look at Hoffmann's professional development as it shows his particular interest for both theoretical and practical medicine. For this I rely on the biography of Hoffmann written by his student Johann Heinrich Schulze as well as on information from the Halle chronologist Johann Christoph von Dreyhaupt. This is followed by a summary of the major aspects of Hoffmann's medical theory based on his early treatise, *Fundamenta Medicinae* (1695), which encompasses the theoretical aspects of physiology, pathology, and therapeutics.

Hoffmann's recommendations on pharmacotherapy are presented in the form of examples from his collection of consultations – the *Medicina consultatoria*, published in 1721–1723 – to assess the influence of his medical theory on his therapeutic practice. Here, I rely on 54 case studies from this source, in which I analyzed the medicines recommended by Hoffmann from a pharmaceutical point of view.[2] In the following, I reexamine the results from that investigation in terms not only of the information about Hoffmann's therapeutic armamentarium, but to demonstrate the relationship between his medical theory and therapeutic practice.

Professional Development[3]

Like Herman Boerhaave (1668–1738) and Georg Ernst Stahl (1659–1734), the physician and professor of medicine from Halle, Friedrich Hoffmann was not only a prominent clinician but contributed importantly to the systematization of medical theory during the early 18th century. He was born on February 19, 1660 in Halle (Saale) as the son of Friedrich Hoffmann the Elder, personal physician to the administrator of the Archbishop of Magdeburg, August von Sachsen-Weißenfels. Hoffmann also served as the town physicus (municipal physician) of

1 I would like to thank my husband, Wolfgang Lanz, for helping me to write this paper, and Antje Matthäus for translating the German text into English.

2 LANZ (1995), in particular, 177–183.

3 Biographical information is from SCHULZE (1741), 223–292 and DREYHAUPT (1755), Vol. 2, 636–637.

Halle. The Hoffmann family descended from a chain of apothecaries who had resided in Halle since the 16th century.

Friedrich Hoffmann's interest in medicine and pharmacy goes back to his childhood, when his father let him attend the lectures on anatomy and chemistry the elder Hoffmann held in his house for medical students from the area. By the time he was twelve years old, he started his own chemical-pharmaceutical experiments under the guidance of his father, and continued on his own after the death of his parents in 1675.

From 1673 to 1678 he was educated in the local Latin grammar school. There he received excellent training in mathematics, which may have contributed to his eventual renown for logic and clarity of exposition.

In 1678 Hoffmann studied medicine at the University of Jena with the famous professor and iatrochemist Georg Wolfgang Wedel, mathematics with Erhard Weigel (1625–1699) and logic and philosophy with Johann Andreas Schmid (1652–1726). He pursued chemical studies at the nearby University of Erfurt in early 1680, where he attended the lectures of the physician and chemist Caspar Cramer. Towards the end of 1680 he returned to Jena, submitted his dissertation to Wedel, and obtained his doctorate in medicine at the end of January 1681. Hoffmann wrote two further medical-chemical treatises in 1681/82 and taught for one year at the University of Jena. Although his lectures on chemistry and medicine were very popular, he left Jena in 1682 and moved to Minden in Westphalia, where for two years he worked as a physician. His patient clientele came largely from the circle of a brother-in-law, a privy councilor and chancellor of Electoral Brandenburg.

In 1684 Hoffmann went on an educational tour of Holland and England, where he met leading scholars. Among these were the botanist Paul Hermann, who was born in Halle but now lived in Holland, and Robert Boyle, whom he met frequently. In November 1684 he returned to Minden and was appointed garrison physician there in 1685. In 1686 the title of court physician was conferred on him by Friedrich Wilhelm, Elector of Brandenburg, who also promoted him to physicus of the Principality of Minden. In 1687 he again visited Holland and Brabant in the company of his brother-in-law.

In 1688 Hoffmann became the official country physician in Halberstadt, where he was in charge of a rural district for six years and cemented his reputation by therapeutic success and several early publications. In 1693, the follower of Friedrich Wilhelm, Friedrich III, offered him the position of the first professor for medicine (*primus*) and natural philosophy at the newly-founded University of Halle, where he was active until his death in 1742. He served as dean of the faculties of medicine and philosophy and was elected vice-chancellor of the University of Halle five times, the last time when he was 81 years old.

Hoffmann's academic reputation was recognized by membership in several of the most prestigious scientific associations of the time, including the Imperial Academy of Naturalists, today called Leopoldina, the Berlin Academy of Science and Humanities, the London Royal Society, and the St. Petersburg Academy of

Science and Humanities. As professor at the Friedrich University in Halle, Hoffmann trained a large number of medical students, many of whom became important court physicians and university professors.

Apart from his teaching functions, Hoffman had always worked as a physician or consultant for several royal courts. His medical advice was not only sought in person but often also in writing. From 1709 to 1712 and again for part of 1734, he suspended his teaching to follow a call to the court in Berlin as a personal physician to the Prussian king, first Friedrich I and later Friedrich Wilhelm I, but returned to Halle instead of staying on as a court physician, in contrast to his former Halle colleague, Georg Ernst Stahl.

Medical Theory: Physiology

According to his biographer and student Schulze, Hoffmann's instruction in both in Jena and Erfurt centered on the iatrochemical theories of the physician Jan Baptist van Helmont (1579 to 1644).[4] Hoffmann's primary professor, Georg Wedel, however, was also familiar with Descartes' natural philosophy and Boyle's corpuscular chemistry. Wedel further advocated the traditional Galenic ideas that all physiological processes in the human body are controlled by the soul, which relied on the animal spirits or *spiritus animales* as an intermediary.[5]

Although Hoffmann had indeed based his inaugural dissertation on the principles of van Helmont,[6] he turned away from iatrochemical theories after further studies in the science and philosophy of nature.[7] Hoffmann's *Fundamenta Medicinae ex principiis naturae mechanicis in usum Philiatrorum succincte proposita* was published in 1695; it was the first comprehensive description of his medical theory in the form of a short textbook for his medical students, written in Latin as customary for academic texts.[8] As Rothschuh has shown,[9] Hoffmann had assimilated Cartesian and corpuscular chemical concepts, especially during his travels to Holland and England, and incorporated them into his teaching. Hoffmann maintained the basic medical principles underlying the *Fundamenta Medicinae*, which he used in his lectures and to which we refer in the following, in his later and major work, *Medicina rationalis systematica*, which was published first in four volumes between 1718 and 1740.[10]

4 SCHULZE (1741), 239.
5 ROTHSCHUH (1976), 190 and 235.
6 DREYHAUPT (1755), vol. 2, 636.
7 SCHULZE (1741), 239.
8 For the most generally accepted and standard English translation of this work, see KING (1971), which the current translation follows to the extent possible.
9 ROTHSCHUH (1976), 235–270.
10 See HOFFMANN (1748), part 1–3. See also MÜLLER (1991).

As suggested by the full title of the *Fundamenta Medicinae,*[11] which at 238 pages is a very succinct volume compared to other medical texts of the period, Hoffmann advocated a theory of medicine based on nature as driven by mechanical principles.[12] His physiology is a self-contained system of iatromechanics that drew on both the physiological and medical knowledge of the 17th century, including the insights offered by macro- and microscopic anatomy, Harvey's theory of the circulation of the blood, Cartesian mechanics, and Boyle's corpuscular chemistry, joined to classical humoral theory and the Greek school of the Methodologists. Speculative elements remained in this edifice where direct observation of natural processes was impossible.

In agreement with Descartes[13] Hoffmann saw the human body as a machine whose functions were maintained by the movement of the three bodily fluids: blood and its serum, lymph, and the nerve fluid, and by the morphologically different particles in these fluids.[14] For Hoffmann, *materia and motus,* matter and motion, were not just the principles of mechanics but also of medicine.[15] According to Hoffmann, blood mixed with the serum consists of numerous differently structured particles that vary in form, size, and weight and hence in mobility. As blood in turn circulates through vessels of various sizes,[16] both size and shape of the blood particles must match that of the respective vessels.

Hoffmann considered lymph an important body fluid because it is produced by the blood and circulates through its own system of vessels, its flow velocity depending on the flow of the blood. It is mainly an aqueous substance that serves to liquefy the blood and dilute the chyle.[17]

The most important bodily fluid, however, was the hypothetical nerve fluid or spirit, the vital spirit of the ancients, which Hoffmann described as the ether. Its extremely fine and subtle consistency permits it to supply all limbs and organs of the human body with blood and enables their motion. The nerve fluid serves

11 Fundamenta Medicinae ex principiis naturae mechanicis in usum Philiatrorum succinte proposita.

12 HOFFMANN (1695).

13 E.g., ROTHSCHUH (1966) and ROTHSCHUH (1978), in particular 240.

14 HOFFMANN (1695), Physiology, chapter III,1, 5; chapter IV, 1, 26, 27. References and paraphrases in the following are from the 238–page octavo volume of the 1695 edition of the Latin Fundamenta by section, and by chapter number and respective number of the proposition (Lehrsatz). As noted, the English version here presented draws on the terminology of King in his translation (1971). We have intermittently used the present tense to present Hoffmann's understanding of nature and physiological and pathological processes in the interest of a smoother flow of the propositions.

15 HOFFMANN (1695), Physiology, chapter II, 1, 2.

16 HOFFMANN (1695), Physiology, chapter IV, 24–27, 54. – Hoffmann's idea of the presence of variously shaped particles in the blood was based on the results of blood analyses by Thomas Willis and Robert Boyle. Hoffmann was also familiar with the microscope, which permitted identifying not only the erythrocytes but also the different crystalline structures of urinary sediments and other chemicals.

17 HOFFMANN (1695), Physiology, chapter V, 1–9.

as mediator and transmitter of perception and emotion; it is responsible for the orderly function of physiological processes.

According to Hoffmann, this nerve fluid is drawn from the blood in the brain and circulates through the very thin hollow ducts of the nerve fibers.[18] It is extremely fine and almost invisible and is possessed of special mechanical attributes. It consists of the very mobile ethereal particles of the air we breathe and of the equally fine liquid that has entered the blood and makes up the blood serum, which hence also should be regarded a spirit.[19] God is the first cause of all motion and thus of the ethereal particles, as matter itself is passive.[20]

Hoffmann paid special attention to the digestion as the site of a major transformation of the individual components of ingested foods. These supply the chyle with smooth, non-acrid but gelatinous and oily, highly mobile globules that are eventually absorbed by the blood and further divided and refined as the blood circulates through the body. Both digestion and secretion support the formation of these blood globules and of nerve fluid particles.[21]

According to Hoffmann, a person is healthy when the bodily fluids, above all the blood, are supplied with both small, highly mobile, globular spirituous particles as well as ethereal or air-like particles, which in turn are the source for nerve fluids and lymph. Normal physiological function requires not only moderate flow of the blood but especially a moderate flow of the nerve fluid, since the latter effects the normal tonus of all motor fibers.[22]

Medical Theory: Pathology

For Hoffmann all physiological functions depended on the intensity with which blood and nerve fluid flowed through their self-contained vascular systems; conversely, an impeded blood and nerve fluid flow was the main cause of morbid phenomena.[23]

The dyscrasia of bodily fluids postulated by humoral pathology as the cause of disease was redefined by Hoffmann as an imbalance of the corpuscles in the body fluids.[24]

As the circulation of the bodily fluids depends on the particles they contain – their quantity, size, and shape – the flow velocities of blood, nerve fluid, or

18 HOFFMANN (1695), Physiology, chapter V, 44–48, 52; chapter VI, 1, 2; chapter VII, 49.

19 HOFFMANN (1695), Physiology, chapter V, 47, 48, 50; chapter VII, 35, 36.

20 HOFFMANN (1695), Physiology, chapter II, 10.

21 HOFFMANN (1695), Physiology, chapter V, 32; chapter VII, 35–38. – When studying blood under the microscope, Hoffmann observed that the little blood globules are particularly mobile and that the blood coagulates when their motion is arrested: HOFFMANN (1695), Physiology, chapter IV, 28–30.

22 HOFFMANN (1695), Physiology, chapter III, 2, 4, 5, 9, 11, 12, 18.

23 HOFFMANN (1695), Pathology, chapter I, 1–5, 28.

24 HOFFMANN (1695), Pathology, chapter I, 8. – Hoffmann sometimes used the term 'corpuscles' to refer to the components of the body fluids he usually called particles.

lymph are variable. Within this mechanical framework, disease is always caused by a disproportionate increase or reduced circulation of the blood, nerve fluid or lymph.[25] Poorly positioned or disproportionately sized particles can also impair the circulatory flow by obstructing vessels. This cannot only obstruct the vessels in which the three body fluids circulate but impede excretion and secretion. The vascular obstruction may also change the direction and intensity of circulation in the unimpeded vessels, which may then be impaired by the increased velocity of the fluids and by solid acrid particles.[26] Abnormal circulation of the nerve fluid changes the tonus of the solid parts, that is the fibers of the vessels and tissue. In turn, an increased fiber tonus resulting from an increased circulation of the nerve fluid produces spasms; reduced circulation of the nerve fluid leads to atony or lack of tonic motion, which causes numerous physical and nervous diseases.

Hoffmann placed particular importance on problems of digestion and excretion that were caused by changes in fiber tonus.[27] While the impaired motion of the three fluids, blood, nerve fluid or lymph, is the immediate cause of all disease, Hoffmann also attributed considerable importance to dietary factors, including the *sex res non naturales* of traditional Galenic dietetics, as they disturb the circulation of blood and nerve fluid.[28]

Medical Theory: Therapeutics

In the last section of his *Fundamenta Medicinae* (1695), the *Therapeutice,* Hoffmann presented his theoretical principles of therapy, which in his terms arose logically from his physiology and pathology. Therapy is meant to be based on both reason (*ratio*) and sound causal premises. It is oriented to health problems that result from the relative constellation of the particles in the bodily fluids (blood, nerve fluid and lymph) and their mobility. The goal of therapy is to change the quantity and shape of the corpuscular components of the blood, as this will correct the abnormal motion of the blood, nerve fluid or lymph.

An important part of therapy is to increase or reduce the motion of the nerve fluid in order to correct an abnormal fiber tonus as well as abnormal circulation of the blood. What is new in Hoffmann's Fundamenta is his attempt to interpret the effects of all medicinal simples available at the time – whether animal, plant or chemiatric simples — in terms of the assumed structure of their particles. With regard to the desired therapeutic effect Hoffmann classified medicinals into four main categories:

Evacuants (medicines that act as laxatives or purgatives, emetics, or sudorifics)
Alterants (medicines that alter the corpuscular particles of the blood),

25 HOFFMANN (1695), Pathology, chapter I, 9, 14–20; chapter V, VI, VII.
26 HOFFMANN (1695), Pathology, chapter I, 21–30.
27 HOFFMANN (1695), Pathology, chapter VII, chapter VIII.
28 HOFFMANN (1695), Pathology, chapter II.

Roborants (medicines that correct the tonic motion or state of the fibers),
Sedatives or *anodynes* (medicines that reduce the increased tonus of the fibers).[29]

Hoffmann classified the alterants into twelve classes of substances, representing all animal, plant, mineral and chemical material medica known at the time (various acids, both volatile and fixed, alkaline substances and salts, both volatile and fixed, waters, essential oils, spirits, resins, mucilagenous substances, fatty oils, minerals). Effects are explained in terms of their differing particle structures (sharp, acrid, needle-pointed, branching, porous, solid, flexible, spherical, air-like), in terms of corpuscular mechanics. The alterants are therefore the most important group of medicines, since they are able to alter both the shape of the particles and the tonus of the fibers. The form of the fluid particles can be altered by absorption, division, dilution, softening or coagulation; the tonus can be changed by mechanically stimulating the fibers and the nerve fluid, which also aids digestion and excretion. Taken together, the inclusive class of medical substances that can be classified as alterants is sufficient to obtain the desired therapeutic effects.[30]

In Hoffmann's opinion, a physician should use few, but well selected medicines, simple rather than compounded. In particular, he should rely on those well known to him in composition and effect from his own dispensing experience. Apart from traditional Galenics, chemiatric preparations should be applied as well.[31]

Therapeutic practice

Hoffmann documented his medical practice in his major work on clinical medicine, in the *Medicina consultatoria*, a collection of his consultant experience published between 1721 and 1739. This 12-volume work, written mainly in German, contains treatment instructions and prescriptions and hence provides detailed insight into his therapies. His medical advice usually follows upon an account of the patient's medical history, which he had received from another physician or the patient by letter. In some cases, though, Hoffmann examined the patients himself; they had either come to Halle or he went to see them personally.[32] The first three volumes of the *Medicina consultatoria*, published between 1721 and 1723, have been the subject of detailed study by this author.[33] In the following, we reexamine 54 case studies from the *Medicina consultatoria,* concentrating on pharmaceutical rather than clinical aspects. Excluded are recom-

29 HOFFMANN (1695), Therapeutics, chapter II.

30 HOFFMANN (1695), Therapeutics, chapter II, 28–39; chapter III, 20, 21, 24 and chapter IV – chapter VI. – On alterants, see also LANZ (1995), 92–105.

31 HOFFMANN (1695), Therapeutics, chapter I, 27, 35.

32 E.g., HOFFMANN (1721a), 229; HOFFMANN (1721b), 152; HOFFMANN (1723), 36.

33 LANZ (1995).

mendations on balneotherapy and mineral waters from various medicinal springs, which Hoffmann held in high regard.

Following Hippocratic-Galenic tradition, Hoffmann's treatment instructions always included recommendations on lifestyle and diet in addition to medical regimens. His occasional recommendation of bloodletting also follows traditional advice.

Based on the 54 patients represented in this study, Hoffmann prescribed an average of six medicines per patient, which include those recommended as alternatives. The prescribed medicines are both simples, containing one ingredient only, and composita of several ingredients.

In accordance with his corpuscular theoretical framework, Hoffmann seems to have preferred liquid medicines; in many cases, these could be prepared without much technical equipment in the patient's home.[34] They included decoctions, teas, laxative drinks, enemas or clysters, broths, oils, whey, one of the elixirs in his armamentarium, and foot baths, sitz baths and full immersion baths augmented by medicinal substances. His more complex liquid medicines were distilled waters, the majority of the elixirs he prescribed, spirits, mixtures, wines, essences, tinctures and syrups, all to be prepared by an apothecary or by Hoffmann himself.

Almost all patients were prescribed a liquid decoction of various drugs, which – often mixed with wine – was to be substituted for other drinks. The medicines described as decoctions,[35] which were supposed to improve the configuration of the particles of the blood and hence its circulation, consisted mostly of the traditionally used parts of plants such as roots, wood, and bark, to which spices containing essential oils were added, such as those distilled from cinnamon and fennel. The decoction could also contain barley, oats or a chemical to optimize the digestive and laxative effects of the mixture.[36] The composition of the medicines and their variations were adapted to the individual constitution and condition of the individual patient.

Decoctions of coffee and chocolate were prescribed for therapeutic purposes as well.[37] Other decoctions were made from plant components, generally mucilaginous substances or essential oils; these were all applied externally, e.g., as an herb bag, compress, or vaporarium.[38]

Teas made of various herbs containing essential oils, bitters, tannins, or mucilaginous substances also formed an integral part of his therapeutic practice. Only occasionally are chemicals such as calcium carbonate or saltpeter added.[39] The reason for this insistence on warm drinks is their positive effect on the mo-

34 LANZ (1995), 120.
35 E.g., HOFFMANN (1723), 126.
36 E.g., HOFFMANN (1723), 126, 136; HOFFMANN (1721a), 85, 187.
37 E.g., HOFFMANN (1721a), 84; HOFFMANN (1721b), 124.
38 HOFFMANN (1721a), 108, 220, 231; HOFFMANN (1721b), 150, 239.
39 E.g., HOFFMANN (1721a), 189; HOFFMANN (1721b), 184, 220; HOFFMANN (1723), 125.

tion of the blood: they serve to dissolve viscous particles, neutralize acrid particles, and then excrete these by stimulating perspiration and urination.[40]

Among the elixirs prescribed by Hoffmann, a balsamic stomach elixir predominates that Hoffmann produced himself. [41] While he kept its composition secret, he recommended it as beneficial for the digestion, the neutralization of acids and the strengthening of the stomach. [42] Since Hoffmann occasionally hinted at the composition of his elixir, we may conclude that it was a vinous extract mainly consisting of essential oils and bitters promoting digestion.[43]

Another remedy often prescribed by Hoffmann also belongs to his own secret remedies. His white *spiritus mineralis*,[44] also called *liquor anodynus mineralis*,[45] is the precursor of a mixture later known as Hoffmann's Drops (*Hoffmannstropfen*), which is still dispensed by many central European apothecaries. Hoffmann probably made it by distilling sulfuric acid with ethyl alcohol; its main component was alcohol and it contained only small amounts of ether.[46] Hoffmann often prescribed this spirit as an analgesic and antispasmodic,[47] on the assumption that because of its extremely fine spirit particles and ethereal components, it was able to enter the blood and hence the nerve fluid and improve their circulation.[48]

Yet another type of medicine prepared and often prescribed by Hoffmann were mixtures he called "my life balm,"[49] the exact composition of which likewise remains unknown. A hint is again found in an advertisement for his secret remedies, which explains that this was a balsamic tonic consisting of fragrant oils and resins that strengthen the head and the nerves ("aromatische … haupt- und nervenstärkende …").[50] Hoffmann recommended this life balm for cases that would benefit from a strengthening of the patient's overall constitution.[51]

Hoffmann used various medicinal wines in his therapy, often in combination with decoctions and powders, to stimulate the digestive system and improve the consistency of the body fluids.[52] In about one third of the 54 cases examined, lukewarm foot baths were recommended. The medicinal substances added, as for

40 HOFFMANN (1695), Hygiene, chapter II, 56.

41 E.g., HOFFMANN (1723), 246.

42 HOFFMANN (1723), 39.

43 HOFFMANN (1723), 51.

44 HOFFMANN (1723), 137.

45 HOFFMANN (1721a), 93 and HOFFMANN (1734), 7.

46 V. GIZYCKI (1952), (1956). An approximation of the recipe is provided in several English language dispensatories of the time, e.g., in WILLIAM LEWIS (1758), 454.

47 E.g., HOFFMANN (1723), 137.

48 HOFFMANN (1695), Therapeutics, chapter V, 24.

49 E.g., HOFFMANN (1721b), 215.

50 HOFFMANN (1734), 4. The term fragrant is taken over here from a comment by WILLIAM LEWIS (1758), who attempted to replicate the recipe, as follows (330): "Thus much is certain, from Hoffmann's own writings, that his balsam was composed of fragrant oils dissolved in a rectified spirit of wine."

51 E.g., HOFFMANN (1721b), 214–215.

52 E.g., HOFFMANN (1723), 162–164.

sitz baths and immersion baths, were potash, camomile blossoms and wheat bran to promote circulation and perspiration as well as counteract spasms and pain.[53]

Hoffmann also advocated the often excessive 18th century practice of cleansing the blood. In some cases he not only recommended laxative drinks or pills to excrete deleterious impurities but also using an enema. Medicines of this type could contain both herbal laxatives and purgative and severely dehydrating chemicals such as Epsom salts (magnesium sulfate).[54]

On the other hand, a household remedy high up on Hoffmann's list for various conditions such as amenorrhea, arthritis, spasms and indigestion were meat or chicken broth, which he often prescribed as a substitute for chemical medicines. These medicinal broths, which Hoffmann also called *alimenta medicamentosa,*[55] were prepared with up to six diuretic and laxative plant components as well as the juice of bitter oranges and sometimes egg yolk.[56] Hoffmann advocated these herbal broths for their multiple therapeutic effects. They served to coat the "sharp-edged, impure salia (saline particles) that accrete in the blood"; they provide the materials necessary for well-balanced bodily fluids, and they facilitate the excretion of urine, sweat and stool.[57]

Solid medicines taken internally in addition to laxative pills were those serving to improve the consistency of the fluids and promote or roborate gastrointestinal tonus. These pills contained extracts from bitter substances (e.g., lesser centaury and wormwood), gum resins and laxatives as well as essential oils.[58] The use of crystalline or pulverized laxative salts, mostly of chemical origin, served the same purpose, i.e. excreting pathogenic particles by facilitating bowel movement and diuresis.[59] His so-called "aperient or opening salt," another one of his secret and frequently recommended remedies, was not only a laxative and diuretic but decreased flatulence and served as a tempering and stimulating medication.[60]

A constant part of his prescriptive regimen for almost all patients was a powder of up to nine constituents of animal, plant, mineral and chemical origins. The majority of these powders absorbed acidity, had aperient or discussant properties and improved peristaltic motion. Hoffmann described them as "precipitating and aperient (*niederschlagende und eröffnende*) powders"[61] or "precipitating powders,"[62] to be used to "temper the acridity and counteract the ebullience of the blood."[63] These powders often contained crab stones or saltpeter[64] and other

53 E.g., HOFFMANN (1721a), 189; HOFFMANN (1723), 97.
54 E.g., HOFFMANN (1721a), 187; HOFFMANN (1721b), 183–184.
55 HOFFMANN (1721b), 193.
56 E.g., HOFFMANN (1721b), 192, 151, 124.
57 HOFFMANN (1721b), 192–193.
58 E.g., HOFFMANN (1721b), 80.
59 E.g., HOFFMANN (1723), 56, 111.
60 HOFFMANN (1721a), 164.
61 HOFFMANN (1723), 255.
62 HOFFMANN (1723), 175.
63 HOFFMANN (1723), 28.

powdered alkaline antacids commonly used at the time for their diuretic and diaphoretic effects.

Additives in the form of various essential oils such as cedar, mace, or cinnamon oil[65] were used not only to improve the taste but also the gastrointestinal tonus. The antacid powders could also contain antimony, mercury or sulfur compounds[66] with strong laxative, diuretic and diaphoretic effects that were thought to eliminate deleterious particles from the blood. Powders with mainly diaphoretic effects, which Hoffmann called "bezoardic powders"[67] were prescribed – in addition to other, laxative and stimulating medicines – for a range of problems, including melancholy,[68] diabetes insipidus,[69] weak memory[70] or colics.[71]

The powders prescribed could be composed of minerals and chemical substances or of drugs from the large store of medicinal plants. These are drugs containing tannin, bitter substances and essential oils, which were supposed to roborate the tonus of the gastrointestinal tract and hence act as a digestive.[72] Considering their multiple pharmacological effects, the frequent recommendation of these powder mixtures makes sense.

Hoffmann's therapeutic practice relied mainly on medicines taken internally. Liniments, cataplasms and therapeutic plasters – all of semi-solid consistency – were recommended for local, external application in the case of circulatory problems, spasms, pain, and inflammations. These medications, too, contained mainly plant parts and essential oils.[73]

As these examples of treatments from his *Medicina consultatoria* show, Hoffmann selected his medicinal substances, mainly but not always simples, from the whole range of the therapeutic armamentarium, in accordance with his own pharmacological theory, and used them singly or in composita. He also recommended his own arcana or secret remedies. The case studies show that all prescriptions took the patient's constitution and medical condition into account. The medications recommended were remedies with whose effects Hoffmann was familiar after long years of practice and probably self-experiment. This is evident from the explanations Hoffmann provided to justify specific recommendations, for example: "[…] and I have found it [a laxative] to be good in many hundreds of people"[74] or "[…] for such incidents I have found nothing better than the use of [...]."[75] Based on the therapeutic success of his intervention, Hoffmann as-

64 E.g., HOFFMANN (1723), 28.
65 E.g., HOFFMANN (1721a), 50, 189; HOFFMANN (1721b), 150.
66 HOFFMANN (1723), 97.
67 E.g., HOFFMANN (1723), 176.
68 HOFFMANN (1721a), 154.
69 HOFFMANN (1721a), 220.
70 HOFFMANN (1721b), 215.
71 HOFFMANN (1723), 136.
72 E.g., HOFFMANN (1721a), 84; HOFFMANN (1721b), 184.
73 E.g., HOFFMANN (1721a), 93–94, 295; HOFFMANN (1721b), 166.
74 HOFFMANN (1723), 197.
75 HOFFMANN (1723), 56.

sumes that his medical theory is valid and the medications he prescribed were suitable for the respective patient and their complaints. He often observed the success of a therapeutic course himself or the patient reported it, and at the end of each consultation the reader was informed in detail.[76]

Conclusion

The relationship between Friedrich Hoffmann's medical theory and practice is characterized by the fact that the latter is the logical consequence of the former. His medical practice followed the corpuscular-mechanical concept of his physiology, pathology and therapeutics, which he published for his medical students at the age of 35. Hoffmann's medical concept no longer focused on the four bodily fluids of Galenic humoral pathology, but on the blood and its corpuscles. These in turn were the source of the lymph and the hypothetical nerve fluid, which like blood and lymph was thought to circulate through its own vascular system. What is new in Hoffmann's medical system is the importance it attributed to the influence of the nerves on physiological function and pathological process. This perspective expands and supplements the previously predominant humoral edifice.

The starting point for Hoffmann's therapeutic practice was the correction of the corpuscular components of the blood to improve the flow characteristics of blood, nerve fluid and lymph. As in traditional humoral therapy, this effect was pursued mainly through pharmaceuticals that promoted excretion, which for Hoffmann meant the removal of particles from the blood that impeded the mechanics of circulation. In pursuit of this effect, Hoffmann's use of common evacuants was not restricted to promoting their depleting effects but was intended to alter the corpuscular structure of pathogenic blood particles by discutient, thinning, and liquefying processes.

These processes not only were to remove the obstruction but also enhanced the flow characteristics of the fluids, improved the tonus of the fibers, and aided digestion. Here, Hoffmann indeed provided new pharmacological explanations for the effects of traditional drugs that are in line with his theoretical framework. Noticeable, on the other hand, are his frequent prescriptions for drugs containing essential oils as well as wines, and which similar to the ethereal component of the blood and nerve fluid were assumed to have effects on the nervous system. The predominance of distilled oils in his composita is a new trend in Hoffmann's medications and directly links them to his theory of a nerve ether. The extremely fine and subtle consistency of both these oils and his own *liquor anodynus mineralis*, the precursor of what became known as *Hoffmannstropfen*, was presumed by Hoffmann to permit penetration of the hollow, tubular nerve fibers and promote a nervous effect. Finally, although he defined the therapeutic effects of all

76 E.g., HOFFMANN (1721a), 221, 231, 234; HOFFMANN (1721b), 166, 221, 248; HOFFMANN (1723), 113.

his medications in terms of corpuscular theory, he predicted these effects from his practical experience, based on patient observations and probably also self-experiment.

His composita are mixtures of few, relatively simple herbal drugs. But he also used pharmaceutical-chemical mixtures as well as his own secret remedies. Noticeably, he recommended new mixtures of commonly used simples, selected and composed on the basis of his pharmacological theory and practical experience from the contemporary armamentarium. This also applies to the preparation of some of his secret remedies or arcana, to the extent to which this can be inferred from occasional hints. Overall, his therapeutic practice follows his medical theory, adapted to the medical condition and constitution of the patient. It thus corresponds to his frequently postulated demand that reason and experience (*ratio et experientia*) should govern clinical practice.[77]

77 E.g., HOFFMANN (1695), Therapeutics, chapter I, 4.
LANZ (1995), 184–207, contains a detailed list of the medications used by Hoffmann (*simplicia* and *composita*).

References:

Dreyhaupt (1755)
Dreyhaupt, Johann Christoph von: Pagus Neletici et Nudzici oder ausführliche diplomatisch-historische Beschreibung des zum ehemaligen Primat und Ertz-Stiffte [...] Herzogthum Magdeburg gehörigen Saal-Creyses und aller darinnen befindlichen Städte, [...] : insonderheit der Städte Halle, Wettin, Lobegün, [...] . 2 Vols. Halle: Waisenhaus, 1755.

Gizycki (1952)
Gizycki, Friedrich von: Liquor anodynus mineralis, Äther und Hoffmannstropfen. In: Die Pharmazie 7 (1952), 303–310.

Gizycki (1956)
Gizycki, Friedrich von: Zur Geschichte des Äthers und der Hoffmannsropfen. In: Veröffentlichungen der Internat. Gesellschaft für Geschichte der Pharmazie N. F. Vol. 8. (1956), 91–98.

Hoffmann (1695)
Hoffmann, Friedrich: Fundamenta Medicinae ex principiis naturae mechanicis in usum philiatrorum succincte proposita. Halle: Salfeld, 1695.

Hoffmann (1721a)
Hoffmann, Friedrich: Medicina consultatoria, worinnen unterschiedliche über einige schwehre Casus ausgearbeitete Consilia, auch Responsa Facultatis Medicae enthalten, und in fünf Decurien eingetheilet, dem Publico zum besten herausgegeben. Part 1. Halle: Renger, 1721.

Hoffmann (1721b)
Hoffmann, Friedrich: Medicina consultatoria, worinnen unterschiedliche über einige schwehre Casus ausgearbeitete Consilia, auch Responsa Facultatis Medicae enthalten, und in fünf Decurien eingetheilet, dem Publico zum besten herausgegeben. Part 2. Halle: Renger, 1721.

Hoffmann (1723)
Hoffmann, Friedrich: Medicina consultatoria, worinnen unterschiedliche über einige schwehre Casus ausgearbeitete Consilia, auch Responsa Facultatis Medicae enthalten, und in fünf Decurien eingetheilet, dem Publico zum besten herausgegeben. Part 3. Halle: Renger, 1723.

Hoffmann (1734)
Hoffmann, Friedrich: Gründliche Anweisung vom nützlichen Gebrauch und zuverläßiger Wirckung einiger bewährten Medicamenten bey vielerley Arten Kranckheiten welche auch zu einer Hauß= und Reise= Apotheck dienlich. Halle: Hilliger, 1734.

Hoffmann (1748)
Hoffmann, Friedrich: Opera omnia physico-medica. Denuo revisa, correcta & aucta, in 6 tomos distributa [...] et per experientiam LVII annorum stabilitae. Part 1–6. Genf: Tournes, 1748.

King (1971)
[Friedrich Hoffmann:] Fundamenta Medicinae, translated and introduced by Lester S. King. London: MacDonald, and New York: American Elsevier, 1971.

Lanz (1995)
Lanz, Almut: Arzneimittel in der Therapie Friedrich Hoffmanns (1660–1742) unter besonderer Berücksichtigung der Medicina consultatoria (1721–1723). Braunschweig: Deutscher Apotheker Verlag, 1995 (Braunschweiger Veröffentlichungen zur Geschichte der Pharmazie und der Naturwissenschaften 35).

Lewis (1758)
Lewis, William (Ed.): The Pharmacopoeia of The Royal College of Physicians at Edinburgh. Faithfully translated from the 4th edition. With useful Notes on the Simple and Compound [...] London: John Nourse, 1758.

Müller (1991)
Müller, Ingo W.: Iatromechanische Theorie und ärztliche Praxis im Vergleich zur galenistischen Medizin. (Friedrich Hoffmann – Pieter van Foreest, Jan van Heurne). Stuttgart: Steiner, 1991 (Historische Forschungen 17).

Rothschuh (1966)
Rothschuh, Karl Eduard: René Descartes und die Theorie der Lebenserscheinungen. In: Sudhoffs Archiv 50 (1966), 25–42.

Rothschuh (1976)
Rothschuh, Karl Eduard: Studien zu Friedrich Hoffmann (1660–1742). In: Sudhoffs Archiv 60 (1976), 163–193; 235–270.

Rothschuh (1978)
Rothschuh, Karl Eduard: Konzepte der Medizin in Vergangenheit und Gegenwart. Stuttgart: Hippokrates-Verlag, 1978.

Schulze (1741)
Schulze, Johann Heinrich: Vernünftige und gründliche Abhandlung von den fürnehmsten Kinderkrankheiten, ausgefertiget von D. Friedrich Hofmann, [...] nunmehro mit dessen Lebenslauf versehen von D. Johann Heinrich Schulzen, [...]. Frankfurt, Leipzig: Reinhard Eustachius Möller, 1741.

MENTORS AND FORMULAE: CONTINUITY AND CHANGE IN EIGHTEENTH-CENTURY THERAPEUTICS

John K. Crellin

In an earlier discussion paper on the Abraham Wagner manuscript – underscoring its value for raising questions about eighteenth-century medical practice, I commented on the role of theory and of clinical experience in Wagner's therapeutics.[1] I suggested that Wagner (1715–1763) drew on and evaluated from his own experiences prevailing medical theories and practices expounded in the array of medical texts he must have read. Moreover, I showed that Wagner was specifically influenced by the teachings of Georg Ernst Stahl (1660–1734) and seemingly recognized trends toward a "gentler medicine" (simpler formulations and relatively mild treatment regimens). The latter included his apparent knowledge of medications from the Halle Orphanage and the Pietist thinking that surrounded them.

This paper extends my earlier account by exploring two topics: (i) Wagner's interest in the remedies of his Silesian teachers/mentors, as distinct from those associated with the Halle Orphanage, and (ii) his own formulation of prescriptions and the extent that they followed trends in the eighteenth century toward simpler formulae. In so doing, I try to make clear that the reputation and formulation of the prescription was just as significant an issue for physicians to evaluate as was theory and clinical experience when choosing the basic medicaments for treating a particular patient.

Mentors

Even a cursory reading of eighteenth-century medical textbooks suggests that published authors and famous teachers were a major factor in a physician's choice of therapies. Leaving aside the hyperboles of the time, the preface to the English translation of *Boerhaave's Aphorisms* is just one reflection of this when noting the "great Number of Physicians [who] recommend themselves highly by

1 CRELLIN (2006 and 2007). For the digitized version of the Wagner manuscript in translation, see "Eighteenth-century Colonial Formularies: The Manuscripts of George de Benneville and Abraham Wagner," College of Physicians of Philadelphia Digital Library. Recent website address: http://www.accesspadr.org/cpp/. Quotations are taken from the English translation on the website. References to this text will be made using the native pagination to enable the user of the physical document to find pages easily, but supplemented with a bracketed physical side number that was used to index the page images of the digitized manuscript, which can be readily consulted on-line. I have retained capitalization of medicines mentioned in the manuscript for ease of identification. Since the German text is not yet available on line, the editors have provided excerpts from the unpublished website transcription by Elisabeth Quast. . – The research underlying this paper was in part supported by the national Library of Medicine, Washington, D.C.

letting the world know, that they were Dr. Boerhaave's Disciples."[2] Yet, aside from the major authorities in eighteenth-century medicine (and various controversies about their therapies), countless physicians also drew on the humbler influences of their apprentice masters, other local practitioners, and perhaps home medicine practices used by their patients. It would add to our understanding of medical practice at the time if we understood more fully how the treatment regimens of such unsung influences were accepted, changed, and ignored, as well as how often mentors served as role models, to use a modern term. Unfortunately, physician manuscripts of the eighteenth century are generally sparse on these matters; the Wagner manuscript is no exception, but it provides hints and suggestions for historians to consider when exploring continuity, change and validation of treatments in the practices of eighteenth-century physicians.

First, it needs to be said that the Wagner manuscript – comprising pages of prescriptions (powders, elixirs, pills, etc) and of treatments for various conditions – is not a case book, a medical diary, or even a commonplace book of medical notes and jottings.[3] Thus, despite many references to medical experiences, the manuscript requires considerable inference about the extent or the nature of Wagner's daily practice. Indeed, just why the manuscript was written is open to debate. Firm interpretation is complicated by uncertainties raised by different handwritings and by apparent errors in the collation of the pages when they were bound. An occasional post-Wagner entry also appears, such as a formula dated 1781 for "Tincture Panchymagog Dr. Benneville," a one-time neighboring practitioner whose possible medical and religious influence on Wagner is beyond the scope of this paper.[4]

The most likely explanation for the compilation is that Wagner intended to distill and pass on his experiences and knowledge (including favorite formulae) to an apprentice, or to a successor in his practice. Whether the latter was his younger brother, Melchior Wagner (born 1725), has not been determined, but the absence of certain details necessary to prepare the formulae almost suggests that he was expecting his advice to be read by someone familiar with his practice.[5]

2 DELACOSTE (1715), unpaginated translator's preface.

3 There is perhaps an analogy to a manuscript of case histories and other notes (1737–1742) compiled by British physician William Brownrigg. See WARD & YELL (1993). Brownrigg's concept of medicine as illustrated in his casebook is interpreted as seemingly conservative depending on the "styles of Sydenham and Boerhaave" (xix). There is no reason at present to think such authorities influenced Wagner in any specific way.

4 George de Benneville is presumably, as Allen Viehmeyer has noted (private communication), the Christian practitioner in Oley mentioned by WAGNER (2005), fol. 11v. See also BERKY (1954), 69, and other pages.

5 It should be noted that a number of entries exist seemingly in a different hand, albeit contemporary to Wagner (that is aside from others added after his death). Judging from the context of some of the different entries, one has to consider that they were entered with Wagner's knowledge, or he merely wrote some of the formulae in a different and clearer hand, cf., for example, WAGNER (2005), fol. 54r. All items referenced in this paper are from a single hand taken to be Wagner's unless otherwise noted.

The influences on Wagner discussed here are three medical practitioners associated with the Schwenkfelder community centered on Harpersdorf, the village of Wagner's birth in lower Silesia.[6] One name stands out, Melchior Hübner (also Heebner; 1668–1738), who was seemingly the primary medical mentor to young Wagner, likely as his apprentice-master (no evidence has been found that Wagner had any formal university education). This was at a time when adherents of the Schwenkfelder faith faced renewed religious persecution. The details that follow on Hübner and Wagner, along with the other two Schwenkfelder practitioners – Martin John, Jr (1624–1707), to whom Hübner was apprenticed, and Wagner's great grandfather, Georg Hauptmann (also Haubtmann; 1635–1722) – indicate a marked impact on Wagner's own practice.

Melchior Hübner

Wagner refers to ten of Hübner's regimens or preparations. In one instance, he noted: "The blessed Melchior Hübner highly recommended Tincture of Tartar against the fever in children, and I have found that it serves well."[7] Despite the testimonial, there is nothing particularly surprising in Hübner's recommendation, for the tincture (presumably tincture of salt of tartar) was widely recognized as a diaphoretic and mild diuretic.[8] In fact, it is noteworthy that, as in other references to Hübner, Wagner first listed what were apparently his own preferential remedies, at least as initial treatments. In this case, Wagner first wrote: "If they have chills, it is good to give them the Halle Digestive Powder prior to the paroxysm, and during the heat Mineral Bezoar Powder or Halle Tempering Powder."[9] These preparations – undoubtedly generally favored ones by Wagner as evidenced by references to them throughout the manuscript (and sometimes rationalized by him on the basis on Stahl's concept of reducing the ebullition of the blood) – were commonly recognized to have actions similar to the tincture recommended by Hübner.[10]

It is appropriate to add that, although Wagner indicated that a laxative might be necessary as part of a fever regimen, nowhere does he promote their vigorous

6 Throughout this discussion, I use the term medical practitioner, rather than physician or doctor. It has become customary to use this term to overcome uncertainties or lack of information on the background, especially education, of those with reputations as healers or practitioners. "Physician" is currently limited to those with known university training. However, it must not be assumed that medical practitioner implies a second class physician or doctor. The latter term was apparently used by local people to describe Wagner. See BERKY (1954), 66.

7 "Der sel[ige] Melchior Hübner rühmet die Tinctur Tartari in den Fiebern der Kinder, welche ich auch gut befunden habe." WAGNER (2005), fol. 48r.

8 QUINCY (1719), 325; JAMES (1747), 675.

9 "Wenn sie Anfälle von Kälte haben, so ist ihnen gut vor dem Paroxysmus das Pulv[is] digestivus hal[ensis] gegeben, und in der Hitze p[ulvis] bezoardicus oder temperans halensis." WAGNER (2005), fol. 48r. Whether the Halle Digestive powder was Pulvis Stomachus has not been determined, cf. WILSON (2000), 75.

10 CRELLIN (2006) for discussion of this influence of Stahl.

usage (as featured in various medical texts at the time), while his use of vomits and blood-letting (also part of well-established antiphlogistic and depletive regimens) was similarly cautious. Wagner seems to have favored relatively simple diaphoretics and tempering powders for fevers just as he favored relatively mild regimens in general.[11] It is, therefore, of interest that many of Hübner's preparations also fit this pattern, a point I return to below.

Hübner, too, as I suspect was the case with Wagner, was perhaps readily open to new treatment possibilities. Wagner wrote that "the blessed Melchior Hübner, Practitioner of Medicine" administered "a Tea of Stinging Nettle Roots to a woman who was swollen up immensely, which immediately restored her and her health. She is now still alive. 1752."[12] Although stinging nettle roots were generally known to physicians as a diuretic, Wagner's remark raises the question whether this was a local home remedy that Hübner felt appropriate to use for dropsy "if it [had] not gone too far."[13] Perhaps, too, Wagner himself was not averse to trying locally popular remedies. For instance, "the common people use only tea of Alexander which has helped many."[14] Maybe this encouraged his use of the tea, at least as a vehicle for his Anti-Emetic Powder to treat convulsions or spasms of the bowel: "Thanks be to God, I have found the following method to have served me well and often in many cases. First two or three doses of my Anti-Emetic powder every hour in a Tea of Alexander. This stopped the vomit."[15]

11 Tempering medicines were associated with the concept of tempering or modifying the temperaments (sanguine, lymphatic, choleric, etc.); although there is also a sense that such medicines were also viewed as sedative in nature; this does not appear to be the case with Wagner's use. This is not the place to examine Wagner's approach to fevers beyond noting that, although he seemingly favored mild treatments, he did not eschew entirely some of the complex formulae of the time such as Stahl's Alexipharmic Essence, or Hübner's Theriac (see also below). Wagner also suggested the use of Peruvian bark on a couple of occasions, but his dosage was relatively small.

12 "Der sel[ige] Melchior Hübner Med[icus] Pr[acticus] hat [.....] einer Frauen welche gewaltig dicke geschwollen gewesen, den Tranck von Brenn=Nessel Wurtzel verordnet, worauf sie so gleich von Stund an gebessert u[nd] völlig zurecht kommen und itzt noch gesund am Leben ist. 1752." WAGNER (2005), fol. 26v.

13 "[...] wenn es noch nicht zu weit kommen gewesen." WAGNER (2005), fol. 26v. For stinging nettle, for example, QUINCY (1719), 99. It is to be noted that a number of nettles have been called "stinging."

14 "Gemeine Leute brauchen nur Thee von Balsam Kraut[.] Das hat vielen gut gethan." WAGNER (2005), fol. 20v.

15 "Ich habe folgende Methode in praxi gottlob vil u[nd] oft dienlich befunden. Erstl[ich] 2 od[er] 3 Doses von meinem Pulver c[ontra] Emetum alle Stunden in Thee von Balsam=Kraut eingegeben. Davon hat das Brechen aufgehöret." WAGNER (2005), fol. 21r. For another example of an appreciation of local usage (for tenesmus, a tendency to want to pass feces): "The common people drink tree oil and consider this good" ("Gemeine Leute trincken Baum Oel und finden solches gut.") WAGNER (2005), fol. 19v. Also, "Mix a dose of one half scruple in warm broth or tea of Yarrow or Alexander, every 3 or 4 or even 5 hours" ("M[ische eine] Dosis [von] ½ Scrupel in warmer Brühe oder Thee von Schafgarbe oder Balsamkraut. alle 3. 4. biß 5 Stunden.") WAGNER (2005), fol. 19r. References also exist

Perhaps the most intriguing of Wagner's references to Hübner is a single preparation designated as "proven" (*probatum est*), which is just one of around twenty formulae Wagner so described throughout the manuscript out of a few hundred recorded.[16] Why were these singled out from others, many of which Wagner judged more circumspectly as "helpful," "very beneficial," and "useful?" The Hübner "proven" remedy – a treatment for "the most serious stage of hot gangrene" – reads:

> Prepare a right sharp lye from hot and glowing embers with coal and Wormwood added, hold the limb above it and finally immerse it. This has proven beneficial even when the limb had lost all sensation and the cold gangrene had set in.[17]

(The description "proven beneficial" is reinforced by the added annotation, *probatum est.*) Hübner's advice is unremarkable, for the use of a caustic (cauterization was an alternative) was a recognized approach for treating the later stages of gangrene, while the inclusion of wormwood rested on its reputation as a discutient (or discussive) when used in external preparations.[18] As with other references to Hübner's treatments in the manuscript, this one follows another – presumably Wagner's own preference – which was also in line with conventional applications of fomentations/compresses compounded from different herbs and resins (with anti-putrefactive and drying properties). It is again noteworthy that Wagner did not mention a vigorous antiphlogistic regimen, though maybe this would have been invoked if the gangrenous condition had become extreme.

Lastly, I notice seven other Hübner preparations mentioned by Wagner. They are Epileptic Powder, Golden Heart Powder, Aromatic Essence, Water against Scabies, Chest Potions, Tincture of Tunica Flowers and his Theriac. No formulae are given for the preparations, although the Chest Potion was seemingly Spirit of Sal Ammoniac with Anise.[19] Not all were prescribed as discrete medicines, for Wagner incorporated, for instance, the Epileptic Powder and Tincture of Tunica Flowers in what were apparently his own extemporaneous prescriptions. In one of these, Epileptic Powder was compounded into a relatively simple formula for "convulsions in a young infant." Wagner's added note illustrates careful clinical observation:

> I have given this several times to a child aged 8 weeks which had had convulsions for several weeks, as many as 10, 12, and up to 14 fits per day. Yeah, as many as 17 on the last

to the use of Virginia snakeroot (once), sarsaparilla (once) and sassafras (twice), all indigenous plants, but these were already long known in Europe.

16 At least one of these "proven" remedies appears to be in a different hand, see WAGNER (2005), fol. 96v.

17 "[...] recht scharffe lauge gemacht Von heisser und glühender Asche mit Kohlen und Wermuth hinein gethan, hernach das Glied drüber end[lich] drein gethan, hat gut gethan. Wenn schon kein Gefühl mehr gewesen und der kalte Brand angefangen hat." WAGNER (2005), fol. 60r.

18 For wormwood, considered something of a panacea, QUINCY (1719), 127.

19 WAGNER (2005), fol. 10v.

day. After use of this medicine, there were 9 fits the next day, 5 the following day, and the next day after that, 2. And in two weeks time, there were no fits.[20]

The Tincture of Tunica Flowers was included in a number of formulae (e.g., Analeptic Potion, Analeptic Julep and the Tempering Julep). A possibility exists that, in specifying Hübner's preparation of the flowers, Wagner tried to ensure the use of a relatively standardized preparation as was apparently the case with other preparations such as his use of Tachenius' Vitriolated Tartar, Balsam of Sulphur prepared "after the art of Boyle,"[21] and, perhaps, John's Elixir of Property (see below).

Martin John, Jr.

Hübner' influence on Wagner's practice extended to passing on remedies from his own mentor Martin John, a widely traveled and well-known Schwenkfelder advocate and medical practitioner, who died in the year of Wagner's birth. Wagner's references seemingly reflected reasonable confidence, for, presumably, Hübner's own positive experiences with the preparations were recognized. Although only one is noticed as "proven," others carry such recommendations as, for a headache: "M John's White Cephalic Water is also a good remedy when put on the forehead."[22] And for "fractures:" "The Fracture Plaster Officinalis of Felix Würz or M[artin] J[ohn], if put on in the beginning, can sometimes distribute these edema, as I have seen myself."[23]

In one of his recommendations for a certain type of "Chill in the Stomach" Wagner mentions both Hübner and John in the same context:

20 "Dieses habe einem Kinde von 8 Wochen ein paar mahl gegeben welches schon einige Wochen Gichter gehabt, endlich täg[lich] 10. 12 biß 14 *fits*. Ja den letzten Tag 17. Hernach nach diesem Gebrauch den nechsten Tag 9. und folgend 5: ferner den nechsten Tag 2. hernach in 2 Wochen keine mehr." WAGNER (2005), fol. 52r. The formula is:
Vitriolated Tartar, scruple ½
M[elchior] Hübn[er] Epileptic Powder, grains 5
Simple Cathartic Powder, grains 5,
Distilled liquid, enough to make 4 doses.
A second formula with Epileptic powder appears in a "vomit." Wagner stated: "When a few weak fits returned [in the above case] subsequently, I again administered the above remedy, and when impending signs of an attack recurred, I administered a vomit." ("Als denn wieder ein paar Wochen drauf hab ihm obiges wieder gegeben und weil es noch ein paar mal gewittert[?], endlich ein Vomitiv.") This included: "Ipecacuanha, grains 3, Saline Cathartic [Powder] grains 4, Vitriolated Tartar, scruple ½, M H Epileptic Powder, grains 5, Elderberry Flower Water. Mix." WAGNER (2005), fol. 52r.

21 The Vitriolated Tartar appears in many places throughout the ms. For Boyle reference, WAGNER (2005), fol. 10r. Various balsams of sulphur are recorded in dispensatories. It has not been determined whether the formula for Compound Balsam of Sulphur (fol. 80v) is the Boyle formula.

22 WAGNER (2005), fol. 2v.

23 "Das Emp[lastrum] fractur. off. Felix Würtzens oder M[artin] J[ohn]s will dieselben[,] im anfang bald aufgelegt, manchmal zertheilen[,] wie ich selbst gesehen habe". WAGNER (2005), fol. 61r.

> But where there only is a cold, and where the patient did not eat much of such harmful things, or has eaten them only in moderation, or has gone on a fast or hunger cure, the patient will only need warming remedies such as Wine, Mead, Aqua Vitae, Stomach Water. Also, prepared and conserved or candied Ginger or Sweet Cane, Martin John's Life Giving Powder, Strong Purgative Powder, Elixir of Property. Also Aromatic Essence of M H, with Peppermint Water after the art can be taken.[24]

Wagner refers to eight Martin John preparations. They are an Aperient Mixture, a draught, Elixir of Property, a Fracture Plaster, Life Giving Powder, Strong Purgative Powder, Tempering Powder, and White Cephalic Water. A couple of points are noted here. First it is unfortunate that Wagner gives details of only two (possibly three) formulae, suggestive, as already said, that the manuscript was to be read by someone familiar with his practice. One formula, for the draught – recommended for "excessive monthly periods" and described as proven – prompts the question as to whether theory or clinical observation was a key factor in its use. The main constituent, Tormentil root, was combined with Juniper berries and boiled in a quart of red wine.[25] This, as with other preparations Wagner recommended for the same condition, had astringent and "binding" properties. While Wagner and his contemporaries commonly rationalized the use of remedies for menstrual bleeding on this basis, Wagner's judgment of the draught as "has also been proven" suggests he was relying, at least in part, on his own clinical experiences. At the same time, the possibility exists that "proven" may need to be read in the context of using the draught as part of a regimen of which he did not give complete details. As Wagner said at the beginning of his recommendations for treating excessive monthly flows:

> Here you must have regard to the difference in natural dispositions, because one person may be sanguine more than others and thus able to lose more blood without harm coming to her. But where it is too strong, help and counsel should be sought because this may lead to serious conditions. [26]

It is unclear whether or not another of Martin John's preparations, his Elixir of Property, is the one Wagner gives in the formulary part of the manuscript. The latter is not noted to be John's, and it must be appreciated that various formulae

24 "Wofern aber nur Verkältung da ist, daß d[er] Mensch entweder nicht viel von dem das ihm schädlich gewesen [ge]gessen, od[er] das er seither schon mässig gewesen, gefastet u[nd] sich aus gehungert hat, So brauche man nur erwärmende Mittel als: Wein, Meth, Aqua Vitae, Magen Wasser, It[em] gegossenen u[nd] eingemachten od[er] uberzogenen Ingwer od[er] Calmus, Martin Johns Lebens Pulver, od[er] Elixir proprietatis It[em] Ess: aromatica M[elchior] H[übner] c[um] aqua menthae S[ecundum] A[rtem] ein genomen." WAGNER (2005), fol. 15v.

25 WAGNER (2005), fol. 44r. The second M. John formula is for an Aperient Mixture: "M[artin] J[ohn]. Rx: Spirit of Salt, 1 drachm, Spirit Sal Ammoniac, drachms 3, mix, 25–30 grains." WAGNER (2005), fol. 87v.

26 "Bey diesem Zustand ist auf den Unterschied der Naturen zu sehen, weil eine Person vor der andern vollblütig und des Geblütes mehr entbehren kan, wenn Er [cj: der Abgang des Bluts] aber zu starck ist, muß Rath gesucht werden, weil er üble Zustände nach sich ziehen kan." WAGNER (2005), fol. 44r.

for the elixir featured in published dispensatories. In fact, questions about the quality of many of these preparations were sometimes raised, and it is not unreasonable to assume that Wagner used the John formula (even when not noted as John's) to ensure consistency of an extemporaneous prescription along the lines I have suggested for other products.[27] Certainly Wagner, as he did with Hübner's compositions, incorporated some of John's into his own preparations: for example, the Tempering Powder in one of his formulae for excessive monthly blood flows,[28] and the Powerful Purgative Powder in a formula for "A Very Strong Purging Powder For a Very Strong Person." (To this, he added: "I have given this to a certain person in one dose who purged without discomfort, not too strongly nor too much."[29])

Georg Hauptmann[30]

In one of the references to the Golden Heart Powder, Wagner notes it has "also been used with much benefit by my blessed great grandfather Georg Hauptmann and the blessed Melchior Hübner,"[31] which perhaps hints that Hübner might have learned it from Hauptmann. Although Wagner was only seven when his great grandfather died, the latter's influence reached him, perhaps not only via Hübner, but also through some writings Wagner possessed or had seen. As Wagner wrote in two places:

> 1. For this [Tincture Against Stones] see Schröder's Apotheken Schatz or the little book I compiled from the writings of the blessed G.H.M.[32]

27 For comment on uncertainty over various formulae, see QUINCY (1719), 390. For reference to Martin John's Elixir of Property see WAGNER (2005), fol. 74v, and to a formula for the Elixir WAGNER (2005), fol. 78r as given here with directions for preparation:
Rx:
Gum Aloes, 1 ounce in Liquor Regenerated Tartar, 6 ounces
Let dissolve, then add Tincture of Myrrh and Saffron with Spirit of Wine, of each 8 ounces and store for use.

28 WAGNER (2005), fol. 44r.

29 "Ein sehr starckes Pulvis purgans: vor eine sehr starcke Person."
"Dieses hab ich einer gewissen Person auf einmahl gegeben, welche ohne Beschwer davon purgiret, und zwar nicht zu starck oder zu viel." WAGNER (2005), fol. 54r.

30 In the manuscript, as in the written German of the period, the name is variously spelled Hauptmann and Haubtmann. In the web edition of the manuscript both GHM and GH have been interpreted as Hauptmann, GHM, the "M" being Medicus.

31 WAGNER (2005), fol. 49r. Two references exist to the use of this remedy for treating children, but without any indication of ingredients. One was said to be "very beneficial" ("hat [...] viel mahl gut gethan") when, during variola and measles, "the children or patients are very restless and the pustules do not fully erupt" ("wenn die Kinder oder Patienten sehr unruhig sind, und die pustulas nicht recht herauß wollen"), WAGNER (2005), fol. 49r. The other instance was for the "wind or colic" ("Wind und Blähungen") after a laxative. WAGNER (2005), fol. 47r,v.

32 "Tinctura c[ontra] Calculum. Siehe in Schröders Apoth[eken] Schatz oder in des sel[igen] G[eorge] H[auptmann] M[edicus] von mir zusammen getragenen Büchlein." WAGNER (2005), fol. 76r.

> 2. I have made this recipe ['Tincture of Antimony with Soluble Tartar'] according to Dr. Rothe and also the instructions of my blessed [great] grandfather G.H.M., paying close attention also to the notes that both Dr. Rothe made in his Chymie and Dr. Neumann in his Chymie.[33]

I have suggested that Wagner's references to preparations of Hübner and John were not necessarily his first choice, and the same applied to Hauptmann's. For instance, in commenting on different tooth powders used by Heister, Stahl and others, he also notes "Georg Hauptmann prescribes cleaning the teeth after eating with water in which a little Spirit of Ammoniac has been dissolved, and the use of the Becher Pills."[34] However, he went on to note another formula that he used in his own practice.[35] He also indicated his own alternative formula for another Hauptmann preparation, Anodyne Pill Mass, perhaps a formula with fewer ingredients reflecting concerns over the even distribution of opium in a multi-ingredient (polypharmaceutical) preparation.[36]

33 "Diese [Tinctura Antimonii tartarisata] habe ich nach D. Rothens auch nach meines sel. Groß Vaters G[eorge] H[auptmann] M[edicus] Beschreibung gemacht, und dabey die Noten in acht genommen, welche D. Rothe in seiner Chymie, u[nd] ferner auch D. Neumann in seiner Chymie beschrieben haben." WAGNER (2005), fol. 76r. Wagner added a note indicating his own experience in making the preparation: "I have found that the Spirit of Anise has extracted a good tincture, or Rectified Spirit of Wine well dephlegmed, but no alkali drawn off, 2 pounds, Oil Anise, 1 drachm. Mix." ("Ich habe gefunden, daß der Spiritus anisi eine schöne Tinctur extrahiret hat, oder spir[itus] vini wohl rectificirt bene dephlegm. aber über kein alcali abgezogen, 2 Pfund. Oli anisi, 1 Drachme. M[ische.]")

34 "George Hauptmann verordnet, die Zähne nach dem Essen mit Wasser[,] darinn ein wenig Salmiack zerlassen, abzuwaschen. nebst dem Gebrauch der becherischen Pillen." WAGNER (2005), fol. 89v.

35 The formula, relatively complex but pleasantly flavored, is included here for convenience:
Washed Crude Tartar, drachm 1
Vitriolated Tartar officinal, drachm [no quantity]
Crude Alum,
Gum Myrrh,
Prepared Crab Eyes, of each drachm ½
Oil of Clove, [deleted: 4 drops]
[Oil of] Rosewood, of each one drop [? quantity not clear]
Mix and make powder. WAGNER (2005), fol. 89v.

36 WAGNER (2005), fol. 8v. Wagner recorded (fol. 65r) a formula for an Anodyne Pill Mass, which I speculate was the more complex one, maybe Hauptmann's and not his:
Rx:
Extract of Opium, drachm 1
[Extract of] Apoplectic Water, drachm ½
Magistral Diaphoretic Antimony
Salt of Coral
Saffron Oriental, of each drachm ½
Double Arcanum, drachm 1
Gold Sulphur of Antimony, drachm 1
Gum Aloes, of each drachm ½
Make a mass with Elixir of Property [Elixir Proprietatis], in sufficient quantity

Whether another Hauptmann preparation, Special Gold Pills, contained opium has not been determined; Wagner noted them as an alternative to Anodyne Pills in treating "gnawing belly aches" in cases of dysentery.[37]

General Comments

What can be said about the collective nature of preparations Wagner linked to his Schwenkfelder mentors, and how did they compare with formulae that Wagner indicated were from Halle, two of which have been mentioned?

The Schwenkfelder preparations that Wagner chose to pass on were, by and large, not unduly complex and, as such, seemingly heralded the simplification of formulae and regimens that quickened pace during Wagner's professional lifetime. This may not be altogether surprising. During the later years of the lives of John and Hauptmann, and certainly during Hübner's time in medical practice, the vigorous, often vituperative, debates over the merits of chemical medicines associated with the name Paracelsus had already lost much vigor, albeit still rumbling along in a variety of publications.[38] Many chemical remedies – invariably simpler in formulation and used in smaller dosages than numerous longstanding Galenical formulations compounded from vegetable and animal products – had entered everyday practice without an overlay of Paracelsian efforts to reform medicine. Physicians were choosing from both chemical and Galenical remedies those they found to be of value, often combining them in formulations. Legacies of controversies were less in the realm of chemical pharmacy (preparing chemical remedies) than in the theoretical concepts within iatrochemistry, which were called upon to rationalize the functioning of the body. Although no evidence has been uncovered so far to suggest that Martin John, Jr. and Hauptmann were specifically influenced by Paracelsian or post-Paracelsian teachings, these found a ready ear among some if by no means all Protestants.[39] Certainly many remedies of the three Schwenkfelders were from chemical pharmacy, for instance, their tinctures, essences, spirits, vitriolated tartar and purified saltpetre. Relevant, too, if further more specific confirmation can be found, are references to Hauptmann as a chymist (*Laborant*), and to a possible exchange of views between John and Hauptmann (described by Wagner as "famous medici") and Christian Sigismund Richter (1672/73–1739), who with his brother Christian Friedrich Richter (1676–1711) was a key figure in the development of the Halle

Make 20 pills from one drachm.
Let the pills be gilded.
Although the formula of the Wagner Anodyne Pill Mass is not identified, Wagner did list a relatively simple Anodyne Powder (fol. 8v), namely: "Opium, prepared, one half ounce, Saffron, best quality, Red Coral, prepared, Pearls, prepared, Sulphur Antimony as third precipitate, of each drachm 1. Mix."

37 "[...] das heftige Leib Schneiden," WAGNER (2005), fol. 19v.

38 For one indication of controversies rumbling on, see DEBUS (2001), 156.

39 For a still helpful discussion on interpretation issues for historians surrounding the evidence to support Paracelsian influence on many Protestants, see ELMER (1989).

Orphanage medicines.[40] At least some of the latter remedies were yet another thread in the trend to what has been called, as already noted, a gentler medicine.[41]

Wagner's own references to the Halle Orphanage medicines – he mentions at least eight – along with invoking Stahlian theoretical ideas is a strong indication of the additional significant influence of much medical thinking that surrounded or emanated from Stahl in Halle. This included "disciples" such as Samuel Carl, Johann Juncker, and Gottfried Rothe to whom Wagner makes one reference each, as well as the commercially prepared medicines of the Halle Orphanage. I suspect that the Halle ambience added to or reinforced his mentors' trend to simplification by adding a framework of Stahlian theory along with what must have been a sense of medical change and reform. At the same time, I am not suggesting that other influences, even if small, were irrelevant in shaping Wagner's practice; for instance, his references to (i) published medical authorities, and (ii) neighboring physicians such as the Moravian John Meyer and, as already noted, the former Huguenot and later Universalist George de Benneville.[42] Further, Wagner referred to the practice of English practitioners, albeit disagreeing with their repeated venesection in treating an outbreak of pleurisy.[43] All this is not to say Wagner accepted the practices of others uncritically, a point we comment on in considering Wagner's own formulations.

40 For reference to Hauptmann as a chemist see HENSEL (1768), 679: "[...] ein alter Chymicus und Practicus medicinae [...]." BERKY (1954), 43, also translates a letter from Wagner who wrote that he was "once told" that both John and Hauptmann had contact with Christian Sigismund Richter in Halle, the co-developer with this brother Christian Friedrich of the Halle Orphanage medications. Unfortunately, Berky does not reference his sources, but he may well have drawn his information from the *Hallesche Nachrichten*, a continuous publication emanating from the Halle Orphanage: see MANN, SCHMUCKER & GERMANN (1886). The letter in question, from Abraham Wagner to Heinrich Melchior Mühlenberg of September 1, 1753, is No. 137 in ALAND (1987).

41 For discussion on the context of "gentler" medicine that is compatible with much of Wagner's practice, WILSON (2000), 184 et seq. For the latest relevant discussion on gentle medicine in general, various papers in TOELLNER (2004).

42 Wagner includes one Meyer formula in his discussion on loss of senses: "Or 3 parts Saltpetre, 1 part Camphor Every two hours during the attack By J.A. Meyer. It is a proven remedy." ("oder 3 theil Salpeter. 1 theil Camph[or] alle 2 Stund in der Hitze --- [...]. Von J.A.Meyer. P[ro]b[atum] est." WAGNER (2005), fol. 4r). On Wagner, see Viehmeyer in this volume.

43 WAGNER (2005), fol. 12r.

General Remarks on Wagner's Medicines

Given the influences described so far, it is appropriate to ask whether or not they are evident in Wagner's own extemporaneous preparations, especially those that he clearly identifies by attaching his own name, initials, or by the use of the possessive. I comment first on quality issues and polypharmaceutical preparations and then Wagner's specific, perhaps new, formulae.

Quality issues and polypharmaceutical preparations

As already indicated, Wagner may have continued to employ some of the preparations of his Schwenkfelder mentors (and of other named authorities) in order to ensure consistent quality of his prescriptions, which, after all, was essential for evaluating clinical effectiveness. At a time when the quality of both the materia medica and of compounded medicines was determined more through assessment of sensory properties and of standardizing ways of preparation – rather than the much later analytical approaches to quality control – Wagner's formulae offer some evidence of concerns with standardizing. For instance, his consistent use of "Purified Saltpetre" as well as references to "best," "good" and "top," quality products such as Myrrh, Diaphoretic Antimony, Opium, Saffron and Theriac, and of certain products such as the already mentioned Tachenius' Vitriolated Tartar.

A particular preparation pointing up quality issues was the popular Theriac, or rather various theriacs. With a history extending back to classical times as a panacea, but especially in the context of an antidote to poisoning or epidemics, theriac remains one of history's best known polypharmaceuticals. In Wagner's time the use of all the theriacs was being questioned because of the great difficulty in formulating the thick unctuous preparations with an even distribution of key ingredients, notably opium.[44] Yet Wagner includes at least one reference to each of the following (invariably as a component in other formulae): Andromachus' Theriac, Hübner's Theriac, and Venetian Theriac, and two references to just Theriac (once as "Theriac, good quality"). Also noted are Spirit of Theriac and Essence of Theriac. The various references hint at copying from diverse sources. Mention of Venetian Theriac is of special interest since it was a recognized synonym for the Andromachus' Theriac, which Wagner also specifically refers to; it maybe that Wagner was just copying a formula from Lorenz Heister for treating "finger worm." Wagner not only noted that "Dr. Heister recommends a solution of Camphor, in particular if some Theriac is dissolved in it and the immersion is made to last several hours,"[45] but also wrote out a formula for Camphorated Spirit of Theriac based on "Venetian Theriac."[46]

44 For some comment on this, JAMES (1747), 721–723.

45 "D. Heister recommendirt Camphor Lösung sonderlich wenn was Theriac darin zerlassen und damit viele Stunden continuiret." WAGNER (2005), fol. 99r. The formula has not yet been located in Heister's writings.

46 The formula is on fol. 75r, though no reference is given to Heister.

Wagner's comments on the latter preparation are worth quoting as a further illustration of the details attached to preparing a medicine to ensure consistency from batch to batch, as well as the need to choose medicines suited to particular patients:

> They can be prepared with and without Camphor because this substance is not tolerated by all dispositions. Some use one half ounce of Camphor for each two pounds of Spirits, which is sufficient. In preparing the Spirit of Theriac without Camphor, one can add about one half drachm for three ounces of Spirit to make the Simple Mixture, which is strong enough. Let it dissolve well before the other spirits are mixed in. Then, for each 9 ounces of Mixture there will be one half drachm of Camphor and for ½ ounce [and] ½ drachm Mixture, barely 2 grains of Camphor.[47]

One especially interesting formula that Wagner indicated as his own – Mineral Bezoar Powder with Precious Stones – is also noteworthy as a complex polypharmaceutical. The formula has all the hallmarks of earlier practices, including the presence of prepared unicorn, and generally seems out of place in the manuscript.[48] However, Wagner does mention its use in an outbreak of Pleurisy in 1748: "With regard to congestion and ebullition of the blood, the Halle Bezoar Powder alone or given together with my Bezoar Powder or the Powder of Precious Stones did good service."[49]

In marked contrast to the polypharmaceuticals are the significant number of formulae – falling within the trend toward simpler medicines – that consist of only four to five ingredients. These are well illustrated by various tempering medicines for which particular formulae were used for different conditions. Two examples are: (i) "Vitriolated Tartar, Purified Saltpetre, and Prepared Crab Eyes

47 "[Diese Arzeneyen] werden mit u[nd] auch ohne Camphor bereitet, weil denselben nicht alle Naturen vertragen können. Von einigen wird zu zwei Pfund Spiritus, eine halbe Unze Camphor verdün[n]et, welches auch genug ist. Wenn der Spir[itus] theriacal[is] ohne Camphor bereitet ist, so kan[n] man zu dem [unleserlich] Spir[itus] zur Mix[tura] Simp[lex] etwan [...] drunter thun, welches starck g[e]nug ist u[nd] erst solviren lassen, ehe man die andern spiritus drunter mischet, so kommt untter 9 Unzen Mixt[ura] ½ Drachme Camphor u[nd] unter ½ Unze Mixt[ura] kaum 2 gr. Camph[or]." WAGNER (2005), fol. 75r.

48 The interesting formula is included here for convenience:
Rx: A Stone Precious 500 times prepared, scruples 5
Pearls, prepared, drachm 1
Red Coral, prepared,
Crab Eyes, prepared,
Philosophic Salt of Hartshorn, prepared
Diaphoretic Antimony, top quality, of each drachms 2
Unicorn, prepared,
Powdered Piony Root, of each drachm 1,
finish with Gold Leaf no 6
Mix. Make a powder. WAGNER (2005), fol. 8r.

49 "Erstl[ich] wegen der Congestion u[nd] Ebullition im Geblüt hat das Hallische Bezoar-Pulver entweder allein oder mit meinem Bezoar P[ulver] oder dem Edelstein Pulver vermischt, gut gethan." WAGNER (2005), fol. 11v.

or Coral, or Prepared Hartshorn;" and (ii) "The Halle Tempering and Mineral Bezoar Powder[s] in a cooling Julep."[50]

One further observation about Wagner's simpler formulae is that they often include more than one principal herb or chemical, perhaps with the intention of synergistic action. Detailed comparative studies of such medicines in pharmacopoeias, dispensatories and textbooks might help clarify the reasoning behind the formulae. For instance, to what extent did they follow what was then the trend – as part of the shift to simplify extemporaneous formulae – to a systematic approach of formulating prescriptions in four parts: (i) a *basis* (the most active ingredient); (ii) an *adjuvans* to promote to assist the action of (i); (iii) a *corrigens* to remove unpleasant or noxious ingredients with impairing their virtues, and (iv) a *constituens* for preparing the medicine into a palatable form?[51]

Wagner's Own Formulae

Any consideration of the reasoning behind Wagner's choice of formulae for a patient must explore those that he specifically identified as his own. Such formulae include an Antihypochondriac Mixture, Bezoar Powder, a Draught and Liniment for Sciatica, Draught for Fever, Dysentery Powder, Expectorant Powder I and II, Lenitive Syrup of Tribus, Mixture For Hearing Difficulties, Discutient Mixture, Mixture against Tussis, Mineral Bezoar Powder with Precious Stones (noted above), and Sudorific Powder. Other Wagner preparations are noted without formulae: Anodyne Pill Mass, Anti-Emetic Powder, Alexipharmic Powder, Elixir of Health, and Theriac.

Leaving aside Wagner's polypharmaceutical formulae such as Bezoar Powder with Precious Stones, many of his prescriptions do not seem overly complex; for instance, the Sudorific Powder prepared from Kermes Mineral, Vitriolated Tartar, Prepared Crab Stones, and Oil of Cinnamon.[52] On the other hand, a number contain at least one component that is a polypharmaceutical. For example, although Wagner's Antihypochondriac mixture contains only five items, one is the Elixir of Health, itself a complex, possibly pleasant-tasting laxative that was probably intended to minimize griping.[53]

50 WAGNER (2005), fols. 2r and 13r.
Other examples of simple formulae include: "Vitriolated Tartar or Double Arcanum [inserted: Cream of Tartar] and Prepared Crab Eyes mixed with a little Saltpetre, all in equal amounts" (fol. 17v); "Double Arcanum or Tachenius' Vitriolated Tartar, Purified Saltpetre, Prepared Crab Stones, of each drachm 1, Cinnabar of Antimony, scruple ½. Mix and make a powder" (fol. 34r); "Healthful Digestive Nitre and Burnt Red Coral, or through addition of mild astringents such as Cascarilla Powder, Anodyne Pills, etc. " (fol. 44r).

51 For this and context, CRELLIN & SCOTT (1970). Wagner's recommendation of administering in a julep (see above) would seem to be the constituens, although since he notes a cooling property, he may be thinking of an adjuvans action. It is noteworthy that relatively few examples of separate external vehicles appear in Wagner's manuscript compared with those in the manuscript of his contemporary George de Benneville, for which see CRELLIN (1997).

52 WAGNER (2005), fol. 55v.

53 WAGNER (2005), fol. 87r.

I sense that a number of Wagner's formulae (and not only those designated as his) were modifications of those he acquired from elsewhere. This might apply to, for instance, the Halle formulae he wrote out in detail – Halle Pills for Obstruction and Halle Bezoar Powder – that do not exactly match what is known of the Halle formulae from elsewhere.[54] Of course, other reasons might account for differences such as Wagner's assumptions about the formulae (supposedly they were secret) or changes in formulae over time that certainly occurred. I might add that various formulae for bezoar powder – primarily used in fevers – existed in dispensatories of the time and Wagner also notes his own.[55] It may be surmised that decisions on which formulae to use rested, in part, on standardizing the quality of the preparation (simpler formulae were easier) as an essential prerequisite in trying to ascertain effectiveness in particular conditions.

Theory and Clinical Experience in Validation

My discussion so far has focused primarily on formulae with only passing mention that, in an earlier discussion, I have suggested Wagner evaluated theory with his own clinical experiences (providing empirical evidence). His conclusions undoubtedly led to the differing judgments that Wagner appends to many of his own formulae. For example, two were described as "proven" and others variously noted as "stopping a vomit," "useful," "restored them [patients]." Unfortunately one can only surmise, in part because we have no indication of the extent of Wagner's practice on which he reached judgments, on the relative weight he attached to theory and to clinical experience, or even the extent to which theory was possibly a rationalization of choices made on the grounds of clinical experience.

54 The two formulae are given here as illustrations:
1. Halle Pills Against Obstructions [Although apparently a simple formula, panchymagogum was a polypharmaceutical]
Rx:
Gum Aloes, ounces 2
Croll[ius]' Extract of Panchymagogum, drachm 1
Prepared Iron Filings, ounce ½
Mix and make into pill to weight 1 grain.
S[ignature, i.e. label]: Pills against constipation
Dose: 3 to 5 grains. (fol. 53v)
2. Halle Bezoar Powder
Rx:
Diaphoretic Antimony
Shell Fish, prepared
Purified Saltpetre
Vitriolated Tartar, of each ounce ½
Cinnabar of Antimony, grains 50
Mix. (fol. 1v)
For differences in the Halle formula, cf. POECKERN (1984), 117–118, 370–371. For an English version based on Poeckern's transcription, see WILSON (2000), Tables 3.1 and 3.2.

55 WAGNER (2005), fol. 11v: "my bezoar powder."

Wagner's two "proven" remedies indicate the difficulty in reaching conclusions on the relative roles of theory and clinical experience. One, a "Mixture For Hearing Difficulties," reads:

Rx:
Essence of Amber, one drachm
Distilled Oil of Anise
[Distilled Oil of] Caraway, of each drops 5
Mix. Of this 3 drops at a time, two to three times daily, dropped into the ear.[56]

Essence of Amber was generally recognized as a deobstructant or discutient for use in a wide range of conditions. (It is noteworthy that Wagner's added note to this formula indicated it could also be used for the same purpose with Halle Discutient Spirit.) The oils could loosen any ear wax contributing to hearing difficulties. It thus seems reasonable to suggest that the validation of this remedy was based on a good level of clinical evidence, supported by the reputation of amber at the time.

In contrast, the second proven remedy cannot be easily rationalized today on empirical grounds. It is the Antihypochondriac Mixture when used for "stabbing pain in the side." The formula given is:

Elixir of Health, drachms 2
Tincture of Rhubarb
Sweet Spirit of Nitre, of each drachm 1
Oil of Anise, drop 1
Mix. The dose 20 to 25 drops.[57]

Given that one ingredient, the Elixir of Health, was a reasonably powerful laxative (I assume it is the one given in the manuscript, although perhaps not in the recommended dose), it is tempting to see this proven remedy as supportive treatment by cleansing the gastrointestinal tract and tempering the blood and very much in line with theoretical conventions of the time.[58]

56 WAGNER (2005), fol. 81v.

57 WAGNER (2005), fol. 87r.

58 A formula for an Elixir of Health is given on fol. 78v; possibly this is Wagner's own formula (cf. his note on fol. 17v). It is copied here, with his note on preparing it, for convenience in showing that, although a laxative, it did not contain senna as did many other formulae for Elixir Salutis circulating at the time; many of these were seemingly derived from the English proprietary preparation, Daffy's Elixir, for which see HAYCOCK & WALLIS (2005), 30–32.
The Wagner recipe is:
Powdered Sucotrine Aloes, ounces 2
Rhubarb, powdered,
White Cichory [Root], of each ounce ½
Anise seed
Liquorice Juice, ounces 2
Salt Regenerated Tartar, [deleted: ounces 4] ounces 2
[Salt] of Sloes, [deleted: ounces 2] ounce 1
Elder Flower Water, pounds 2

Formulation as a Part of Validation

The Wagner manuscript is clearly tantalizing for many reasons. Just as soon as one feels confident in seeing an overall trend to, say, simpler and relatively gentler remedies, then relatively complex ones are noted. The manuscript offers a feeling for the shifts in therapies from the old to the new. There is, too, a complex coexistence between theory and clinical experience, although the latter was an evident monitor of the theory when evaluating the outcome of a treatment. The monitoring was also linked, as suggested in the discussion so far, to standardizing formulae as far as possible.

Given this, the continued use of well-known, complex remedies is noteworthy, although a commonplace in medical practice in general. It suggests Wagner would not readily "let go" of remedies for which a long history offered strong validation. Continuing existence also applies to various simpler remedies from his Schwenkfelder mentors; their secondary place in many of his recommendations hints that allegiance to Schwenkfelder practice was a factor behind this, although consideration has also to be given to Wagner's own positive experiences, the additional explanatory Stahlian framework, and their role in standardizing preparations. Furthermore, continued use has to consider a patient's confidence in long-standing remedies, while there was no point in dispensing with the old unless newer remedies were demonstrated as superior in some cases, at least to Wagner's satisfaction.

The Practitioner-Patient Relationship

Mention has just been made of the issue of patients' confidence, and any discussion of the interplay of theory, clinical experience, and assessments of effectiveness of treatments has to consider the nature of the practitioner-patient relationship; especially significant is the possible role of the practitioner in enhancing what is widely recognized nowadays as an important component of any therapy, namely a placebo action. Hence any analysis of Wagner and his manuscript needs to ask the question posed for some time by historians: "What did doctors really do?"[59]

The question is sharpened by the fact that, at face value, the manuscript may be viewed as fitting the pattern of what can be called reductionism in eighteenth-century medical writings — that is the approach, or apparent approach, to a disease as a chemical, physical or mechanical derangement that demanded a medi-

Spirit of Wine Regular 2 [twice distilled?], pound 1
Make elixir according to the art.
Note: The salts are each dissolved and filtered. Mix into one pound of Elder Flower Water, [several words deleted] then pour into the spirits, then the species [plant material] added and let them be extracted from this mixture. The Liquorice Juice can be added last.
Another recipe given on the same page is in a different hand and has been added later in 1776. It contains senna and is compared to a preparation sold by the Bartram [sic: Bertram] pharmacy in Philadelphia.

59 For a recent emphasis in the American setting, see FLANNERY (1999).

cal treatment. It was an approach that took attention away from other less tangible notions such as superstition/magic, or soul (that perhaps allowed the embodiment of God), or a person's mind and spirit as factors in the nature and outcome of a disease. (Wagner mentions God only once and then almost incidentally in terms of "Thanks be to God" that he had one useful remedy for what was presumably a difficult problem.[60]) One aspect of trends toward reductionism, too, was to limit the number of variables when trying to establish cause and effect in treatment, something that I feel Wagner was aware of through his efforts to standardize treatments.

However, what may seem to be reductionist cannot be assumed to reflect Wagner's actual approach to patients, especially in view of his acquaintance with Stahl's animism and his own religious convictions. Although a full discussion of this matter is beyond this article, general comments are appropriate. Physicians have always been able to benefit patients in various ways. Given Wagner's deep sense of spirituality as a Schwenkfelder, did he ignore, say, the spiritual needs of his patients? Or does, in fact, the manuscript reflect a compartmentalizing of knowledge – a pragmatic way to approach clinical situations? Is it possible that Wagner saw himself as just recording one aspect of how to benefit fellow creatures? Perhaps he was in tune with a comment in John Tennent's popular colonial publication, *Every Man His Own Doctor: or The Poor Planter's Physician* (of which there were many editions from 1734 including one in German) that spelled out ways of helping patients:

> There are Three Ways of benefiting our Fellow Creatures. We may be useful to their Souls, by good Instruction, and good Example. We may be helpful to their Bodies, by feeding the Hungry, clothing the Naked, and prescribing easy Remedies to the Sick: We can aid them in their Fortunes, by encouraging of Industry, by relieving the Distrest, and doing all the kind Offices we are able, to our Neighbours.[61]

If the manuscript indeed reflects a compartmentalizing of knowledge – and much precedent for this already existed in medical writings, especially those that focused on medical treatment – how might Wagner have approached patients? It has always to be remembered that a physician's success – financial or otherwise – has always depended on an ability to develop trusting relationships with patients. Unfortunately, we have no information on numbers of Wagner's patients to indicate his level of success or how much income he derived from medicine (maybe farming was his primary means of livelihood), whether he was viewed as an authoritative or a father figure, and so on. Nor do we have any real understanding of the extent to which his own views on the body and soul matched those of his patients and how between them care and treatment of a condition was negotiated.[62] However, he was a Schwenkfelder and spiritualist, and there is

60 WAGNER (2005), fol. 21r.

61 TENNENT (1734), 3–4.

62 For one sense of negotiation between patients and one physician, but likely to be representative of others see an account of a physician roughly contemporary to Wagner, Johann

every reason to believe that he felt his medical care described in the manuscript was linked to spiritual care.[63] It is reasonable to suggest that he viewed treating the body as also sustaining the soul, and providing an "environment" for spiritual rebirth or regeneration.[64]

Undoubtedly, it was not the purpose of his manuscript, dealing with bodily symptoms and pharmaceutical therapies, to point out such matters. Nor was it the purpose to deal with counseling patients when there might be a need to remind them of other ways of nourishing the soul, or to take responsibility for their health or physical ills in line with the growing trend of popular literature on such matters. Yet I suspect there were good reasons why Wagner was able to establish trusting relations with patients, and thereby enhance the therapeutic relationship and the positive effects of medications. It is unclear whether he recognized this was a factor in his clinical experiences.

Storch, also influenced by Stahl: DUDEN (1991). Her view (e.g., 87) is that "the doctor did not work from his findings, but from the expression of suffering in the patients' complaint."

63 It is also possible that Wagner, in writing the manuscript, felt he was contributing to sustaining the Schwenkfelder tradition in the New World. Among others, HUCHO (2002) has noted the role of Schwenkfelder women in sustaining transatlantic bonds that, in turn, helped to sustain larger central European cultural and medical traditions.

64 For the relationship between physical healing and spiritual rebirth in Halle Pietism, see HELM (2006), 24–25. For a sense of Wagner's spiritual depth, see BERKY (1954). I argue that Wagner was undoubtedly acquainted with the Stahlian view of a holistic, self-determined organism, a unity of body and soul, just as he was acquainted with Stahl's medical theory. Furthermore, many of Wagner's therapeutic recommendations were in line with the general Stahlian-Pietist approach to care, namely to support the healing power of nature, or for Stahl the soul, and to strengthen the body by the conservative use of many relatively simple remedies. The literature on Stahl is vast, but for a summary of theory and therapeutics, see HABRICH (1991) and KONERT (1997), especially 26–27.

References

Aland (1987)
Aland, Kurt (Ed.): Die Korrespondenz Heinrich Melchior Mühlenbergs. Aus der Anfangszeit des deutschen Luthertums in Nordamerika, Vol. 2: 1753–1762. Berlin, New York: de Gruyter, 1987.

Berky (1954)
Berky, Andrew S.: Practitioner in Physick. A Biography of Abraham Wagner 1717 [sic] – 1763. Pennsburg: The Schwenkfelder Library, 1954.

Crellin (1997)
Crellin, John K.: How Shall I Take my Medicines? Dosages and other Matters in Eighteenth-Century Medicine. In: Caduceus 13 (1997), 39–50.

Crellin (2006)
Crellin, John K.: Theory and Clinical Experience in Eighteenth-Century Extemporaneous Prescriptions – a Reciprocal Relationship? In: Pharmacy in History 48 (2006), 3–13.

Crellin 2007
Crellin, John K.: Reductionist Trends in Eighteenth-Century Therapeutics: a Discussion on Two Medical/Pharmaceutical Manuscripts. In: Pharmaceutical Historian 37 (2007), 26–34.

Crellin & Scott (1970)
Crellin, John K.; Scott, J. R.: Pharmaceutical History and its Sources in the Wellcome Collections. III Fluid Medicines, Prescription Reform and Posology, 1700–1900. In: Medical History 14 (1970), 132–153.

Debus (2001)
Debus, Allen: Chemistry and Medical Debate: van Helmont to Boerhaave. Canton: Science History Publications, 2001.

Delacoste (1715)
Delacoste, Jean: Boerhaave's Aphorisms Concerning the Knowledge and Cure of Diseases. London: Cowse and Innys, 1715.

Duden (1991)
Duden, Barbara: The Woman Beneath the Skin. A Doctor's Patients in Eighteenth-Century Germany. Cambridge: Harvard University Press, 1991.

Elmer (1989)
Elmer, Peter: Medicine, Religion and the Puritan Revolution. In: French, Roger; Wear, Andrew (Eds.): The Medical Revolution of the Seventeenth Century. Cambridge: Cambridge University Press, 1989, 10–45.

Flannery (1999)
Flannery, Michael A.: What do doctors really do? In Search of a Therapeutic Perspective of American Medicine. In: Journal of Clinical Pharmacy and Therapeutics 24 (1999), 151–156.

Habrich (1991)
Habrich, Christa: Characteristic Features of Eighteenth-Century Therapeutics in Germany. In: Bynum, William F.; Nutton, Vivian (Eds.): Essays in the History of Therapeutics. Amsterdam: Rodopi, 1991 (Clio Medica 22), 39–49.

Haycock & Wallis (2005)
Haycock, David Boyd; Wallis, Peter John (Eds.): Quackery and Commerce in Seventeenth-Century London. The Proprietary Medicine Business of Anthony Daffy. London: The Wellcome Trust Centre for the History of Medicine at UCL, 2005.

Helm (2006)
Helm, Jürgen: Krankheit, Bekehrung und Reform. Medizin und Krankenfürsorge im Halleschen Pietismus. Tübingen: Verlag der Franckeschen Stiftungen im Niemeyer Verlag, 2006 (Hallesche Forschungen 21).

Hensel (1768)
Hensel, Johann Adam: Protestantische Kirchen=Geschichte der Gemeinen in Schlesien Nach allen Fürstenthümern, vornehmsten Städten und Oertern dieses Landes, [...] in acht Abschnitten [...]. Leipzig, Liegnitz: David Siegert, 1768.

Hucho (2001)
Hucho, Christine: Female Writers, Women's Networks, and the Preservation of Culture. The Schwenkfelder Women of Eighteenth-Century Pennsylvania. In: Pennsylvania History 68 [1] (2001), 101–130.

James (1747)
James, Robert: Pharmacopoeia Universalis: or a New Universal English Dispensatory. London: Hodges, 1747.

Konert (1997)
Konert, Jürgen: Academic and Practical Medicine in Halle During the Era of Stahl, Hoffman and Juncker. In: Caduceus 13 (1997), 23–38.

Madden (2004)
Madden, Deborah: Contemporary Reactions to John Wesley's Primitive Physic. Or the Case of Dr. William Hawes Examined. In: Social History of Medicine 17 (2004), 365–378.

Mann, Schmucker & Germann (1886)
Mann, Wilhelm Julius; Schmucker, B. M.; Germann, Wilhelm (Eds.): Nachrichten von den vereinigten deutschen evangelish-lutherischen Gemeinen in Nord-America, absonderlich in Pensylvanien. Allentown, PA: Brobst, Diehl & Co., 1886.

Poeckern (1984)
Poeckern, Hans-Joachim: Die Hallischen Waisenhaus-Arzeneyen. Leipzig: Edition Leipzig, 1984 (Bibliotheca Historico-Naturalis Antiqua).

Quincy (1719)
Quincy, John: Pharmacopoeia Officinalis & Extemporanea. London: A. Bell, 1719.

Tennent (1734)
Tennent, John: Every Man His Own Doctor. Or The Poor Planter's Physician. Williamsburg: William Parks, 1734.

Toellner (2004)
Toellner, Richard (Ed.): Die Geburt einer sanften Medizin. Halle: Verlag der Franckeschen Stiftungen zu Halle, 2004.

Wagner (2005)
Wagner, Abraham: Remediorum Specimina aliquot ex Praxi A. W. [Manuscript Book of Medical Recipes and Observations]. In: Eighteenth-century Colonial Formularies. The Manuscripts of George de Benneville and Abraham Wagner. The College of Physicians of Philadelphia Digital Library.
Recent website address (access date: June 23, 2008): http://www.accesspadr.org/cpp/.

Ward & Yell (1993)
Ward, Jean E; Yell, Joan (Eds.): The Medical Casebook of William Brownrigg, M.D., F.R.S. (1712–1800) of the Town of Whitehaven in Cumberland. London: Wellcome Institute for the History of Medicine, 1993 (Medical History Supplement 3).

Wilson (2000)
Wilson, Renate: Pious Traders in Medicine. A German Pharmaceutical Network in Eighteenth-Century North America. University Park, PA: Penn State University Press, 2000.

THE TRANSMISSION OF MEDICAL AND PHARMACEUTICAL KNOWLEDGE TO COLONIAL NORTH AMERICA

Renate Wilson

In its thematic focus on the interaction between eighteenth century theory and practice, this volume has been able to include a rare transatlantic context – two manuscripts in North American archives attributed to two European medical practitioners from radical religious backgrounds. The author of the *Medicina Pensylvania*, George de Benneville, was of French Huguenot extraction, reared in England but with medical training in apparently radical medical settings in Germany.[1] Abraham Wagner, who collated his observations from a rural practice together with numerous recipes in a manuscript entitled *Remediorum specimina aliquot ex praxi A.W*, was an active Schwenckfelder dissident from a lively and longstanding Silesian medical tradition, which included the manufacture of chemical cures. He and his coreligionists were expelled first from Silesia and then from the estates of Count Zinzendorf.[2] Both men incorporated the therapeutic traditions of the seventeenth and early eighteenth century on an eclectic basis into their receptures and, both implicitly and explicity, their therapeutic advice and practice. Both used the High German of the period (*Schriftdeutsch*), intermixed with Latin terminology and nomenclature as the main narrative language of their manuscripts, addressed to and reflecting cooperation with their Anglophone, German, and Dutch copractitioners in North America.

The manuscripts have been known to exist but have been little described or analysed in the medical historiography of the North American colonial period.[3]

I will suggest some of the reasons for this neglect in this paper, prominently among them two major themes of the eighteenth century as it played out on the North American shores: (1) The contest for linguistic dominance and medical tradition in the scientific discourse of the New Republic. (2) The relative place of sectarian or dissident medical practitioners vs the standard bearers of the

1 For these, see HABRICH (1991), HABRICH (1997), and HABRICH (2002).

2 For biographical detail and the religious background, see the contribution of Allen Viehmeyer; for the traditions invoked in Wagner's clinical notes and receptures, see John Crellin in this volume and a previous paper, CRELLIN (2006); for the genealogy of the Paracelsian portions of the de Benneville manuscript, see Jole Shackelford, also in this volume. Work on these manuscripts was undertaken with the objective of providing digitized and transcribed versions for a website, now accessible at "Eighteenth-century Colonial Formularies: The Manuscripts of George de Benneville and Abraham Wagner," College of Physicians of Philadelphia Digital Library. Website address: http://www.accesspadr.org/cpp/.

3 The research underlying this paper was in part supported by the National Library of Medicine, Washington, D.C.

Enlightenment, in particular its Scottish version.In particular, partly because of their assumed adherence to Stahlian medical concepts, the anglophone North American medical establishment of the second half of the eighteenth century does not seem to have wished to acknowledge the presence of highly trained and skilled European medical practitioners in their midst. And the historiography of American colonial medicine has followed suit, leaving German medical practice in the colonies to the ethnohistorians.[4]

Both manuscripts reflected the contemporary state of the use of medicinals in therapy – that is, ample and occasionally discordant prescriptions for the relief from pain and illness and cure, rather than medical theory. The de Benneville manuscript, which like its companion by Abraham Wagner originated in one of the heavily German-language regions of the colonies, is in fact bilingual (German – English), suggesting its intended use in a multicultural medical setting. Most likely, this was a Philadelphia pharmacy filling prescriptions and apparently coowned during the 1750s by de Benneville, Moses and Isaac Bartram, and Thomas Say.[5] The manuscript by Abraham Wagner exists only in German, although the author's interaction with his English-language co-practitioners again included the pharmacists Moses and Isaac Bartram and a pragmatic awareness of English medical literature, in particular William Lewis' *New Edinburgh Dispensatory,* as evident from a number of cross-references in the text.[6]

The two men respresented very different geographic and social strata, but were joined by their inclusion in the pervasive web of radical evangelical dissidence, many of whose members, including medical practitioners, migrated to North America in the first half of the eighteenth century. Their work, and the history of their relative neglect, suggest several questions that deserve fuller treatment in both colonial American and nineteenth century American medicine.

I will first turn to the generic antecedents of these two texts and their place in the long tradition of German medical and pharmaceutical writing, both in

4 For the rejection of Stahlian medicine by William Cullen, the influential tutor of many of the colonial physicians trained in Edinburgh, see CULLEN (1784), XI-XXV. For the persistent relegation of German and other non-English vernacular or national languages to ethnic and religious domains, see AMORY (2000), 28–30, by the otherwise immensely knowledgeable Hugh Amory.

5 There is no well documented record of his proprietorship or a silent partnership in this pharmacy on Race Street, although there is indirect evidence that he was a partner of Thomas Say sr., who first coowned with and then sold the establishment to Isaac and Moses Bartram in the late 1750s. See MÜLLER-JAHNKE (1988), BAIRD (2003). I thank Joel Fry of Bartram Gardens for this elusive information. De Benneville's financial position can be traced through several deeds, his will, and surveys showing his properties to the north of Philadelphia and real estate sold after his death. These included holdings in the Race Street section on the commercial riverfront in Philadelphia. His family gravesite still exists and is maintained under a family Trust.

6 For the definitive overview and summary of editions of this much published work, see COWEN (2001).

terms of genre and language of discourse. In this discussion, the development of *Fachprosa* or *artes* literature in the organization and transmission of medical knowledge will be of greater concern than explicit medical theory.

Second, we should inquire into the place and fit of these two manuscripts within the medical practice of their new, largely and insistently Anglophone environment, taking into acount that in eighteenth century North America, Latin was no longer the dominant language of medical and therapeutic discourse.[7] Both de Benneville and Wagner clearly stood in a long tradition of Latin and German medical bilinguality, and their compilation and transmission of therapeutic sources in the German vernacular should be examined within a professional rather than a popular framework.[8]

The Manuscripts and Their Vernacular Antecedents

Much of the discussion of the growth of national vernaculars in medicine[9] during the early modern period has been in terms of elite academic culture, set off against the growing differentiation of professional and technical languages. Other points of departure of relevance in our context are the culture of the common man or woman as active consumers of medical knowledge, and the orientation of many post-Reformation medical writers to the biblical vernacular of evangelical Christians and their rejection of heathen (i.e. classical) knowledge traditions.[10]

7 REINHOLD (1984), in particular chapters 2 and 4, and the literature cited there.

8 For the importance of this distinction in the American setting, see COWEN (2001), 233–260, COWEN (1985) and COWEN & WILSON (1997).

9 This heading is adapted from RIHA (1992b) as providing focus on the propositions raised here. In the following, I draw on her categorization and development of medical and related genres in RIHA (1992a) as providing a sophisticated framework for categorizing our manuscripts in terms of both structure and content. While the main period for her work and that of the Würzburger Research Institute is the period 1300–1600, the larger framework is from the beginning of the "[…] 12th century to the threshold of the Enlightenment." RIHA (1992a), 3. I thank Professor Riha for facilitating my access to these sources. An important overview of German medical texts for the early modern period is by TELLE (1982), whose catalogue of the famous Herzog August Bibliothek exhibition provides a rich sampling of titles and of genres.

10 There is a large and still growing literature on this subject that informs itself from multiple paradigms. For an insightful introduction to the problem, see EAMON (1994), in particular 9–11, which includes a good discussion of Elisabeth Eisenstein's seminal work on the importance of the print culture for the differentiation of secular knowledge and communication by authors otherwise firmly committed to their beliefs; EISENSTEIN (1997). For a different perspective of interest in our context, see OGILVIE (2005). For outstanding examples and a summary of the extensive English research on this question, which reflects the closeness of the medical vernacular and medical reform to British religious and political issues of the seventeenth century, see above all WEBSTER (1975) and WEAR (2000), in particular Part 2.

Ortrun Riha and Gundolf Keil have outlined the growth of a language of information that translated and adapted late medieaval and early modern academic medicine into the German vernacular.[11] Their work and that of other mediaevalists suggests that this trend started much earlier than is still generally assumed and antedates by several centuries the turn from Latin by Paracelsus and many of his followers in the sixteenth century.

Briefly, while Latin remained the major European academic language throughout the eighteenth century and beyond, the various technical medical and pharmaceutical texts in the European vernaculars (what may be called *landessprachliche medizinische Fachprosen*) had gained importance at least since the arrival of the printing press in the fifteenth century and go back well into the Middle Ages.[12] By the late seventeenth century, in most Western European cultures (Eastern Europe being an exception until the nineteenth century) vernacular receptures, *Arzneibücher*, tracts, compendia and eventually dispensatories stood side by side with the Latinate pharmacopoias compiled by academic physicians and territorial and municipal authorities. Most still belonged to the various genres established at the end of the Middle Ages and, as pointed out by Riha and others,[13] used or adapted accepted techniques of transcription over the whole range of selective and free adaptation and author attribution. This slow but eventually pervasive development permitted and was driven by the various waves of transmission of classical medical texts in increasingly free translations and compilations of different sources. By the late sixteenth century, the scholastic and humanist canons had been augmented by the texts emanating from the schools of Paracelsus and his followers.

In other words, in contradistinction to much of the periodization of German belles lettres and political literature, the end of the seventeenth century to roughly 1750 might be considered an end point rather than the beginning for vernacular medical publications transmitting Latin sources. The major exception was the continuing prevalence of academic Latin at the universities and in disciplines like the theory of mathematics, natural history and philosophy.[14]

The *Medicina Pensylvania*, standing at the end of this period, is a trenchant example. While at first sight its building blocks may seem heterogeneous and joined without a convincingly stated or obvious theoretical rationale, they

11 RIHA (1992a) and RIHA (1992b), KEIL (1987).

12 Here, the German literature is particularly fruitful if often difficult to access: see for example, RIHA (1992a) and RIHA (1992b), KEIL (1987), TELLE (1979), TELLE (1982), FRIEDRICH & MÜLLER-JAHNKE (2005); also, EAMON (1994), EAMON & KEIL (1987).

13 See in particular RIHA (1992a), 7–18, 23.

14 A helpful general overview is provided by PÖRKSEN (1983), 227–258, who largely concentrates on the period 1500–1800. For very detailed investigations, see also KUHN (1992), wo addresses some of the more recent English language literature, and HABERMANN (2001), who provides a valuable analysis of levels of style in the early modern *Fachsprache*.

contain clearly recognizable, distinct[15] and necessary elements. The deviations in sequence and emphasis from traditional compilations provide a glimpse into the probable priorities of the author or compiler and his intended and multiple audience.

To summarize, the *Medicina Pensylvania* is a large bilingual compendium,[16] apparently written down by a local scribe on the instruction of the author from a large selection of sources and bringing together on roughly 150 facing German-English folios

- a German-only introduction addressed to the reader;
- a trilingual (Latin, German, English) listing of materia medica clearly adapted from standard but unidentified sources, with a few intriguing clinical caveats;
- a lengthy dispensatory with detailed but traditional information on the types and manufacture of medicinal preparations, both simple and complex. This appears to be the most modern of the various building blocks. It corresponds in many ways to the 1753 and 1765 editions of the *New Edinburgh Dispensatory* by William Lewis, although there are a number of differences in both sequence and formulation of recipes from the Lewis scheme;[17]
- a uroscopy tract and portions of a discourse on tartars and spagyric diseases that we have been able to trace to a series of *Drei Tractätlein* by Johann Hayne published first in 1620 and then several times over the seventeenth century.[18] Here, clearly, the German is the *Urtext*, and the English translation and adaptation may well be the author's own (see Shackelford in this volume for a detailed discussion);

15 Again, see RIHA (1992a), on the different ordering of textual building blocks (*Textbausteine*) in these works. More specifically for de Benneville, see WILSON & SAVACOOL (2001).

16 DE BENNEVILLE (2005). For de Benneville, there is a German-English facing page digital version in addition to the English text with a transcription. Except for the excerpts from the Hayne tracts, we are still limited by the lack of a fuller understanding of where the German version preceded the English or vice versa, and if more than one author was involved.

17 We owe the identification of the LEWIS (1753) and LEWIS (1765) Dispensatories as a partial model for the English version to the late David L. Cowen, who identified differences and similarities and additional sources, including the BROOKES (1765) Dispensatory, in a number of private communications. As COWEN (2001) noted, Lewis and other English writers drew on these but also on many other European sources. A full comparison of the English and German versions in the de Benneville compendium and their specific sources is still outstanding and an important research desideratum for the history of North American therapy.

18 Note that the introduction *ad lectorem benevolum*, presented only in German, is drawn from Johann Schröder's introduction in HAYNE (1663). De Benneville omits all learned classical references in Schröder's otherwise identical if longer text. For an early mention of the 1620 printing, see TELLE (1982), unpaginated exhibit from Georg Draudius, Bibliotheca Librorum Germanicorum Classica, Vol. 3, 1625.

- an intervening and large alphabetical glossary of complaints and diseases (with Latin names governing the alphabetization in both German and English) and specific recipes and treatments, to which is attached a traditional section on women and small children. As in the dispensatory, the individual entries by type of complaint contain dosage prescriptions and caveats against certain procedures and substances, such as bleeding and the use of laxatives and a panacea. They appear to complement the dispensatory component and may well have been added to address a more general public.

Throughout, there is no attribution of sources.[19] However, inferences as to which of the two facing versions served as model are relatively easy in the dispensatory section.[20] The progress from medicinal simples to composita follows fairly closely the 1753 and 1765 *New Dispensatory* editions of William Lewis, although buttressed here and there by more direct reliance on major collections like Quincy's 1720 and 1736 edition of the *London Pharmacopoia* and Lewis' 1749 edition of the *Edinburgh Pharmacopoia.*[21] The English version is fluent in most but by no means all cases. Although in terms of content, Lewis like his predecessors and contemporaries on the continent drew from multiple earlier sources, which are often cumbersome and didactic, the particular innovative format used by Lewis is replicated to a good extent in both the German and the English versions of the de Benneville. It is in fact this relatively modern and economical format that points to the Lewis dispensatory as a model and template, indicating in turn a good awareness on the part of the compiler of the *Medicina Pensylvania* of the current state of the art and the expectations of the medical community in the colonies.

The German sources are less easy to pinpoint; at least in terms of chronology, a 1768/1772 German translation, published by Brandt in Hamburg,[22] of the Lewis dispensatory is an unlikely basis of the German text. Among the numerous German candidates, Johann Schröder's *Pharmacopoia physica* and one of the editions of the Augsburg Pharmacopoia with Johann Zwelfer's commentary suggest themselves as likely sources.[23] Again, however, this raises questions of antecedent and origin: Both Schröder and Zwelfer originally wrote in Latin and then were translated into the vernacular in numerous and ever expanding versions. But we found in none of these older sources a parallel to the

19 For the famous publisher Christian Egenolff's practice, see EAMON (1994), chapter 3, 108–12, in particular 110.

20 DE BENNEVILLE (2005), fol. 1–65 [040–169].

21 QUINCY (1720), QUINCY (1736), LEWIS (1749).

22 LEWIS (1768/1772).

23 We have not been able, however, to verify Zwelfer as a direct soure, as suggested by W.-D. Müller-Jahnke (private communication).

very efficient Lewis format – who more or less had poured old wine into new and very serviceable bottles.[24]

Despite the abridged text of the Paracelsian inclusions – the astralis, tartar and uroscopy sections – therefore, de Benneville's pragmatic sense of the needs of North American pharmacists and dispensing physicians seems to have governed his choices – both omissions and inclusions – to a good extent. And it may well be that even the lengthy uroscopy was a more pragmatic inclusion than is readily apparent. According to Benjamin Rush,[25] uroscopy vessels were still to be found in numerous Philadelphia households in the 1760s and possibly beyond, and de Benneville may have wished to provide appropriate instruction in the proper uses of this diagnostic procedure.

By contrast, both precedents for and attributions in the Wagner manuscript – *Remediorum specimina aliquot ex praxi A.W.* – are both less complex in terms of its components and more revealing of its antecedents.[26] This relative ease of classification is in part due to the fact that, at least as it has come over to us after 200 years, the work appears intended for a narrower audience, mainly Wagner's own circle of colleagues and successors. If in fact it was written for eventual circulation or publication, it was left in a far less finished state than the de Benneville manuscript. On the other hand, it suggests an effort to integrate an experience-based account of practice and treatment in a small rural practice with a reservoir of current and traditional recipes that reflects a more traditional format. Also, its component parts are fewer and relatively easy to distinguish, despite subsequent attempts to reorganize and intertwine their sequence.

Briefly, there is (1) a tradititional medical scheme classifying afflictions by site or organ of the body, largely based on the author's own case notes and patient observations, and (2) a substantial compendium of recipes. In both sections, the sources are fully acknowledged, including the author's own preparations; the sequence of the medications is the one used in official pharmacopoias and public and private dispensatories, that is by type of preparation and their use for specific or general conditions. The medical scheme runs in the standard classes, from head to toes, with special classes for women and children and exanthemous diseases of the skin and limbs, including those

24 Among likely sources, Lémery's *Cours de Chymie* offers little to suggest a direct model: LÉMERY (1683). A fuller investigation than has been possible of the sources for Lémery's *Pharmacopée universelle* might offer a more definitive answer: LÉMERY (1697). Some of the similarities might be fortuitous or simply reflect the spirit of the times, such as the disdain of the medical qualities of tinctures of gold. Note however that de Benneville offers about four of them.

25 In his *Inquiry into the Comparative State of Medicine in Philadelphia between the years 1760 and 1766, and the year 1809*, Rush observed: “Great reliance was placed upon the powers of nature, and critical days were expected with solicitude, in order to observe the discharge of the morbid cause of fevers from the system. This matter was looked for chiefly in the urine, and glasses to retain it were a necessary part of the furniture of every sick room.” RUSH (1809), 396.

26 Cf. the observations by John Crellin in this volume.

due to injuries and accidents frequent in a rural practice. Fevers and generalized internal conditions occupy their separate classes, but many of the subheadings under these are left without text – possibly for lack of patients on whose condition observations could be made.

Of specific interest in terms of actual medical practice in the colonies are case stories or clinical notes, often dated by year, with brief descriptions of individual patient complaints and treatments, but also of general afflictions like a 1748 outbreak of pleurisy. Reported treatments include a moderate to modest level of venesection, use of many of the prescriptions listed, most likely prepared by Wagner and his successor, and numerous treatments such as plasters and infusions.[27]

The recipes are multiple, occasionally duplicative, and arranged in classifications employed by *Wundärzte* or surgeons since the Middle Ages but still to be found in Lorenz Heister's famous Chirugia of 1719.[28] The catalogue runs in standard sequence from pills and powders to potions and plasters for exanthema and external conditions, such as burns, frostbite, gangrene, and erysipelas and skin infections of various types. As customary, extemporaneous recipes for potions, pessaries, ointments, plasters and waters, in standard order, are given for a range of disparate conditions. The final page, although bearing the inscription *Finis*, seems not in fact to have been the last page; there is a carry-over "Re…" for which there is no corresponding page.[29] It is followed by a lengthy prayer, in a different hand. We note that this is the only instance of a formal appeal to the Deity throughout the manuscript. The narrative language, as noted, is German throughout. Eighteenth century pharmaceutical notation and Latin nomenclature are used for the recipes, and occasionally Latin technical phrases occur in the text.

It is not apparent from the manuscript why and when author or collator decided to change tack. In other words, despite the fact that the title (*remediorum specimina*) and the beginning and ending sections offer receptures from a very wide range of sources, including famous recipes from the Halle Orphanage, [30] we

27 While the recipes are not parsimonious in ingedients and number, it would require a separate numerical analysis of dosages and use in specific treatments to determine where Wagner stood in terms of 18th century polypharmacy. He does not offer any theoretical suggestions in this respect. This question is taken up briefly by CRELLIN (2006).

28 KEIL (1987), 234; HEISTER (1719). Interestingly, Lorenz Heister becomes an increasingly frequent source for surgical treatments and diagnoses in the latter part of the Wagner manuscript. We do not know from which edition in which language Wagner or his successor worked.

29 WAGNER (2005), fol. 99v.

30 For the multiple references to the Halle recipes, which were supposed to be jealously guarded proprietary secrets, the reader should search the website images and transcription. Also, see CRELLIN (2006). The possible link between the Richter brothers as manufacturers of these medications and Wagner and his Silesian mentors is being investigated by the author and her colleagues. For a brief reference to this connection, see letter 137 in ALAND (1987).

can only infer the purpose for this attempt at intertwining clinical materials from a rural practice with a full *Rezeptarium*. In view of the scarcity of such materials from actual colonial practice, however, we must be grateful for these therapeutic sections, however incomplete, *stichworthaft*, they may be. We may conclude, at least at this stage of our research, that the author intended a practical compendium of clinical histories joined to a *Rezeptarium* that would permit trained practitioners to adapt German practice to a new setting, informed both by traditional knowledge and local observations.

The section concerning birthing and nursing problems and diseases of childhood suggests a practice supervising deliveries, with a large amount of therapeutic suggestions for adverse circumstances.[31]

In summary, we are faced with two medical and pharmaceutical compendia from the North American colonial period conveying clinical and technical knowledge and experience and procedural information. The compendia each address two different audiences – the larger medical and pharmaceutical community of providers in Philadelphia and its outlying areas, and the smaller group of medical providers centering on the Schwenkfeld settlements to the northeast of Philadelphia. Despite their formal and structural differences, both manuscripts draw on comparable and traditional fonts of knowledge. While the nomenclature and technical notation is still oriented to medical Latin, with the Paracelsian exceptions noted, in the bilingual text by de Benneville in particular, the emphasis is not on the use of the vernacular to make a Latin text comprehensible to a lay audience. Instead, the choice of parallel English and German narratives appears to have been intended to bridge a true gap in understanding and professional communication between practitioners working in two living languages.

The Language of Medical Discourse in a Bilingual Medical Market: Eighteenth-Century North America

In the preceding, I have tried to trace generic and classificatory patterns of two medical compendia written or collated in North America at the end of the early modern period. In part, these well established European patterns represented the transition from Latin to the national vernaculars, driven by market forces and the developing hierarchy of medical providers during the early modern period.[32] There is little doubt that many North American practitioners, with or without academic qualifications and including our dissident friends Wagner and de Benneville, were sufficiently fluent in Latin to read original sources as well as translations. These practitioners would have included the many clerics of the

31 WAGNER (2005), fol. 37r–44v: "*Die 8. Classe, von denen besonderen weiblichen Kranckheiten.*"

32 For a cogent and definitive description of these changes in England, see COOK (1986) and COOK (1996).

established churches, whether Anglican, Lutheran, or Presbyterian, who practiced medicine up and down the coast of the 13 colonies. On the other hand, these and the small class of largely Southern landed gentry and the graduates of Harvard University represented a small market niche. North America did not have – and apparently did not seem to need until well into the modern period – a reservoir of reasonably learned civil servants at the levels of provincial and municipal authority – the cadres of early modern bureaucracy and diplomacy in Europe, who wrote in Latin, if poorly, until well into the eighteenth century.

We should ask, then, if there was any room left in the British North American colonies for the one quality that had set Latin apart from the European vernaculars of the early modern period – access by all educated men and women to the lingua franca of natural science and philosophy.[33] But even in Europe, medical authors and their publishers moved freely back and forth between the languages by mid eighteenth century at the latest. Heister's *Chirurgia*, for instance, was a 1740 translation from German into Latin;[34] Caspar Neumann's chemical works, as noted by William Lewis in his 1759 translation,[35] were bilingual, depending on the context and the audience. Lewis himself, in his 1744 *Pharmacopoiea Reformata*,[36] is a perfect example of this mixture, with all recipes in Latin and all narrative in English.

By the late eighteenth century, the therapeutic discourse in the United Kingdom had largely left Latinity behind. Thus, Andrew Duncan Sr., the famous Edinburgh physician, in 1783 used an unpublished English translation by William Lewis to disseminate "the practical part of Frederick Hoffmann's medicina rationalis systematica" as an invaluable tool, despite its tendency to polypharmacy:

> Their [the works of Fr. Hoffmann] voluminous size, joined to the circumstance of their being written in the Latin language, they have been less extensively useful in Britain than might have been otherwise the case.[37]

The growing German pharmaceutical discursive literature, including its journals,[38] had by now fully turned to the vernacular. On the other hand, as shown elsewhere,[39] many of the scholarly books that the German North

33 See on this, among others, PÖRKSEN (1983), 244–245.

34 HEISTER (1740).

35 NEUMANN (1759). I quote from the Lewis preface: "The works published by Neumann himself consist chiefly of dissertations on particular subjects; some in Latin and inserted into the transactions of different societies and academies [...] others in the German and printed separately."

36 LEWIS (1744).

37 This statement is attributed to his father by A. Duncan, Jr. in the preface to the 1805 edition of the New Dispensatory: DUNCAN (1805). Note, that Duncan addresses practical therapeutics, not theory.

38 For a valuable overview, see FRIEDRICH & MÜLLER-JAHNKE (2005), 545–570. For a case study from the latter part of the eighteenth century, see SEILS (1995), 144–152, and the sources and contributors to the *Journal der Physik* cited there.

39 WILSON (2000) and WILSON (2008).

American market ordered through Halle Pietist sources were both in the original Latin and in German translations, suggesting a period where both publishers and a traditional public remained in transition.

More specifically, then, we should ask what governed the choices of the language of medical discourse in North America, a society with different culturally and socially defined medical markets? Who determined which books in what language would be either imported or printed in a country where printing resources – fonts and presses – were scarce, shipping costs large, and demand diffuse and limited? It may be safe to say that in an era of printing abundance in Europe, few important classical or early modern medical texts had remained untranslated.[40] But in North America, who were the agents whose choices determined which version would be imported, whether brought over as part of the libraries of medical practitioners, or promoted by the publishers in Boston and Philadelphia before the Revolution?[41]

For the medical literature accessible to and imported by the German educated lay readership prior to roughly 1815, the standard and magisterial work by Robert Cazden can now be updated by more detailed findings.[42] The Francke Orphanage Institutions, which were heavily invested in the book and bible trade, furnished their North American clerics and customers, through privileged English channels before the Revolutionary War and later through Holland and Hamburg, with a wide range of learned works in both Latin and German. As early as the 1750s, there are titles suggesting learned and utilitarian inclinations among a necessarily small but likely influential group among the reading public, regardless of cost. One early example in the medical field is Johann Jacob Schmidt's *Bibl. historicum, geographicum, physicum, metem, et medicum* (sic), a well known, expensive and learned five volume work relating physics, geography, medicine, mathematics and history to the scriptures that grew out of the Protestant attempt to retain the primacy of Christian religion in the evolving natural sciences.[43] Another order for two sets came in 1756[44] and orders resumed after

40 For Scotland and in particular Edinburgh, the signal tower for American practitioners of medicine, see the list of primary sources used by RISSE (2005), where even the Latin works by the Edinburgh greats were all available in translation.

41 The most recent full treatments of this subject are by AMORY & HALL (2000), who largely omit technical and medical literature, and, for the middle colonies, GREEN (2000). Amory points out that not only North American printers were considered unwelcome competitors the metropolitan printing establishment, but also their closer and Anglophone cousins, the Irish and Scots: AMORY (2000), 31.

42 CAZDEN (1984). Cazden as well does not address technical and medical literature as their own genres. For the period of interest here, see chapter 1, and his insightful summary. For more recent and specific findings for German printers and imprints in the period before and after the Revolution, see ROEBER (2000), WILSON (2000), and WILSON (2008), from which I have drawn material in the following.

43 AFSt/M 4G6 fol. 79, 28 August 1753. The German title is "*Biblischer Medicus* ...," "*Biblischer Historicus* ...", "*Biblischer Physicus* ...", etc. See also DEHMEL (1996).

44 AFSt/M 4G6, 1756, fol. 113–114, Lit A.

the Revolutionary War. By the end of the 1750s, a Halle vicar in Philadelphia had ordered all parts of Ernsting's *Nucleus Totius Medicinae Quinque Partes*, a large pharmaceutical dispensatory, requested by "a member of the congregation."[45] Several orders for Lorenz v. Mosheim's multivolume and costly *History of the Church* also date to this period. In the 1790s, the scholarly scion of the Lutheran Pietist Mühlenberg family, Gotthilf Heinrich Ernst Mühlenberg and his medical and botanical colleagues, including Kasper Wistar, William Bartram, and Adam Kuhn, concentrated on the new branches of natural investigation, above all the immense transatlantic, still largely Latinate scholarly exchange of post-Linnean classificatory schemes that attempted to integrate American into European botany.[46] Learned books also went to the burgeoning community of Moravian travellers in the sciences and medicine.

Additionally, there were orders for both Latin and the progressively vernacular *Fachliteratur* from the Erlangen publisher Palm, including 60 copies each of 1787 Johann David Schöpf's treatise on minerals *(Beiträge zur Mineralogischen Kenntnis des Östlichen Theils von Nord-Amerika und seiner Gebürge*), his *Materia medica Americana*, and his 1788 travels through North America. An order of 25 copies covered an unidentified treatise on opium (*vom Mohnsaft*), and several titles by the medical reformer Wilhelm Hufnagel. In terms of language, a mixed lot indeed.

George de Benneville, a presumably trilingual physician with a profound knowledge of the botanical and chemiatric manufactures of the time, had probably understood the needs of this market and of his most immediate audience, that is, druggists, pharmacists, and prescribing physicians. He responded to the needs of the pharmacy business by a carefully scripted bilingual (but not French) dispensatory, accessible to the trade and still oriented to Latin nomenclature for cross reference. Producing a Latin version would not have been user friendly in this environment. Instead, he fell back on the continuous translation and retranslation of dispensatories, tracts, and similar genres throughout the early modern period, offering two equally valid vernacular versions derived from analogous models in the pharmaceutical lingua franca of the eighteenth century, with Latin nomenclature, reflecting a long tradition of equivalent vernacular use.

45 AFSt/M 4G6 1744–60, fol. 5, no date. Handschuh listed the work with all part titles and provided the following information in a not uncommon mixture of German and Latin: "pars 1 continent lexicon et dispensatorium oder vollkommenen und allzeit fertiger Apotheker, etc., darinnen alle und jede Stücke so wirklich in den Apotheken zu finden ihrer Gestalt und Gehalt, Herkunft etc auch was daraus zu machen ist, und wird die Composita auf das beste daraus zu bereiten erklart worden sind dabey auch nach dem Alphabet die Kunstworter und viele andere Namen mehr folgen. [...] Helmstedt, 1741," sold at Braunschweig and Leipzig in the Meisser bookstore.

46 This material is from WILSON (2008). G. H. E. Mühlenberg's large correspondence with European and North American botanists is now being edited by the present author and her colleagues.

As noted, we have not at this point been able to determine the specific source for his therapeutic pescriptions offered in the glossary of diseases and their treatments and for specific prenatal, perinatal and postnatal symptoms and procedures, which include instructions to the midwife for birthing assistance.[47] Their source is not apparent and their linguistic origin, with titles and thus alphabetical order again organized by Latin nomenclature, is not readily apparent. They may well not come from one source but have been be collated from several sources, inluding possibly the author's own case notes.[48] In other respects, however, and as noted previously, a specific word and line comparison would be required for a fuller assessment.

As collated, the prescriptions in this section prominently include chemiatric medicinals (most recipes start in fact with the admonition to take "panacea" in addition to a laxative), which would date their version in the de Benneville glossary to the seventeenth century. They integrate these, however, with the full panoply of botanical materia medica and time-honored warnings and admonishments, such as for the traditional restrictions on phlebotomy by age and on the use of panacea (in de Benneville's case probably an antimony preparation) and strong laxatives in debilitated patients. Overall, the therapies mix galenic and chemiatric prescriptions, as customary in both German and English *Arzneibücher* and receptures of the late early modern period.

Evidence of actual eighteenth century practice can be found in the trilingual inventory of *materia medica* at the beginning of the manuscript[49] where concern for patient safety in terms of precise dosages for anodynes, purges and emetics breaches the three-column format; for reasons not obvious to this author, the vomits and purges are in English, and the anodynes in German (see Figure 1 on next page).

For the Wagner compendium, changes in nomenclature apparently added later to the manuscript suggest an increasing distance of American rural practice from Latin sources, such as the addition of German indications for specific remedies (*Ohren Schmertzen, vor die lauffende Gicht*) to the Latin names[50] and the occasional introduction of English measures, such as gill and pint in the section on infusions and decoctions.[51] This supports the assumption that the manuscript was eventually used by a successor or successors no longer easily familiar with Latin terminology.

It should be clear from the foregoing that neither the *Medicina Pensylvania* nor the Wagner observations and recipes were intended as lay self-help texts on the model of *The Poor Planters Physician* by John Tennent (1734), a German

47 See DE BENNEVILLE (2005), fol. 66–132 [170–303].

48 I thank Michael Stolberg for this suggestion.

49 DE BENNEVILLE (2005), [015–037] (unnumbered fols.).

50 WAGNER (2005), fol. 81v, 83r.

51 WAGNER (2005), fol. 88r; see also 25v, 63r, 96v.

Vomits, The Doses	Grains:
Crocus Metallorum, dose	3
Mercurius Vitæ	3
Tartarum Emeticum	6
Turpetum Minerale	6
Vitriolum Album	15
Vitrificatum Antimonium	6
Gummi Gutta	15
Panacæa Antimonii	12

Purgers, The Doses	Grains:
Manna, dose from 1 to 4 Ounces	
Aloe Socotrina	30
Rhabarbarum in Substance	30
Senna in Substance	30
Scammonium in Substance	16
Jalapium in Substance	30
Resina Jalapii	16
Helleborus Niger	15
Mercurius Dulcis	20
Colocynthis	10

Them that purges or vomits must be kept warm and from sleeping. And so often it works, drink Flax Seeds tea upon it. If it works too strong, drink Sweet Oil or a little spirit.

Anodyna **Pulvis**	Grains:
Opium Cydoniatum dose	1
Laudanum Opiatum, dose	2
Laudanum Hystericum dose	3
Pulvis Anodynus dose	5
Crocus Substant[ia] dose	20
Sem[ina] Papaver dose	20

Schmertz stillend Mitteln **Gutta**	Drops:
Tinctura Opicydon[iatum] dose	8 to 15
Tinctura Crocii dose	20 to 30
Laudanum Hystericum dose	20 to 30
Theriaca Anodyna dose	20 to 30
Balsamum Anodynum dose	20 to 30

To Ease Pains

Die Schmertz stillend Artzeney müßen mit Vorsichtigkeit gebrauchet werden. Man muß nicht über die Dosis schreitten vornemlich die Dropfen von 8 biß 15 oder von 20 Dropfen biß 30 in schwachen Thee oder in den Dranck

Figure 1: Considerations of safety and appropriateness of dosages: Instructions on the use of anodynes, purges and emetics in colonial Philadelphia, DE BENNEVILLE (2005), [031] and [032] (unnumbered fols.)

translation of which was also published for the growing German-language medical market by Benjamin Franklin in 1736.[52]

On the other hand, as for other early modern medical genres, the distinction between self-help texts for male and above all female heads of households that are part of the early modern *Hausväterliteratur* (the economiae or husbandry texts) on the one hand and those intended for the rural and eventually the colonial practitioner was never quite as clear cut as this terminology implies. In the case of our compendia, the assumed date for completion of the de Benneville manuscript (1770) might well indicate the intent to tap the demand for the manuals of medical advice by William Buchan (published in Philadelphia in 1774) and S.A. Tissot (an English translation was published in Philadelphia in 1771), which dominated the medical self-help market in North America until the 1790s, when homegrown texts began to emerge.[53] The work by Tissot (originally published in French) was current in British North America in both English and German versions, having grown from earlier traditions of *Arzneibüchlein* which attempted to offer simple and relatively inexpensive versions of standard recipes. In fact, when charged with providing a manual of medical instructions for their mission settlements, the Moravian physicians at the Barby center in Germany reported that most of their practitioners were working from the Tissot manual, and considered an earlier and more elaborate text, the *Kurze und deutliche Unterricht* by Christian Friedrich Richter, as too complex for local settings.[54] None of the medical men at Barby even mentioned the early modern manuals of instruction by both male and female authors, which not only addressed a female audience of consumers but presupposed considerable expertise and equipment for the preparation of medicinals from both the traditional materia medica and chemiatric components. In the abundant self-help literature of late eighteenth century North America, the female experimenter had given way to the female head of household as an intermediary between physician and patient.[55]

Medical Dissidence, Medical Theory, and the Religion of the Physician

In concluding this discussion of the choices made by German-language physicians in communicating their medical knowledge and traditions to their North American colleagues and successors in practice, I will briefly raise the question of the relationship between religious and medical dissidence. In other

52 TENNENT (1734). The translation did not find much of an audience because it was set in Roman type.

53 BUCHAN (1774), TISSOT (1771). For a recent discussion of English self-help texts, see ROSENBERG (2003), in particular the contribution by HORROCKS (2003).

54 See for this WILSON (2007).

55 For North America, see MURPHY (1991). The more general omission of female pharmaceutical practice outside midwifery and its relegation to the *Hausväterliteratur* (the *oeconomia*) is only slowly being addressed from what are in fact quite abundant sources. See SZASZ (2004); FISSELL & COOTER (2003).

words, what was the place and reception of unorthodox views in religion and medicine in the North American colonial environment?

American medical historiography has without much hesitation merged the two for the German sects which came over. This is in contrast to the large and sophisticated English literature on the complementarity of medical dissidence and *religio medici* (the religion of the physician) for the period between roughly 1550 and 1690.[56]

For Wagner and de Benneville, who grew up and practiced in the eighteenth century, we can proceed from a few givens: Both were from dissident *religious* communities which had been segregated from the governing academies and their orthodoxies, whether Roman Catholic, Lutheran, or Calvinist-Reformed. In Germany at least, these dissident communities remained outside the academic discourse and realities of power. *Medical dissidence*, however, in terms of the controversy between the followers of Galen and Paracelsus, often flourished under the patronage systems of territorial princes and Imperial counts, and in several cases established its own centers of academic learning.[57] In contrast to the seventeenth century, in particular in the United Kingdom, there was no pervasive juncture in the politically fractured Germanies between the path to the godly state and the reform of medical theory and practice, despite the roots of these reforms in the utopian central European movements of men like Comenius and Andreae.[58]

While de Benneville's medical training remains a matter of speculation,[59] he is known to have corresponded with the radical Pietist Gerhard Tersteegen and belonged to the radical circles, medical and otherwise, around the Pietist physician Samuel Carl at the Wittgenstein court and the refuge of the Marquis de Marsay in the Wetterau.[60] In North America, he seems to have made sure that he remained outside the purview of the Philadelphia fashionable and medical elite but accumulated considerable assets and established a family of some standing in the community. In general he seems to have worn the mantle of Nicodemism decried by August Hermann Francke.[61] His careful, traditional and eclectic

56 For wide ranging discussions, and a full survey of the literature on this topic, see WEAR (2000); FRENCH & WEAR (1989), in particular the contributions by Peter Elmer and Andrew Cunningham: ELMER (1989), CUNNINGHAM (1989); GRELL & CUNINNGHAM (1996), in particular chapter 1, and WEBSTER (1975).

57 MORAN (1990), MORAN (1991).

58 For the meeting of these medical and social utopias in England, see WEBSTER (1975). COOK (1996) is one of the few to argue against the omnipresence of this juncture, at least for the Royal College of Physicians. For the medico-philosophical debates, see most recently SHACKELFORD (2004).

59 WILSON & SAVACOOL (2001); see also DE BENNEVILLE (2005), introductory text: *About the Medicina Pensylvania and George de Benneville.*

60 For the German and transatlantic context of radical spiritualist writers whom de Benneville and the Sauer family apparently frequented, see SCHRADER (1989).

61 FRANCKE (1707a), FRANCKE (1707b), FRANCKE (1744). Cunningham suggests a similar attitude for Sydenham: CUNNINGHAM (1989).

therapeutic practice is reflected in the many different dosages and vehicles of ingestion such as herbal teas in his recipes, both in the dispensatory section and in the glossary of diseases and treatments.[62] Whether the inclusion of the uroscopy materials was to put a venerable if dying practice on what for him was still a sound traditional and theoretical footing is open to question until we know more about the persistence of this practice than the retrospective observation by Benjamin Rush.[63]

De Benneville clearly was not much interested in the newer theories of medicine and physiology, whether these came from the Germany of Friedrich Hoffmann and Georg Ernst Stahl or from England or France. His polypharmacy would have displeased the reform-minded physician of the latter part of the eighteenth century, but as Andrew Duncan noted, the traditional treasures of seventeenth century pharmacy were not easily discarded in view of the lack of acceptable alternatives.

This is in some contrast to Wagner, whose lineage is much more transparent. His sources for his courses of treatment even more than the extemporaneous recipes include a clear selection from the post-medieval chymiatric medical canon, proceeding over several centuries: Robert Boyle and Johann Joachim Becher are mentioned once each, Otto Tachenius and Adrian Mynsicht have roughly 5 mentions each of their standard eponymous preparations. Other references go back as far as Johann Agricola (d. 1580), David Ludovicus, (d. 1680), Franciscus Josephus Burrhus, whose balsam is cited several times as *Balsam Burrhi* (Balsam of Burrhus), and François de la Boë (Sylvius). These may all be references, however, cited mainly to validate the author's knowledge.

In terms of practice, Wagner rarely mentions Georg Ernst Stahl's theories of medicine, but, as noted by John Crellin, they are ever present in the courses of treatment described, as are those of Stahl's teacher Georg Wolfgang Wedel in Jena.[64] Beyond the seventeenth century and its medical dissenting traditions, Stahl's students Johann Samuel Carl (1677–1757) and Johann Juncker (1679–1759) appear with only a few preparations, although as noted the plentiful references to the Halle Orphanage medications suggest previous and possibly current contacts with the Orphanage in Halle. In the latter part of the Wagner manuscript, practical sources predominate, with multiple references to Lorenz Heister's *Chirurgia*[65] and to the chemist Caspar Neumann. There is little theory, then, contemporary or arcane, nor much in the way of religion. Wagner makes

62 CRELLIN (1997) remarks on the numerous teas suggested, among which fennel is conspicuous.

63 See note 24 above.

64 It is possible that many of the Stahl recipes in fact were copied from Gottfried Rothe's introduction to chemistry: ROTHE (1727). Rothe's book appeared in numerous editions from 1719 to the 1750s, including an English translation in 1749. According to KRAFFT (2002), 161, Rothe was a student of Stahl and his work was representative of the Stahlian tradition.

65 Apparently a desk copy of one of the multiple German editions.

only one explicit reference to Friedrich Hoffmann,[66] and none to Hermann Boerhave or, for that matter, the classic authors, nor to van Helmont or to Paracelsus.

The second possible confluence of religious and medical dissidence might be found in the author's own preparations and those of his Silesian mentors: George Hauptman Medicus, who was the author's grandfather or great grandfather; Martin John the Younger, a famous religious dissident and defender of the rights of the Schwenkfelders at the court of Vienna; and Melchior Hübner (Heebner), who emigrated to America in 1727 after period of residence in Görlitz and became Wagner`s mentor. By the time of the last Schwenkfelder emigration in the 1720s, Silesia was poor and exhausted after a century of religious warfare. But it had been a flourishing territory until the first decades of the seventeenth century. How and in which medical framework did Wagner's mentors practice? We still know little of the rules and regulations of their practice, since Silesia as an Habsburg *Erbland* lay outside the legal structures of the Empire.

Martin John the Younger is known to have travelled widely in Europe and to have visited spiritualists like Johann Georg Gichtel in Holland and even Philipp Jakob Spener in Frankfurt. An antiheretical Latin tract[67] described Martin John as a self-professed physicus and in particular a provider of botanicals. According to an anonymous source, he and George Hauptmann were able to travel because of their income from their cures.[68] We do not know the nature of these *Curen,* how they were provided and who paid for them, or whether they were even part of a commercial manufacture. It remains to be shown if and how aspects of this Silesian trade were similar to that described by Peickert as far back as 1932 and more recently by Bernschneider-Reif.[69]

Specifically, among the providers of medicines outside the German medical hierarchy were a large number of *Olitätenhändler* and *Laboranten* (oil men and chymists) who worked in the impoverished areas of Thuringia and the Erzgebirge.[70] This medical fringe, to use the term famously coined by William

66 Wagner (2005), fol. 20r.

67 Our attention was drawn to this quote by WEIGELT (1973), notes 173–176, 222. See LIEFMANN (1698), B iv: v: "Medicinam profitebatur ac Botanices imprimis."

68 "[...] (ihrer) Honorare [...] da Martin John mit seinen Curen sehr glücklich und hin und wieder bekannt geworden." WEIGELT (1973), 225.

69 PEICKERT (1932). For recent research conducted at the Institute for the History of Pharmacy at the University of Marburg, see BERNSCHNEIDER-REIF (2004), 157–161, whose valuable work is paraphrased here. The geographic scope of her work is concentrated on Thuringia, thus excluding both the Erzgebirge and neighboring Silesia, but my reading of the sources in the Francke Archives that she quotes clearly indicate a wider geographical scope. See WILSON (2000), chapter 3.

70 For their presence in a more fully integrated medical system in the Duchy of Braunschweig-Wolfenbüttel, a more prosperous area a little further to the west, see LINDEMANN (2000). According to her sources, even here peddlers and oil men (*Olitätenhändler*) were well known, particularly on the eastern borders of the duchy. LINDEMANN (2000), 162–163.

Bynum and Roy Porter,[71] included both small manufacturers and itinerant peddlers who were indispensable providers of medicines to the rural populations in poorly served areas. They offered both botanicals and a number of chemical preparations produced in their laboratories, which until the eighteenth century appear to have been not all that different from more conventionally manufactured medications. But these people, although doubtless medical irregulars, may or may not have belonged to pockets of religious dissidence, and their manufactures and practices may well have been local phenomena. In other words, their transgression of the boundaries of medical hierarchies was an economic phenomenon by men and women likely to have been oblivious of the theoretical and religious disputes of early modern medicine.

Summary

By the middle of the eighteenth century, the question of medical dissidence in Paracelsian-Helmontian terms had become moot in terms of any causal relationship with religious dissidence. The debate had assumed Enlightenment overtones and if anything, medical disidents were the ones whose theories were now based on tradition rather than reform.[72] In our case, we may wish to reformulate the question by examining the relationship between theory and therapeutic practice in a rural environment where practitioners were remote from academic discourse.[73]

Both de Benneville and Wagner accommodated their medical existence to – and prospered in – a welter of sectarian communities freed from European constraints. There was, with some exceptions, a nonhierarchical medical environment where academic vanities, so distasteful to most spiritualist practitioners, could be easily avoided but where the manufacture and therapeutic recommendation of complex and simple preparations seem to have been profitable assets. De Benneville married into an established Huguenot family in the Philadelphia region, the Bertholets, soon after his arrival and was the progenitor of a socially and economically well established clan which produced several physicians, first his son George, and extending to a surgeon serving during the Civil War. Wagner married but had no children. For his practice and that of his successors in particular, the transition in rural North American practice to a physician-poor and eclectic environment is another research desideratum.[74]

Their relations with the colonial medical establishment, largely its German contingent in the area north of Philadelphia, suggest a preference for the

71 Bynum & Porter (1987); Porter (1988), 1–26.

72 Physicotheology being one example. See for this Krafft (1999) and Ogilvie (2005).

73 For early 19th century debates in the United States, see Vogel & Rosenberg (1979) and Rosenberg & Golden (1992).

74 See, most recently, Berman & Flannery (2001).

traditions of their mentors but easy interaction with other practitioners.[75] Wagner's notes include a recipe from George de Benneville, one by a neighboring Moravian physician from Bethlehem, Johann Adolph Meyer, and a reference to Isaac and Moses Bartram, apothecaries from the famous family of botanists and naturalists in Philadelphia.[76] On the other hand, there is the disapproving mention, common among Central European practitioners in colonial North America, of excessive bloodletting by their English or Scottish colleagues.[77]

In all, on the evidence of their manuscripts and despite obvious and large differences in therapeutic approach, both authors worked within the parameters of mid-century eighteenth century practice. But in view of what we know of the open boundaries of this practice, particularly in a non-hierarchical setting, it would be begging the question to argue that the sources in the manuscripts of either de Benneville or Wagner unequivocally linked them to the alchemical and hermetic heritage described by Jon Butler for New England and Robert E. Cazden for the German printers in North America.[78] There is little to indicate a specifically spiritualist or religious provenance for Wagner's remedies or for his sources, nor is this obvious for the Paracelsian inclusions by de Benneville.

On the other hand, there is little doubt of the full and continuing dedication of our authors to their religious beliefs. Christa Habrich describes a similar intensely emotional and compassionate attitude for de Benneville's occasional correspondent, the spiritualist and medical practitioner Gerhard Tersteegen, but she comes to similar conclusions about the medical and therapeutic framework of his practice. Tersteegen's major medical sources were the popular writings of Johann Samuel Carl rather than the "[...] *theosophisch-alchimistische Anthropologie, vita animalis et morbis medicina* [...]" of Johann Conrad Dippel, which had been translated into German in 1736.[79]

75 This interaction, despite the possible emergence of enlightenment chauvinism, reflected the reception of German and Austrian medical thought in Edinburgh. See for an example of Cullen's influence on Benjamin Smith Barton, EWAN & EWAN (2007).

76 See WAGNER (2005), fol. 63r for de Benneville, and fol. 78v for the Bartrams, and fol. 16v for an otherwise unidentified English Dispensatory. For Meyer, see MEIER (1976).

77 For the seventeenth century English debate on this practice, see again WEAR (2000), in particular 378–387. However, neither de Benneville nor Wagner ruled out phlebotomy. For another colonial voice, this time from a student of Johann Juncker, see WILSON (1993) and JONES & WILSON (1995), introduction.

78 CAZDEN (1984), chapter 1, in particular 18–21, which summarizes the works on magic and alchemy discussed by BUTLER (1979), and Seidensticker in ARNDT & ECK (1989). For the tradition of the works advertised by the Lancaster publisher Reinhold, see EAMON (1994), chapter 4. We leave it to further research to determine the antecedents and significance of the alchemical manuscripts left by de Benneville in the Schwenkfelder archives, as described by Jole Shackelford in this volume.

79 HABRICH (1997), 169. For some of the rare personal testimonials to de Benneville as a spiritual healer and practitioner of medicine, see Allen Viehmeyer in this volume.

Thus, the medical texts discussed in this paper present themselves to the reader not so much as part of a dissident medical tradition but, at their different levels, reflect the web of manifold and interacting European transmissions of therapeutic knowledge into North America. If our writers seem impervious to developments in the numerous theoretical debates of the century, this may well be a reflection of their personal lifecourse. Wagner had died in 1763, and de Benneville was almost 70 years of age when the *Medicina Pensylvania* was assembled, if we are to accept the dating of the manuscript to 1770. The authors' therapeutic preferences sought to integrate their continental European antecedents into North American practice. For this, they adopted the bilinguality of their new environment, which was lateral – English and German – instead of hierarchical, as in Europe – from Latin into the vernacular. Absent the dicta of academic settings, they wrote for their bilingual medical markets. They relied on longstanding precedents in the assembly and dissemination of therapeutic information in the vernacular, and on the continuous exchange, across European national and linguistic boundaries, of pharmaceutical knowledge and tradition that had in turn been driven by the medical markets of the early modern period and its print culture.

Unpublished Sources and References

Archiv der Franckeschen Stiftungen zu Halle / Missionsarchiv (AFSt/M)
AFSt/M 4G6 1744–60
AFSt/M 4G6, 1756 Lit A
AFSt/M 4G6

Aland (1987)
Aland, Kurt (Ed.): Die Korrespondenz Heinrich Melchior Mühlenbergs. Aus der Anfangszeit des deutschen Luthertums in Nordamerika, Vol. 2: 1753–1762. Berlin, New York: de Gruyter, 1987.

Amory (2000)
Amory, Hugh: Reinventing the Colonial Book. In: Amory, Hugh; Hall, David D. (Eds.): A History of the Book in America, Vol. 1: The Colonial Book in the Atlantic World. Cambridge: Cambridge University Press, 2000, 26-54.

Amory & Hall (2000)
Amory, Hugh; Hall, David D. (Eds.): A History of the Book in America, Vol. 1: The Colonial Book in the Atlantic World. Cambridge: Cambridge University Press, 2000.

Arndt & Eck (1989)
Arndt, K. J. R.; Eck, Reimer C. (Eds.): The First Century of German Language Printing in the United States of America. A Bibliography Based on the Studies of Oswald Seidensticker and Wilbur H. Oda. Göttingen: Niedersächsische Staats-und Universitätsbibliothek, 1989.

Baird (2003)
Baird, Eleanora Gordon: Moses Bartram's Account Book, 1778–1788. Notes made by a Philadelphia Apothecary. Bartram Broadside, Spring 2003.

de Benneville (2005)
de Benneville, George: Medicina Pensylvania Or The Pensylvania Physician. In: Eighteenth-century Colonial Formularies. The Manuscripts of George de Benneville and Abraham Wagner. The College of Physicians of Philadelphia Digital Library.
Recent website address (access date: June 23, 2008): http://www.accesspadr.org/cpp/.

Bernschneider-Reif (2004)
Bernschneider-Reif, Sabine: Das Laienpharmazeutische Olitätenwesen im Thüringer Wald – (adelige) Frauen als Laboranten und ihre Rezeptbücher. In Wahrig, Bettina (Ed.): Arzneien für das "schöne Geschlecht". Geschlechterverhältnisse in Phytotherapie und Pharmazie vom Mittelalter bis zum 19. Jahrhundert. Stuttgart: Deutscher Apotheker Verlag, 2004, 151–168.

Berman & Flannery (2001)
Berman Alex; Flannery, Michael A.: America´s Botanico-medical Movements. Vox populi. New York: Pharmaceutical Products Press, 2001.

Brookes (1765)
Brookes, Richard: The General Dispensatory. Containing a Translation of the Pharmacopoeias of the Royal Colleges of Physicians of London and Edinburgh, together with that of the Royal

Hospital of Edinburgh [...] (2nd edition, with large additions). London: Printed for J. Newbery, in St. Paul's Church-yard, and R. Baldwin, in Pater-noster Row, 1765.

Buchan (1774)
Buchan, William: Domestic Medicine; or, The Family Physician. Philadelphia: Crukshank, 1774.

Butler (1979)
Butler, John: Magic, Astrology, and the Early American Religious Heritage, 1600-1760. The American Historical Review 84 (1979), 326–328.

Bynum & Porter (1987)
Bynum, William; Porter, Roy: Medical Fringe and Medical Orthodoxy. London: Wellcome Institute for the History of Medicine, 1987.

Cazden (1984)
Cazden, Robert E.: A Social History of the German Book Trade in America to the Civil War Columbia, SC: Camden House, 1984.

Cook (1986)
Cook, Harold J.: Decline of the Old Medical Regime in Stuart London. Ithaca: Cornell University Press, 1986.

Cook (1996)
Cook, Harold J.: Institutional Structures and Personal Belief in the London College of Physicians. In: Grell, Ole Peter; Cunningham, Andrew (Eds.): Religio Medici. Medicine and Religion in Seventeenth-Century England. Aldershot, UK: Scholar Press, 1996, 91–114.

Cowen (1985)
Cowen, David L.: "Zum Dienst des gemeinen Mannes, insonderheit für die Landleute." The Domestic and Veterinary Medicine Books Printed in Colonial North America and the United States in the German Language. In: Orbis Pictus. Kultur- und pharmaziehistorische Studien. Festschrift für Wolfgang-Hagen Hein zum 65. Geburtstag. Frankfurt/Main: Govi-Verlag, 1985, 43–66.

Cowen (2001)
Cowen, David L.: Pharmacopoeias and Related Literature in Britain and America, 1618–1847. Aldershot, UK: Ashgate Publishing, 2001.

Cowen & Wilson (1997)
Cowen, David L.; Wilson, Renate: The Traffic in Medical Ideas. Popular Medical Texts as German Imports and American Imprints. In: Caduceus. Vol. 13, 1 (Spring 1997, special issue: Eighteenth Century Traffic in Medicines and Medical Ideas), 67–80.

Crellin (1997)
Crellin, John K.: How Shall I Take My Medicine? Dosages and Other Matters in Eighteenth-Century Medicine. In: Caduceus. Vol. 13, 1 (Spring 1997, special issue: Eighteenth Century Traffic in Medicines and Medical Ideas), 39–50.

Crellin (2006)
Crellin, John K.: Theory and Clinical Experience in Eighteenth-Century Extemporaneous Prescriptions – a Reciprocal Relationship? In: Pharmacy in History 48 (2006), 3–13.

Cullen (1784)
Cullen, William: First Lines of the Practice of Physic. For the Use of Students in the University of Edinburgh. Vol. I. Edinburgh and London: Elliot, 1784.

Cunningham (1989)
Cunningham, Andrew: Thomas Sydenham. Epidemics, Experiment and "The Good Old Cause." In: French, Roger K.; Wear, Andrew (Eds.): The Medical Revolution of the Seventeenth Century. Cambridge: Cambridge University Press, 1989, 164–190.

Dehmel (1996)
Dehmel, Gisela: Die Arzneimittel in der Physikotheologie. Münster: Lit Verlag, 1996.

Duncan (1805)
Duncan, Andrew, Jr.: The Edinburgh New Dispensatory. […] Worcester, Mass.: Isaiah Thomas, Jr., 1805.

Eamon (1994)
Eamon, William: Science and the Secrets of Nature. Princeton: Princeton University Press, 1994.

Eamon & Keil (1987)
Eamon, William; Keil, Gundolf: 'Plebs amat empirica.' Nicolas of Poland and His Critique of the Medieval Medical Establishment. In: Sudhoffs Archiv 71 (1987), 180–196.

Eisenstein (1997)
Eisenstein, Elisabeth: The Printing Press as an Agent of Change. Communications and Cultural Transformations in Early-modern Europe. 2 vols. Cambridge [u.a.]: Cambridge University Press, 1997.

Elmer (1989)
Elmer, Peter: Medicine, Religion and the Puritan Revolution. In: French, Roger K.; Wear, Andrew (Eds.): The Medical Revolution of the Seventeenth Century. Cambridge: Cambridge University Press, 1989, 10–45.

Ewan & Ewan (2007)
Ewan, Joseph; Ewan, Nesta Dunn: Benjamin Smith Barton. Naturalist and Physician in Jeffersonian America. St. Louis: Missouri Botanical Garden Press, 2007.

Fissell & Cooter (2003)
Fissell, Mary; Cooter, Roger: Exploring Natural Knowledge. Science and the Popular. In: Porter, Roy (Ed.): Eighteenth-Century Science. Cambridge: Cambridge University Press, 2003 (Cambridge History of Science 4), 129–158.

Francke (1707a)
Francke, August Hermann: Nicodemus, Oder Tractätlein von der Menschen-Furcht, Deren Beschreibung Ursachen […] Zu Pflantzung der wahren Furcht Gottes […]. 3. Aufl. Halle: Waisenhaus, 1707.

Francke (1707b)
Francke, August Hermann: Nicodemus: or, a Treatise against the Fear of Man. […] Written in High Dutch by Augustus Franck, […] With a preface Written by Josiah Woodward, […] to which is Added a Short History of Pietism (2nd edition). London: Downing, 1707.

Francke (1744)
Francke, August Hermann: Nicodemus, or, A Treatise Against the Fear of Man [...]; Rendered into English from the High-Dutch and Dedicated to the Honorable Society for Reformation of Manners. Boston: Rogers and Fowle, 1744.

French & Wear (1989)
French, Roger K.; Wear, Andrew (Eds.): The Medical Revolution of the Seventeenth Century. Cambridge: Cambridge University Press, 1989.

Friedrich & Müller-Jahnke (2005)
Friedrich, Christoph; Müller-Jahncke, Wolf-Dietrich; (Schmitz, Rudolf): Geschichte der Pharmazie,Vol. 2: Von der Frühen Neuzeit bis zur Gegenwart. Eichborn: Govi, 2005.

Green (2000)
Green, James N.: English Books and Printing in the Age of Franklin. In: Amory, Hugh; Hall, David D. (Eds.): A History of the Book in America, Vol. 1: The Colonial Book in the Atlantic World. Cambridge: Cambridge University Press, 2000, 248–298.

Grell & Cunningham (1996)
Grell, Ole; Cunningham, Andrew (Eds.): Religio Medici. Aldershot, UK: Ashgate Publishing, 1996.

Habermann (2001)
Habermann, Mechthild: Deutsche Fachtexte der frühen Neuzeit. Naturkundlich-medizinische Wissensvermittlung im Spannungsfeld von Latein und Volkssprache. Berlin: Walter de Gruyter, 2001.

Habrich (1991)
Habrich, Christa: Characteristic Features of Eighteenth-Century Therapeutics in Germany. In: Bynum, William F.; Nutton, Vivian (Eds.): Essays in the History of Therapeutics. Amsterdam: Rodopi, 1991 (Clio Medica 22), 39–49.

Habrich (1997)
Habrich, Christa: Heilkunde im Dienst der Seelsorge bei Gerhard Tersteegen. In: Kock, Manfred (Ed.): Gerhard Tersteegen – Evangelische Mystik inmitten der Aufklärung. Köln: Rheinland-Verlag GmbH, 1997, 161–180.

Habrich (2002)
Habrich, Christa: Johann Samuel Carl (1677–1757) und die Philadelphische Ärztegemeinschaft. In: Lehmann, Hartmut; Schrader, Hans-Jürgen; Schilling, Heinz (Eds.): Jansenismus, Quietismus, Pietismus. Göttingen: Vandenhoeck & Ruprecht, 2002 (Arbeiten zur Geschichte des Pietismus 42), 272–289.

Hayne (1663)
Hayne, Johann: Drey underschiedliche newe Tractätlein. Deren Erstes von astralischen Kranckheiten Das Andere, von tartarischen Kranckheiten [...] Das Dritte, begreifft in sich das Fundament [...] wie man die Urinen des Menschen [...] künstlich iudiciren erkennen möge (2nd edition). Frankfurt/M.: Thomæ Matthiæ, 1663.

Heister (1740)
Lorenz Heister: Institutiones chirurgicae in quibus quicquid ad rem chirurgicam pertinet, optima et novissima ratione pertractatur […].Venetiis: Apud Franciscum Pitteri, 1740.

Heister (1719)
Lorenz Heister: Chirurgie, in welcher alles, was zur Wund-Artzney gehöret, nach der neuesten und besten Art gründlich abgehandelt, und [...] die neuerfundenen und dienlichste Instrumenten [...] vorgestellet werden. Nürnberg: Hoffmann, 1719.

Horrocks (2003)
Horrocks, Thomas A.: Rules, Remedies, and Regimens. Health Advice in Early Amerrican Almanacs. In: Rosenberg, Charles (Ed.): Right Living, the Anglo American Tradition of Self-Help Medicine and Hygiene. Baltimore, MD: Johns Hopkins University Press, 2003, 112–146.

Jones & Wilson (1995)
Jones G. F.; Wilson R. (Eds. and transl.): Detailed Reports of the Salzburger Emigrants Who Settled in America. Vol. 18 (1744–45): Camden, ME: Picton Press, 1995.

Keil (1987)
Keil, Gundolf: Organisationsformen des medizinischen Wissens. In: Wolf, Norbert Richard (Ed.): Wissensorganisierende und wissensvermittelnde Literatur im Mittelalter. Kolloquium December 5–7, 1985. Wiesbaden: Ludwig Reichert Verlag, 1987, 221–245.

Krafft (1999)
Krafft, Fritz: "Die Arznei kommt vom Herrn und der Apotheker bereitet sie". Biblische Rechtfertigung der Apothekerkunst im Protestantismus; Apotheken-Auslucht in Lemgo und Pharmako-Theologie. Stuttgart : Wissschaftliche Verlagsgesellschaft, 1999 (Quellen und Studien zur Geschichte der Pharmazie 76).

Krafft (2002)
Krafft, Fritz: Johann Christian Wiegleb und seine Rolle bei der Verwissenschaftlichung der Pharmazie. In: Friedrich, Christoph; Müller-Jahncke, Wolf-Dieter (Eds.): Apotheker und Universität. Die Vorträge der Pharmaziehistorischen Biennale in Leipzig [...] 2000 und der Gedenkveranstaltung "Wiegleb 2000" [...] in Bad Langensalza. Stuttgart: Wissenschaftliche Verlagsgesellschaft, 2002, 151–196.

Kuhn (1992)
Kuhn, Michael: De nomine et vocabulo. Der Begriff der medizinischen Fachsprache und die Krankheitsnamen bei Paracelsus (1493–1541). Heidelberg: Universitätsverlag C. Winter, 1992.

Lémery (1683)
Lémery, Nicolas: Cours de chymie, contenant la maniere de faire les operations qui sont en usage dans la medecine, par une methode facile […] (5th rev. edition). Paris: Estienne Michallet, 1683 (multiple editions until the 1760s).

Lémery (1697)
Lémery, Nicolas: Pharmacopée universelle, contenant toutes les compositions de pharmacie qui sont en usage dans la medecine […]. Avec un lexicon pharmaceutique. Paris: Laurent d'Houry, 1697 (multiple editions until the 1760s).

Lewis (1744)
Lewis, William: Pharmacopoeia reformata: or, An Essay for a Reformation of the London Pharmacopoeia, [...]. London: R. Willock, 1744.

Lewis (1749)
Lewis, William: The Pharmacopoeia of the Royal College of Physicians At Edinburgh. London: John Nourse at the Lamb, opposite Katherine Street in the Strand,1749.

Lewis (1753)
Lewis, William: The New Dispensatory [...] The Whole interspersed With Practical Cautions and Observations. Intended as a Correction, and Improvement of Quincy. London: John Nourse, opposite Catharine Street in the Strand, 1753.

Lewis (1765)
Lewis, William: The New Dispensatory [...] The whole interspersed with practical cautions and observations (2nd edition corrected, with large additions). London : printed for J. Nourse, 1765.

Lewis (1768/1772)
Lewis, William: Neues verbessertes Dispensatorium oder Arzneybuch, in welchem alles, was zu der Apothekerkunst gehöret, nach den Londoner und Edinburger Pharmacopeen mit practischen Wahrnehmungen und Bemerkungen vorgetragen wird. Theil 1–2. Hamburg: Brandt, 1768/1772.

Lindemann (2000)
Lindemann, Mary: Health and Healing. Baltimore, MD: Johns Hopkins University Press, 2000

Liefmann (1698)
Liefmann, Gottlieb: Dissertatio Historica de Fanaticis Silesiorum et Speciatim Quirino Kuhlmanno. Wittenberg: Christian Schrödter, 1698.

Meier (1976)
Meier, Louis A.: Early Pennsylvania Medicine. A Representative Early American Medical History, Montgomery County, Pennsylvania, 1682–1799. Boyertown, Pa.: Gilbert Printing Co., 1976.

Moran (1990)
Moran, Bruce T.: Prince Practitioners and the Direction of Medical Roles at the German Court. Maurice of Hessen-Kassel and His Physicians. In: Nutton, Vivian (Ed.): Medicine at the Courts of Europe. London: Routledge, 1990, 95–116.

Moran (1991)
Moran, Bruce T.: The Alchemical World of the German Court. Occult Philosophy and Chemical Medicine in the Circle of Moritz of Hessen (1572–1632). Stuttgart: Franz Steiner, 1991.

Müller-Jahncke (1988)
Müller-Jahncke, Wolf-Dieter: Die Medicina Pensylvania des George de Benneville. In: Völker, Arina (Ed.): Dixhuitieme. Zur Geschichte von Medizin und Naturwissenschaften im 18. Jahrhundert. Halle: Universität Halle-Wittenberg, 1988 (Wissenschaftliche Beiträge der Martin-Luther-Universität Halle-Wittenberg 20), 121–133.

Murphy (1991)
Murphy, Lamar Riley: Enter the Physician. The Transformation of Domestic Medicine, 1760–1860. Tuscaloosa: University of Alabama Press, 1991.

Neumann (1759)
The Chemical Works of Caspar Neumann [...] / Abridged and Methodized, with Large Additions [...]. By William Lewis. London: W. Johnston, G. Keith, A. Linde, P. Davey, B. Law, T. Field, T. Caslon, and E. Dilly, 1759.

Ogilvie (2005)
Ogilvie, Brian W.: Natural History, Ethics and Physico-Theology. In: Pomata, Gianna; Siraisi, N.G. (Eds.): Historia, Empiricism and Erudition in Early Modern Europe. Cambridge, MA: MIT Press, 2005, 75–104.

Peickert (1932)
Peickert, Heinz, Geheimmittel im deutschen Arzneiverkehr: Ein Beitrag zur Wirtschaftsgeschichte der Pharmazie und zur Arzneispezialitätenfrage. Leipzig: Edelmann, 1932.

Pörksen (1983)
Pörksen, Uwe: Der Übergang vom Gelehrtenlatein zur deutschen Wissenschaftssprache. Zur frühen deutschen Fachliteratur und Frachsprache in den naturwissenschaftlichen und mathematischen Fächern (ca. 1500–1800). In: Schlieben-Lange, Brigitte; Kreuzer, Helmut (Eds.): Fachsprache und Fachliteratur. Göttingen: Vandenhoeck & Ruprecht, 1983 (Zeitschrift für Literaturwissenschaft und Linguistik 13, 51/52), 227–258.

Porter (1988)
Porter, Roy: Before the Fringe. 'Quackery' and the Eighteenth-Century Medical Market. In: Cooter, Roger (Ed.): Studies in the History of Alternative Medicine. New York: St. Martin's Press, 1988, 1–27.

Quincy (1720)
Quincy, John: Pharmacopœia officinalis et extemporanea. Or, a Complete English Dispensatory, in Four Parts (3rd edition, with large additions). London: A. Bell, 1720.

Quincy (1736)
Quincy, John: Pharmacopœia officinalis & extemporanea. Or, a complete English Dispensatory, in Four Parts (10th edition, much enlarged and corrected). London: Thomas Longman, 1736.

Reinhold (1984)
Reinhold, Meyer: Classica Americana. The Greek and Roman Heritage in the United States. Detroit: Wayne State University Press, 1984.

Riha (1992a)
Riha, Ortrun: Wissensorganisation in medizinischen Sammelhandschriften. Wiesbaden: Dr. Ludwig Reichert Verlag, 1992.

Riha (1992b)
Riha, Ortrun: Ortolf von Baierland und seine lateinischen Quellen. Hochschulmedizin in der Volkssprache. Wiesbaden: Dr. Ludwig Reichert Verlag, 1992.

Risse (2005)
Risse, Guenter B.: New Medical Challenges During the Scottish Enlightenment. Amsterdam: Rodopi, 2005 (Clio medica 78).

Roeber (2000)
Roeber, A. Gregg: German and Dutch Books and Printing. In: Amory, Hugh; Hall, David D. (Eds.): A History of the Book in America, Vol. 1: The Colonial Book in the Atlantic World. Cambridge: Cambridge University Press, 2000, 298–313.

Rosenberg (2003)
Rosenberg, Charles (Ed.): Right Living, the Anglo American Tradition of Self-Help Medicine and Hygiene. Baltimore, MD: Johns Hopkins University Press, 2003.

Rosenberg & Golden (1992)
Rosenberg, Charles E.; Golden, Janet (Eds.): Framing Diseases in Cultural History. New Brunswick, NJ.: Rutgers University Press, 1992.

Rothe (1727)
Rothe, Gottfried: Gottfried Rothens [...] gründliche Anleitung zur Chymie, darinnen [...] auch die Praeparationes derer besten chymischen Medikamenten aus der berühmtesten Medicorum, sonderlich Ludovici, Wedelii, Stahlii &c; Schriften [...] aufrichtig gewiesen wird (3. Aufl.). Leipzig: Caspar Jacob Eyssel, 1727.

Rush (1809)
Rush, Benjamin: Inquiry into the Comparative State of Medicine in Philadelphia between the years 1760 and 1766, and the year 1809. In: Medical Inquiries and Observations, Vol. 4. Philadelphia: Kimber and Conrad et al., 1809, 383–427.

Schrader (1989)
Schrader, Hans-Jürgen: Literaturproduktion und Büchermarkt des radikalen Pietismus. Johann Heinrich Reitz' "Historie Der Wiedergebohrnen" und ihr geschichtlicher Kontext. Göttingen:Vandenhoeck und Ruprecht, 1989.

Seils (1995)
Seils, Markus: Friedrich Albrecht Carl Gren in seiner Zeit, 1760–1798. Heidelberg: Heidelberger Verlagsanstalt, 1995 (Heidelberger Schriften zur Pharmazie und Naturwissenschaftsgeschichte).

Shackelford (2004)
Shackelford, Jole: A Philosophical Path for Paracelsian Medicine. The Ideas, Intellectual Context, and Influence of Petrus Severinus (1540/2–1602). Copenhagen: Museum Tusculanum Press, 2004.

Szasz (2004)
Szasz, Ildiko: Pharmazeutische Literatur für Frauen von Brunfels bis zu den Damen-Konversationslexika. In: Wahrig, Bettina (Ed.): Arzneien für "das schöne Geschlecht". Geschlechterverhältnisse in Phytotherapie und Pharmazie vom Mittelalter bis zum 19. Jahrhundert. Stuttgart: Deutscher Apotheker Verlag, 2004, 135–150.

Telle (1979)
Telle, Joachim: Wissenschaft und Öffentlichkeit im Spiegel der deutschen Arzneibuchliteratur. Zum deutsch-lateinischen Sprachenstreit in der Medizin des 16. und 17. Jahrhunderts. In: Medizinhistorisches Journal 14 (1979), 32–52.

Telle (1982)
Telle, Joachim: Arzneikunst und der "gemeine Mann". Zum deutsch-lateinischen Sprachenstreit in der frühneuzeitlichen Medizin. In: Ausstellungskatalog der Herzog August Bibliothek, Vol. 36. Wolfenbüttel, 1982, 43–50.

Tennent (1734)
Tennent, John: Every Man His Own Doctor, or: The Poor Planter's Physician. Williamsburg: Parks, 1734.

Tissot (1771)
Tissot, Samuel Auguste: Advice to the People in General, with Regard to Their Health. Philadelphia: Sparhawk, 1771.

Vogel & Rosenberg (1979)
Vogel, Morris J.; Rosenberg, Charles E. (Eds.): The Therapeutic Revolution. Essays in the Social History of American Medicine. Philadelphia: University of Pennsylvania Press, 1979.

Wagner (2005)
Wagner, Abraham: Remediorum Specimina aliquot ex Praxi A. W. In: Eighteenth-century Colonial Formularies. The Manuscripts of George de Benneville and Abraham Wagner. The College of Physicians of Philadelphia Digital Library.
Recent website address (access date: June 23, 2008): http://www.accesspadr.org/cpp/.

Wear (2000)
Wear, Andrew: Knowledge and Practice in English Medicine, 1580–1680. Cambridge: Cambridge University Press, 2000.

Webster (1975)
Webster, Charles: The Great Instauration. Science, Medicine and Reform, 1626–1660. London: Duckworth, 1975.

Weigelt (1973)
Weigelt, Horst: Spiritualistische Traditionen im Protestantismus. Die Geschichte des Schwenckfeldertums in Schlesien. Berlin: Walter de Gruyter, 1973.

Wilson (1993)
Wilson, Renate: Piety and Commerce in Colonial Georgia. In: Georgia Historical Quarterly 77 (1993), 336–366.

Wilson (2000)
Wilson, Renate: Pious Traders in Medicine. A German pharmaceutical network in 18th century North America. University Park, PA: Penn State University Press, 2000.

Wilson (2007)
Wilson, Renate: Moravian Physicians and their Medicine in Colonial North America. European Models and Colonial Reality. In: Gillespie, Michelle; Beachy, Robert (Eds.): Pious Pursuits. New York: Wehrhahn, 2007, 65–82.

Wilson (2008)
Wilson, Renate: The Second Generation. Pietist Clergy, Commerce, and the Commerce Scientifique in the New Republic, 1780–1820. In: Grabbe, Hans Joachim (Ed.): Halle Pietism, Colonial North America, and the Young United States. Stuttgart: Steiner, 2008 (in print).

Wilson & Savacool (2001)
Wilson, Renate; Savacool, Jacob Woodrow: The Theory and Practice of Pharmacy in Pennsylvania. Observations on Two Colonial Doctors. Pennsylvania History 68 (2001), 31–65.

Part IV:
Religion and Society in Eighteenth Century Medicine

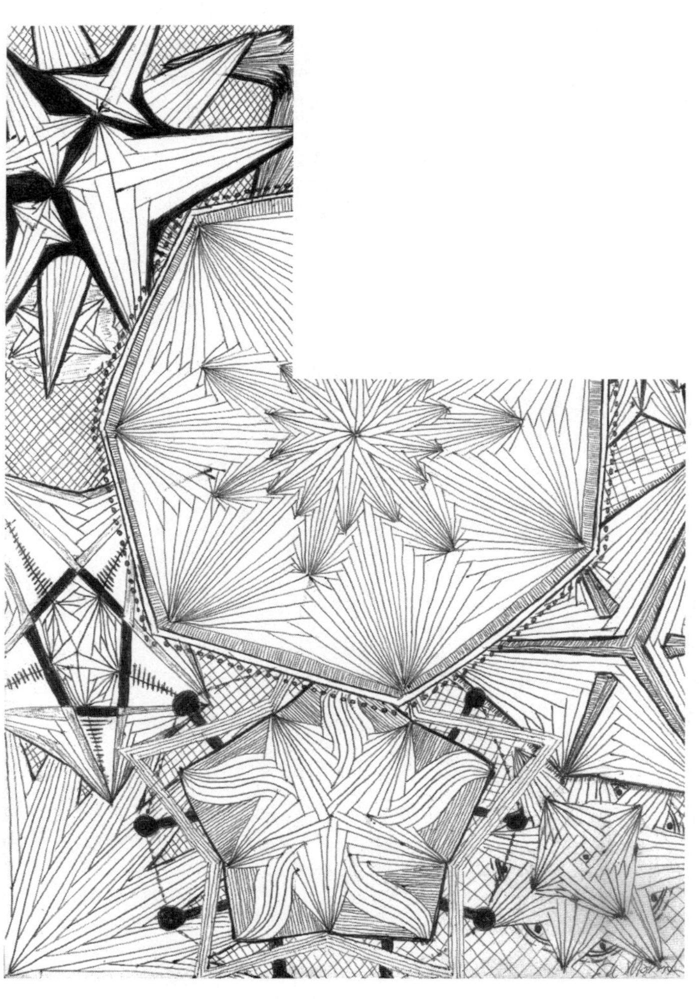

„ … DENN BIST DU NICHT BEY IHR MIT DEINER KRAFFT ZUGEGEN, SO HILFT KEIN DIPTAM NICHT, UND KEINE PANACEE.“ – MEDICINA THEOLOGICA ALS KONSEQUENZ DER THEOLOGIA MEDICINALIS IM PROTESTANTISMUS

Fritz Krafft

Vorbemerkungen

„Wie soll ich aber dir, o grosser Artzt! nun danken“, fragt 1725 der wohl bedeutendste Arzt-Dichter im Umfeld der Physikotheologie Daniel Wilhelm Triller (1695–1782),[1] damals Landphysicus und Apotheker in Merseburg, später Leibarzt des Erbprinzen von Nassau-Saarbrücken und Professor der Medizin in Wittenberg, in einem Gedicht über eine gerade überstandene Fiebererkrankung und dankt dann schließlich Gott auch dafür, dass er „so großen Segen / Der Artzeney geschenkt“ habe; „denn bist du nicht bey ihr mit deiner Krafft zugegen, / So hilft kein Diptam nicht, und keine Panacee“.[2] Krankheit und Schmerz könnten daraufhin vom Menschen ertragen werden, und sie müssten es auch, um in der Ewigkeit von Gott erlöst werden zu können.

Erst Gottes ‚Krafft‘ und Absicht verleihen demnach den ‚Arzneien‘ ihre heilende Wirkung. Und die Physikotheologie des 18. Jahrhunderts, die im Sinne Martin Luthers von einer Providentia Gottes ausging, die ständig und überall (nicht nur beim Schöpfungsakt) gegenwärtig ist, sodass sogar seine Existenz aus deren bemerkbarem Vorhandensein erschlossen werden könne, hat Gott die zu spezifischen Arzneien zu verarbeitenden Kräuter jeweils dort wachsen lassen, wo eine mit ihnen zu heilende Krankheit auftritt (oder irgendwann einmal auftreten wird).[3]

Diese Überzeugung geht in Deutschland dann im letzten Drittel des Jahrhunderts zurück, und die nach 1711 einsetzende Flut physikotheologischer Schriften versiegt hier (anders als im angelsächsischen Sprachraum) fast schlagartig. Das hängt sicherlich ursächlich damit zusammen, dass Immanuel Kant (1724–1804), dessen *Allgemeine Naturgeschichte* von 1755 noch gänzlich physikotheologisch orientiert gewesen war und teleologische Beweise geführt hatte, 1763 mit seiner Schrift *Der einzig mögliche Beweisgrund zu einer Demonstration des Daseyns Gottes* in einem wesentlichen Punkt der Argumentation der Physikotheologen den Boden entzog, indem er den ‚physikotheologischen‘ Gottesbeweis endgültig als scheinbar erwies, da die empirischen Erfahrungen, von denen er ausgehe,

1 Siehe DEHMEL (1996), 179–186.

2 TRILLER (1725), 122.

3 Siehe DEHMEL (1996) und KRAFFT (1996). – Bei Philipp Melanchthon hatte es nur geheißen (*De sympathia et antipathia*, CR 11, 925), dass Gott gegen jede Krankheit „jeweils eigene Heilmittel gesetzt hat“ („sua quaedam remedia opposuit“; ähnlich auch *De medicinae usu*, CR 12, 224) – auch gegen künftig entstehende; siehe dazu HOFHEINZ & BRÖER (2003), 80.

lediglich auf einen Weltbaumeister, nicht aber auf einen Schöpfer führen könnten; folglich sei „Physikotheologie eine mißverstandene physische Teleologie“.[4] Kant proklamierte dann 1781 in der *Kritik der reinen Vernunft* abschließend einen ausschließlich kausalen Wissenschaftsbegriff, innerhalb dessen die Natur material als der Inbegriff aller Erscheinungen und formal als die apriorische „Gesetzmäßigkeit der Erscheinungen in Raum und Zeit“ fungiert, sodass allein dadurch empirische Erkenntnis von der Natur möglich werde, dass wir „die Folge der Erscheinungen, mithin alle Veränderung, dem Gesetz der Kausalität unterwerfen“.[5] Damit war der ‚Natur‘ als Objekt der Naturwissenschaft, Pharmazie und Medizin jegliche finale (teleologische) Komponente genommen und war daraufhin auch die Möglichkeit einer teleologischen Beweisführung innerhalb der Wissenschaften zumindest im deutschsprachigen Raum nicht mehr gegeben. Von Gott Erschaffenem konnte innerhalb seines kausalen Gefüges nur mehr schwer ein anthropozentrisch zu deutender Zweck unterstellt werden – wenn auch gerade in den Biowissenschaften noch heute immer dann, wenn man in Beweisnot gerät, in unpräziser Sprechweise so getan wird, als ob diese Kausalität in ihr nicht gelte, sondern weiterhin die aristotelische, in der die *causa finalis* (die ‚Zweckursache‘: Gott habe erschaffen / Die Natur habe eingerichtet, damit ...) eine mindestens ebenso wichtige Rolle spielte wie die *causa efficiens* (die ‚Bewegungsursache‘).

Wir müssen uns aber auch umgekehrt davor hüten, die moderne, ausschließlich kausale Denkart im Sinne Kants schon der vorkantischen Naturwissenschaft und Medizin zu unterstellen und mit ihr vermischte teleologisch-theologische Denkweisen als unangemessen zu eliminieren. Selbst wenn man nämlich aus der Sicht der modernen Pharmakologie den nicht empirisch bestätigten Arzneimitteln eine tatsächliche Heilwirkung absprechen wollte, so bliebe doch die ungeheure Suggestivwirkung erhalten, die mit ihnen zusätzlich zu der Überzeugung von der Richtigkeit der ihnen zugrunde liegenden Medizin(theorie) über den christlichen Glauben verbunden werden konnte.

Was aus späterer Sicht als schlauer Werbetrick erscheinen könnte, scheint jedenfalls aufrichtige Überzeugung gewesen zu sein, wenn August Hermann Francke (1663–1727) regelrecht ‚verkündete‘, dass seine Gebete erhört und sein Gottvertrauen belohnt worden seien „durch das Eingreifen Gottes“, der die von der Waisenhaus-Apotheke vertriebenen neuen Arzneien in seiner allweisen Providentia dem Waisenhaus zur jeweils rechten Zeit in die Hände gegeben und geschenkt habe, auf denen deshalb ein besonderer göttlicher Segen ruhe und die eine heilende Wirkung selbst dort entfalteten, wo andere Mittel versagten.[6] Der Arzt und Apotheker der Franckeschen Anstalten Christian Friedrich Richter

4 KANT (1902-1923), Kritik der Urteilskraft, A 405.

5 KANT (1902-1923), Kritik der reinen Vernunft, B 234.

6 Siehe insbesondere FRANCKE (1701) und FRANCKE (1709), weiterhin vor allem den Vorbericht bei RICHTER (1705); generell dazu POECKERN (1984) (hier 15–39 die Kritik an C. F. Richters Behauptungen und Fähigkeiten durch seinen Konkurrenten G. H. Neubauer [1666–1726]); DEHMEL (1996), 38–46, WILSON (2000), 15–96, HELM (2004).

(1676–1711)[7] hat dieses dann im Vorbericht zu seinem *Kurtzen und deutlichen Unterricht von dem Leibe und natürlichen Leben des Menschen* 1705 wiederholt und gleichzeitig über die speziellen Waisenhaus-Medikamente und ihre Heilerfolge berichtet.[8] – Hier war es also der Hallesche Pietismus, der mit Hilfe des Netzes anderer philanthropischer Zirkel im protestantischen Europa das geistige und wirtschaftliche Fundament für einen blühenden Arzneimittelhandel lieferte, dessen Gewinne wieder in die Stiftung zurückfließen konnten. Er weitete sich über das protestantische Deutschland[9] hinaus in Europa und sogar in Nordamerika aus; Renate Wilson hat in ihrem Buch *Pious Traders in Medicine* das von Halle ausgehende dortige ‚pharmazeutische Netzwerk' und dessen Voraussetzungen aufgearbeitet.[10]

Aber nicht um diese enge Verknüpfung zwischen christlichem Glauben und gottgegebenem speziellen Arzneimittel geht es mir in diesem Zusammenhang, sondern vielmehr um die dabei anklingende Vorstellung, dass Gott dem Menschen nicht nur einzelne Arzneimittel, sondern die Kunstfertigkeit überhaupt verliehen habe, aus den von ihm erschaffenen Kräutern und Simplicia Arzneien zu bereiten (die Kunst des Apothekers also von Gott verliehen sei) – und um die auf dieser Basis entstandene eindrucksvolle Ikonographie zur Unterstützung dieser Aussagen, die Christi Heilsgeschehen mit der Tätigkeit des so aufgewerteten Apothekers sinnbildlich veranschaulicht.

Die von Gott dem Menschen verliehene Apothekerkunst (*Jesus Sirach*)

Julius Bernhard von Rohr (1688–1742), der möglicherweise während seines Studiums bei Christian Wolff in Halle mit Franckes *Paedagogium* in Berührung gekommen war, zumal er sich seinen Lebensunterhalt mit Unterricht verdienen musste, hatte diese Thematik in seiner 1740 erschienenen Physikotheologie, der ersten Physikotheologie der Pflanzen überhaupt, im dritten Buch, das „Vom Nutzen der Kräuter" handelt und gleichsam eine „Pharmaco-Theologia" darstellt, natürlich zur Rechtfertigung der Apothekerkunst anschneiden müssen.[11] Das Werk trägt den im Aufbau für physikotheologische Werke typischen Titel: *Phyto-Theologia, oder Vernunft- und Schriftmaeßiger Versuch, wie aus dem Reich der Gewächse die Allmacht, Weisheit und Guete und Gerechtigkeit des großen Schoepfers und Erhalters aller Dinge von den Menschen erkannt und sein allerheiligster Name hiervor gepriesen werden möge.* In § 16 heißt es mit vielen

7 Zu C. F. Richter siehe ALTMANN (1972).

8 Siehe RICHTER (1705), Theil IV, 1. Kapitel (395–452).

9 Zu damit durchaus verbundenen Problemen (etwa ökonomischer Art) siehe beispielhaft HELM (2001).

10 WILSON (2000), generell TOELLNER (2004).

11 Zu J. B. von Rohr und seiner *Phytotheologie* siehe vor allem DEHMEL (1996), 70–85; DEHMEL (1996), 123–162 bringt unter dem Titel *Pharmaco-Theologia* ein kommentiertes Faksimile des ersten Kapitels des dritten Buches.

wörtlichen Anklängen an den Anfang des 38. Kapitels des *Ecclesiasticus* (*Jesus Sirach*) in Martin Luthers Übersetzung:

> Ein ieder hat Ursache, der göttlichen Vorsorge Lob und Preiß abzustatten [*Jesus Sirach* XXXVIII, 6], daß sie nicht nur denen Menschen aus dem Reich der Pflantzen so viel Hülffs-Mittel wider mancherley Beschwerden zugeordnet [2, 4, 13], sondern ihnen auch die Wissenschafft verliehen, sie auf so mancherley Weise nach den Regeln der Apothecker-Kunst zu verändern [6] [...]. Ihre Kräffte werden auf diese Weise weit besser heraus gezogen, als wann sie nur sonst genossen, oder bloß abgekocht werden. [...] Wie vielen würden die besten Tugenden und Kräffte mancher Pflantzen unnützlich seyn, wann GOtt nicht den Menschen die Wissenschaft verliehen hätte, die Artzneyen nach eines ieden Natur einzurichten [6], und dasjenige, was mancher vor das allerwidrigste achten würde, ihnen zu benehmen.[12]

Die besten ‚Wirkkräfte' der Pflanzen wären folglich unnütz, wenn Gott dem Menschen nicht die ‚Wissenschaft' beziehungsweise ‚Apotheker-Kunst' verliehen hätte, den Pflanzen die heilenden ‚Kräfte' (‚Wirkstoffe' würden wir heute von einer anderen medizinisch-pharmazeutischen Basis aus sagen) zu entziehen und daraus individuelle Arzneien zu bereiten. Damit scheint Rohr auf die von Paracelsus (1493/1494–1541) initiierte Chymiatria anzuspielen – wie es auch in der 1618 erlassenen zweiten Fassung der Medizinalordnung für das Kurfürstentum Mainz geschah, wenn sie in einem ergänzten Passus des Eingangskapitels bemerkte:

> Und dieweil bey unsriger jetzigen Zeiten die löbliche Kunst der wahren Chymiae, welche eine sonderbare Gottesgab des Allmächtigen ist, durch welche aus den Arzneyen fürnemblich aber den vegetabilibus und Minerabilibus die reineste, zarteste Kräften und Essentiae extrahirt, von ihrem groben Cörper abgeschieden und nutzlich zur Erhaltung und Wiederbringung menschlicher Gesundheit usurpirt werden; Wollen wir auch solche Kunst und dessen Medicamenta legitima bey unsern Medicae Doctoribus und Apotecke[r]n hinfüro leyden und gestatten [...].[13]

Und auch Kurfürst und Erzbischof Johann Schweickhart von Kronberg (1553–1626, ab 1604 Kurfürst) stellte seine Ordnung unter das Motto zweier Verse aus dem 38. Kapitel des *Jesus Sirach*,[14] von deren von der *Vulgata* abweichenden Formulierung zwei Halbverse hier von besonderem Interesse sind: „Est enim a Supremo Medicina" („Denn vom Höchsten ist die Medizin"), und: „Dominus ex terra condidit Medicamenta" („Der Herr fügte aus Erde Medikamente zusammen" oder: „erschuf sie aus Erde"). Der Text der *Vulgata* lautete dagegen: „(2) A Deo enim omnis medela" („Denn von Gott ist jegliche Heilung"), und „(4) Altissimus creavit de terra medicamenta" („Der Höchste hat aus Erde Medikamente

12 ROHR (1740), 444. – Die anklingenden Verse aus dem Buch Jesus Sirach sind jeweils in eckigen Klammern hinzugefügt.

13 Reformatio und erneuerte Ordnung deren Apotecken [erlassen von Erzbischof Johann Schweickhart von Kronberg], Mainz 1618 [erste Fassung 1605], 2; ediert in DADDER (1961), 199–327, hier 202.

14 DADDER (1961), 201. „Ecclesiastici cap. 38 [2 et 4]: Est enim a Supremo Medicina, et a Rege stipendium accipiet: Dominus ex terra condidit Medicamenta, et vir prudens non contemnet eam."

erschaffen“) – von Gott dem Menschen verliehen wurde demnach gemäß Schweickhart nur die spezielle chymiatrische Kunst des Extrahierens; und in diesem Punkt übernimmt die Ordnung sicherlich einen entsprechenden Passus aus der von Landgraf Moritz kurz zuvor (1616) erlassenen Medizinalordnung für Hessen-Kassel.[15]

Martin Luther, der ja einen Bibeltext schaffen wollte, den seine Zeitgenossen aus ihrem Leben und Erleben heraus verstehen sollten, hat die ersten Verse unter Verwendung auf jahrhundertelanger Entwicklung des Apothekerstandes und seiner Kunst beruhender zeitgenössischer Begriffe[16] wie folgt übersetzt:

> (1) Ehre den Artzt mit gebürlicher Verehrung / das du jn habest zur not. (2) Denn der Herr hat jn [das heißt den Arzt, nicht also: die Medizin] geschaffen / und die Ertzney kompt von dem Höhesten / und die Könige ehren jn [= den Arzt]. (3) Die kunst des Artzts erhöhet jn / und macht jn gros bey Fürsten und Herren. (4) Der Herr lesst die Ertzney aus der Erden wachsen / und ein Vernünfftiger veracht sie nicht. (5) Ward doch das bitter Wasser süsse / durch ein Holtz [im Wunder von Mara, *Exodus* 15, 25] / Auff das man seine krafft erkennen solte. (6) Und er hat solche kunst den Menschen gegeben / das er gepreiset würde in seinen Wunderthaten. (7) Damit [nämlich mit seinen ‚Wunderthaten‘ wie diesem Holz] heilet er und vertreibt die schmertzen / und der Apotheker macht Ertzney draus. […] (9) Mein Kind / wenn du kranck bist / so verachte dis nicht / sondern bitte den Herrn / so wird er dich gesund machen.

Luthers *Sirach*-Übersetzung erschien 1532; Leo Jud war ihm 1529 mit seinen *Apocryphi* zuvorgekommen, in denen auch erstmals der Begriff „Apotheker“ eingeführt worden war:

> Der Herr hat die artzney von der erd geschaffen [noch entsprechend der Vulgata] / und der weiß würt kein scheüen drab haben […]. Der Herr hat den menschen weyßheit und verstandt geben / das man jn eere in seinen wunderthaten. Mit denen heylt er [nämlich Gott] nun die menschen / und nimpt jre schmertzen hyn / von denen machet der Apoteker ein vermischung […].[17]

Hieran schloss sich Johan Dietenbergers katholische Übersetzung ursprünglich an, wenn er 1534 schrieb: „[…] von denen machet der Apoteker ein Vermischung […]“,[18] während er sich ab der durchgesehenen Ausgabe von 1540 eher wieder Luther anschließen sollte: „[…] von denen machet der Apotheker süsse artzney und salb der gesundheit […]“.[19]

Zur Zeit der Abfassung der biblischen Bücher hatte es diesen ‚Apotheker‘-Beruf noch gar nicht gegeben, und die moderne Einheitsübersetzung tilgt ihn denn auch wieder aus dem Text. In der Septuaginta stand für „Apotheker“ μυρεψός / „Salbenmischer“, in der *Vulgata* richtig und zeitgemäß wiedergegeben

15 Nach DÜBBER (1969), 271, sind die entsprechenden Inhalte hier erstmals in eine Medizinalordnung aufgenommen und speziell auf die hessischen Bedürfnisse zugeschnitten worden.

16 Siehe dazu KRAFFT (1999), 33–43.

17 Leo JUD (1530), vj: „Der weiß mann / Ecclesiastes genannt“ [dritte Ausgabe, erstmals Basel: Chr. Froschauer d. Ä., 1529].

18 DIETENBERGER (1534) – ohne Verszählung.

19 DIETENBERGER (1540) – ohne Verszählung.

mit *unguentarius*, was dem hierfür im Hebräischen verwendeten Begriff *rokeach* entspricht, dem Hersteller von Räucherwerk und heiligem Salböl, die nie als Arzneimittel verwendet wurden. Eine nicht so schöne, aber eher historische Übersetzung des griechischen Textes würde lauten:

> Gott hat auch den Arzt erschaffen; denn von Gott stammt jegliche Heilung. [...] Der Herr ließ aus der Erde die pharmaka [das sind jegliche Formen von in der Regel ambivalent wirkenden Stoffen, Gewächsen und Tieren] wachsen, und ein Vernünftiger wird sich ihnen nicht verschließen. Wurde nicht durch ein Holz das bittere Wasser süß gemacht, auf dass die Menschen seine Kraft erkennen? Und er selbst hat den Menschen die Wissenschaft gegeben, damit er in seinen Wunderwerken [nämlich den pharmaka] gepriesen werde. Mit ihnen heilt er und wird den Schmerz aufheben; und der Salbenmischer wird mit ihnen eine Mixtur (μίγμα) machen.[20]

In Antike und frühem Mittelalter waren es die Ärzte gewesen, welche die *pharmaka* bereiteten und anwendeten; das Wissen um deren Wirkung habe Gott ihnen eingegeben, damit die Wunderwerke seiner Schöpfung durch sie gepriesen würden. Der Arzt ist gleichsam nur der Vermittler von Gottes Wirken durch die *pharmaka*, mit denen die mittels Gebet erreichte Heilung durch Gott eingeleitet und verstärkt werden soll – vergleichbar dem hippokratischen Arzt, der mit den *pharmaka* die ‚Heilkraft der Natur' *(vis medicatrix naturae)* nur unterstützen kann.[21] Daran zeigt sich, dass der Verfasser dieser um 200 v. Chr. entstandenen Spruchweisheit, Ben Sira aus Jerusalem, Jude nach Religion und aufgeklärter hellenistischer Grieche nach Kultur war. (Jüdische) Religion, Arzt(kunst) und (Arznei-)Mittel bilden eine durch tiefe Religiosität geprägte Einheit in Gott und seinen Werken.

Der ‚Apotheker' war als zu ihrer Zeit geläufiger Begriff erst durch die Übersetzungen von Leo Jud und Martin Luther in die Bibel und speziell in das Buch *Jesus Sirach* eingeführt worden, sodass die gebotene Verehrung des von Gott eingesetzten Arztes und seiner Kunst jetzt auch auf den Apotheker, der zu dieser Zeit die Arznei bereitete, und dessen Kunst übertragen werden konnte. Aber es ist dann erst die Formulierung Luthers, die Gott zwar den Arzt erschaffen lässt, nicht aber die fertigen Arzneimittel, vielmehr die ‚Arzneien' aus der Erde wachsen lässt und damit (entsprechend dem Septuaginta-Begriff „pharmaka") die durchaus wunderbaren Pflanzen und Minerale als Simplicia (entsprechend dem auf Weisung Gottes süßmachenden Holz) meint, die als solche noch nicht der Heilung und Schmerzlinderung für den Menschen dienen können, sondern nur, wenn Gott sich ihrer durch Vermittlung des Arztes bedient oder/und der Mensch daraus mittels der ihm von Gott verliehenen Apothekerkunst ein Arzneimittel bereitet.

20 Der lateinische Text der Vulgata differenziert dann frei vom Text, also interpretierend, die letzte Aussage: „Mit diesen wird er heilend den Schmerz vertreiben, und der Salbenmischer wird *pigmenta suavitatis* [süß duftende Salböle] und *unctiones sanitatis* [Salben für die Gesundheit] anfertigen."

21 Vgl. NEUBURGER (1926), 6.

Zu Luthers Zeit waren die Berufe von Arzt und Apotheker bereits getrennt; und ein nahes und wohlbekanntes Beispiel war für ihn der befreundete, hoch gebildete und wohlhabende Maler Lucas Cranach d.Ä. (1472–1553), dessen Reichtum nicht zuletzt auf dem Betreiben einer Apotheke in Wittenberg beruhte, für die er 1520 wegen seiner Verdienste als kurfürstlich-sächsischer Hofmaler ein Privileg erhalten hatte. Aber ein Cranach macht noch nicht den Apothekerstand aus, und der stand als Mitglied der Krämerzunft in denkbar schlechtem Ruf. Eine Gleichstellung des Apothekers mit dem Arzt war damit noch nicht erreicht. Dazu bedurfte es neben der scheinbar biblischen Rechtfertigung von Apotheker und Apothekerkunst seiner sozialen Aufwertung; und hierfür war die Akademisierung einer ‚wissenschaftlichen' Arzneibereitung zu Beginn des 17. Jahrhunderts die entscheidende Voraussetzung, nachdem der ‚Apotheker' und seine Kunst in der protestantischen Erbauungs- und Hausväterliteratur im Anschluss an Martin Luthers *Jesus Sirach* als verehrenswerte Gottesgabe begründet worden war.

Martin Luther hatte wieder ein verstärktes Augenmerk auf die apokryphen Schriften, die „Bücher, so der heiligen Schrift nicht gleich gehalten, und doch nützlich und gut zu lesen sind", gelegt. Von diesen schätzte er die *Weisheit Salomonis* und das *Buch Jesu Sirach* besonders hoch. Letzteres spielte dann auch innerhalb der von Luther neu belebten *Theologia medicinalis*, der ‚medizinischen Theologie', eine tragende Rolle in Verbindung mit dem sogenannten Heilandsruf aus dem *Matthäus-Evangelium* (11,28): „Kommt her zu mir alle, die ihr mühselig und beladen seid [oder in der katholischen Version: die ihr mit Arbeit und Mühen (oder auch: Krankheiten) beladen seid], ich will euch erquicken." Diese Werbung Christi, seiner Gemeinschaft in Gott, seinem Vater, beizutreten, begründet ja letztlich das Evangelium und die Christenheit als diese Gemeinschaft; und sie bilden auch die Grundlage der konfessionellen Werbung zur Zeit der Glaubensspaltung, bei Martin Luther und den Lutheranern, bei den römischen Katholiken und bei den Calvinisten.

Zur veranschaulichenden Umschreibung dessen, was der Mensch in dieser Gemeinschaft zu erwarten hat, wurde schon im Neuen Testament auf der Grundlage der rational-wissenschaftlichen Medizin des Hellenismus metaphorisch auf das Begriffsfeld Arzt/Arznei/Apotheke (letzteres noch im ursprünglichen Sinne eines bloßen ‚Arzneidepots') zurückgegriffen und Christus in Konkurrenz zum antiken Heilgott Asklepios zum ‚Heilenden' schlechthin, zum ‚Heiland' gemacht. Die nachträgliche Ausdehnung der Metaphorik der *Theologia medicinalis* auf das Alte Testament ist allerdings auch wieder erst ein Werk der Lutherübersetzung. *Exodus* 15,26 lässt sie Jahwe, den Gottvater der Christen, sich dem Volk Israel mit den Worten „ich bin der Herr, dein Arzt" offenbaren, als Begründung dafür, dass er dem Volke nicht die Krankheiten schicke wie den Ägyptern – was so keinen Sinn ergibt; die *Vulgata* hatte denn auch geschrieben: „ego sum Dominus sanator tuus" / „ich bin dein Herr, der dich gesund erhält".

Luther übernahm dann von den Kirchenvätern die Vorstellung, dass die Heiligen Schriften eine ‚Apotheke' (geistlicher) Arzneien seien, weil das Wort

Gottes die wichtigste Arznei in der göttlichen Therapie sei;[22] und er bezeichnet gelegentlich auch schon Christus als den Apotheker,[23] der dieses Arzneidepot verwaltet und Arzneien herausgibt, nimmt dabei aber auf *Jesus Sirach* 38 noch keinen Bezug. In einer Predigt von 1530 hatte er aber bereits diesem Text entnommen, dass Arznei, Medizin und Arzt von Gott erschaffen, ein *donum Dei* seien.[24] In seiner *Pestschrift* greift er dann auf Formulierungen der eigenen Übersetzung zurück, wenn er jenen, die im Vertrauen auf Gott nichts gegen ihre Krankheit tun, entgegnet: „Solchs heist nicht Gott trawen, sondern Gott versuchen. Denn Gott hat die ertzney geschaffen und die vernunfft gegeben, dem leibe für zustehen und sein [zu] pflegen, das er gesund sey und lebe."[25]

Die Nachfolger Luthers haben sich dann bis tief ins 17. Jahrhundert intensiv darum bemüht, in diesem Sinne „der Verachtung der Heilkunst aus vermeintlich frommen Gründen entgegenzuwirken",[26] und haben sich dazu immer wieder auf *Jesus Sirach* berufen, zum Teil im Kontext einer ausführlichen speziellen Exegese dieses für die Hausväter-Literatur vorbildhaften Buches, auch nachdem Medizin und Pharmazie gewaltige Fortschritte erfahren hatten. Als Beispiel hierzu mag die Auslegung der *Sapientia Salomonis* des Ulmer Superintendenten Conrad Dieterich (1575–1639) dienen, über die er 1627 im Druck erschienene Predigten im Ulmer Münster gehalten hatte:

> Es hat Gott besondern Kräutern / Wurtzeln / Oelen / besondere Krafft inn der Natur mit getheilet / daß sie den Menschen in Tränken / Pulvern / Pflastern vnnd Vberschlägen / so durch der Medicorum Kunst und Wissenschafft darauß praeparirt vnnd gemacht werden / heylen vnnd gesund machen können / will auch / daß der Mensch deren zu seiner Gesundheit gebrauchen soll / wie dann die Medicin vnd Artzneykunst für ein besondere Gab Gottes gehalten vnd gerühmet in der Schrifft / Syr. 38. 1. seq. Aber es hat weder Kraut noch Pflaster die Krafft zuhelffen von sich / sondern von deß Herrn Wort / der jhnen solche durch sein Wort mitgetheilet. Ebenmessig weder der Medicus noch Artzt die Kunst zuheylen von sich / oder in sich / sondern von deß Herrn Wort / Gnad vnd Segen / so er darzu gesprochen.[27]

Das ist zeitgemäß umgesetzter Luther.

Die älteste monographische *Sirach*-Auslegung stellt Caspar Huberinus' (1500–1553) 1555 posthum erschienener *Spiegel der Haußzucht – Jhesus Syrach genant* dar, der das Wohl von Leib und Seele gleichermaßen anspricht und zum 38. Kapitel ausführt,[28] dass man sich nur an einen professionellen Arzt wenden

22 Siehe jetzt STEIGER (2005), 19; 39–41.

23 STEIGER (2005), 42–47; STEIGER (2003).

24 LUTHER (WA), Band 30/II, 580,9–581,9; vgl. auch M. Luther, Tischreden, Nr. 360. – Zur Thematik siehe auch TOELLNER (1994); Belege für Medizin und Apothekerkunst als *donum Dei* bei STEIGER (2005), 13 (Fußnote 44, bei Luther), 82–83 (mit Fußnote 257); zu Philipp Melanchthon, der die Medizin zu den von Gott verliehenen „heroischen Tugenden" zählte (*De Hippocrate*, CR 11, 503 f.), siehe HOFHEINZ & BRÖER (2003), 80, Fußnote 50.

25 LUTHER (WA), Band 23, 365, 5–8.

26 STEIGER (2005), 85.

27 DIETERICH (1627), Band 2, 867; zitiert nach STEIGER (2005), 83.

28 HUBERINUS (1555), fol. 193–196; zitiert nach STEIGER (2005), 103.

dürfe, da Arzt und Arzneikunst gleichermaßen von Gott erschaffen seien; Gott habe der Natur die Heilkräfte „eingestiftet“, sodass „ein jeglichs“ Gewächs, Tier und Mineral „jhre sondere natur / art und wirckung“ hätten. Zur Nutzung dieser ‚schlummernden Kräfte‘ habe Gott die Medizin und Arzneikunde gestiftet, und der Mensch habe sie deshalb auch zu nutzen; in erster Linie solle er jedoch „nach der Geystlichen / vnd hymlischen / artzney trachten / nemlich / nach dem hymlischen artzet / vnnd Apotecker“. Hier wird also in Anlehnung an Luthers Andeutungen ausdrücklich von Christus nicht nur als ‚himmlischem Arzt‘, sondern auch als ‚himmlischem Apotheker‘ gesprochen, dessen ‚geistliche‘ Arzneien Priorität vor den ‚leiblichen‘ hätten.

Ausführlicher und fachgerechter sind die Ausführungen von Luthers einstmaligem Schüler und Hausgenossen Johannes Mathesius (1504–1565) in seinem erstmals 1586 posthum erschienenen *Syrach Mathesij*, in dem der Auslegung des 38. Kapitels breiter Raum eingeräumt wird: Über die Argumente von Huberinus hinaus wird hier betont, dass Gott als oberster Arzt, als *Consiliarius*, durch das Gebet hinzuzuziehen sei, sodass Leibesarzt (der die *causae secundae* appliziere) und Seelenarzt (als *causa prima*) gemeinsam praktizierten.[29] Mathesius bezeichnet das 38. *Sirach*-Kapitel als Loblied nicht nur auf die medizinische Wissenschaft und den Ärztestand, sondern auch auf die von Gott verliehene Kunst des Apothekers. Deren Ausübung befolge ein Gebot der Nächstenliebe, verehre dadurch zugleich Gott den Schöpfer und sei folglich ein Gottesdienst, sodass der Apotheker selbst in dieses göttliche Geflecht einzubeziehen sei. „Das reden wir zum trost den Apoteckern“, heißt es ausdrücklich, und im Zusammenhang mit der Exegese von Vers 4 („Der Herr lesst die Ertzney aus der Erden wachsen / vnd ein Vernünfftiger veracht sie nicht“) fordert Mathesius sogar:

> Freylich solt man diesen Spruch an alle Apotecken schreiben / damit man nicht allein die Artzney für Gottes Güte vnd nützliche Gabe erkenne / sondern auch Gott in seinen Creaturen erkenne vnd preise.[30]

Dieser Aufruf erfolgte hier aber wohl nicht zum ersten Mal; denn schon der 1568 eingeweihte Apotheken-Flügel des Rathauses in Hannover trug über dem Portal der Apotheke eben diesen Vers: „Der Herr läßt die Artzney auß der Erden wachsen // und ein Vernünfftiger verachtet sie nicht.“[31] Auch hatte er in der Fassung von Leo Jud schon auf dem Titelholzschnitt der ab 1537 mehrfach gedruckten *Hauß apoteck* mit Auszügen aus Hieronymus Brunschwygs Laienarzneibuch gestanden.[32] Und selbst der erzkatholische Kurfürst Schweickhart hatte ihn ja als Motto seiner Medizinalordnung verwendet.

Eine neue Wendung erhalten die Berufung auf und Rechtfertigung durch *Jesus Sirach* schließlich 1588 durch das *Paradeißgärtlein* des lutherischen Pre-

29 Siehe vor allem MATHESIUS (1586), Theil II, 115v und 116r.

30 MATHESIUS (1586), Theil II, fol. 116v.

31 Siehe GUTMANN (1975), 14–19; siehe auch KRAFFT (1999), 120–122.

32 BRUNSCHWYG (1538). Vgl. dazu KRAFFT (2001), 185–186.

digers in der Wetterau Konrad Rosbach (geb. 1535),[33] das Rohrs *Phyto-Theologie* gleichsam in nicht-physikotheologischer Form vorwegnimmt, insofern es aus dem 38. Kapitel die gottgefällige Anwendung auch der ‚geistlichen Arznei' ableitet und die arzneiliche Wirkung der Pflanzen auf beiderlei Verwendung ausdehnt, gemäß dem Prinzip,

> daß wir auß den sichtbaren vnd wolbekandten Creaturen die vnsichtbare vnnd von Natur vnbekandte Geheimnuß vnnd Haußhaltung Gottes zu vnserer Lehr / Trost / Vermahnung vnd Besserung betrachten / vnd daher zur Danckbarkeit / Glauben / Lieb / Hoffnung / Gedult vnd allen Christlichen Tugendten gereitzet werden solle.[34]

Das Buch stellt in Holzschnitten Pflanzen vor, denen jeweils botanische und arzneikundliche Informationen sowie eine an einer Bibelbezugsstelle orientierte Beschreibung der ‚geistlichen' Eigenschaften beigegeben werden.

Die Möglichkeit, aus den sichtbaren und bekannten Creaturen das unsichtbare und von Natur unbekannte Geheimnis in Gottes Vorsehung erkennen zu können, scheint der paracelsischen Signaturenlehre entnommen zu sein – und damit der Chymiatrie als besonderer Form von Apothekerkunst, auf die dann insbesondere im 17. Jahrhundert häufig die Vorstellung von einer ‚Gottesgabe' eingeengt wurde.

Die akademische und soziale Aufwertung der Apothekerkunst

Dieser Abgrenzung entgegenwirken sollte noch das Medizin- und Pharmazie-Programm, das der 1611/12 errichtete Erker der Rats-Apotheke in Lemgo darstellt – wiederum unter dem Motto von *Jesus Sirach* 38. Ein aus den Versen 2, 7, 9, 10 und 12 als Versatzstücken gebildeter, durch bauliche Vorgaben in vier Sätze gegliederter Text läuft hier als Schriftband unterhalb des Giebels um. Die erste Hälfte beinhaltet die Hinwendung zu Gott, die zweite die Hinwendung zum Arzt. Jeder der vier Sätze besteht wiederum aus zwei Halbsätzen[35]:

> Wenn du krank bist, so bitte den Herrn [das heißt: so bete zum Herrn],
> Und lass ab von [den] Sünden, so wird er dich gesund machen.
> Danach lass den Arzt zu dir kommen, denn der Höchste hat ihn geschaff[en],
> Die Arznei kommt vom Herrn, und der Apotheker bereitet sie.

Diese Berufung auf das Buch *Jesus Sirach* zur Rechtfertigung der Anwendung von ärztlicher und ausdrücklich auch pharmazeutischer Kunst bei gleichzeitiger Berücksichtigung religiöser Gepflogenheiten protestantischen Glaubens weist nun insofern etwas Besonderes und Neues auf, als sie erstmals ausdrücklich

33 Siehe hierzu KRAFFT (2003), 77–78.

34 In der unpaginierten Vorrede des Auftraggebers, des Frankfurter Verlegers J. Spieß, zu Rosbach (1588), a vj^{v}. – Von dem Werk erschien 1613 in Frankfurt eine neue Ausgabe.

35 Generell zum Erker sowie zu Inschrift und Figurenfries siehe KRAFFT (1999), 75–122; zur kunsthistorischen Einordnung darüber hinaus KRAFFT (2002).

verknüpft wird mit dem neuen Programm einer nach zwei Richtungen orientierten Medizin und Pharmazie, der Verknüpfung von traditioneller, auf Hippokrates und Galenos zurückgehender humoralpathologischer Medizin mit der neuen, von Paracelsus initiierten Chymiatria auf chemischen Grundlagen, die, durch Bildzitate eindeutig bezeugt, für den in dieser Apotheke agierenden Apotheker reklamiert wird. Auf einem eindrucksvollen Porträtfries zwischen den beiden Geschossen sind nämlich von links nach rechts zehn Ahnherren beider Medizinen in Hochreliefs abgebildet: Dioskurides und Aristoteles an der linken Schmalseite (sie repräsentieren die antiken Grundlagen), Rhases, Galenos und Hippokrates in der linken Hälfte der Frontseite (sie stellen die Hauptvertreter der traditionellen Medizin dar) sowie Hermes Trismegistos, Raimundus Lullus und Geber in der rechten Hälfte der Frontseite (sie repräsentieren die alchemisch-hermetischen Lehren), sodann Andreas Vesalius und Paracelsus an der rechten Schmalseite als Repräsentanten der neuesten Medizin. Dabei soll Paracelsus auf den drei Vertretern der hermetischen Lehren fußen; denn diese vier Porträts sind bis ins kleinste Detail genaue Relief-Umsetzungen der vier Porträtmedaillons in den Ecken des von dem Prager Hofstecher Aegidius Sadeler (um 1570–1628) geschaffenen Titelkupfers zu Oswald Crolls (um 1560–1608) 1609 posthum in Frankfurt erschienenem Buch *Basilica Chymica*, das auch in späteren Ausgaben und in der deutschen Übersetzung mit übernommen wurde.[36] Und in diesem Werk wird die paracelsische Heilmittellehre von ihrem philosophisch-esoterischen Überbau weitgehend befreit, gleichsam entmystifiziert, und erstmals durch eindeutige chemische Vorschriften nachvollziehbar und praktisch anwendbar und damit auch lehrbar gemacht.

Daraufhin konnte Johannes Hartmann (1568–1631), als ihm 1609 die erste und lange Zeit einzige Professur für *Chymiatria* übertragen wurde, die Landgraf Moritz von Hessen-Kassel eigens für ihn an der Universität Marburg zusammen mit einem Laboratorium eingerichtet hatte, dieses Werk paracelsischer Arzneibereitung seinem theoretischen und erstmals auch praktischen Unterricht zugrundelegen; 1611 veranstaltete er eine aufgrund der Erfahrungen bei der Nutzung annotierte *Editio secunda* mit demselben Titelkupfer. Besonders der praktische Unterricht zog zahlreiche Interessenten aus ganz Europa zu Hartmann; ein Labortagebuch bezeugt für das Studienjahr 1615/16 insgesamt 18 Teilnehmer, von denen sich ein großer Teil für beide Kurse eingeschrieben hatte – eine für damalige Verhältnisse ungeheuer große Anzahl.[37] Hartmann betonte allerdings immer wieder, dass er gemäß den beiden Bestandteilen des Wortes ‚Chymiatria' beide ‚Medizinen' lehre und miteinander verknüpfe, die Chymia im Sinne von Crolls Modifizierung paracelsischer chemischer Lehren und die Iatria oder Medicina im Sinne hippokratisch-galenischer Humoralpathologie. In dieser Form galt die Einrichtung der Professur vielen für vorbildlich und nachahmenswert; und der

36 Siehe dazu im einzelnen KRAFFT (1999), 93–116; eine Bibliographie der verschiedenen Ausgaben der *Basilica Chymica* einschließlich vieler Titelblätter bieten KÜHLMANN & TELLE (1996), 253–297.

37 Zu Einzelheiten vgl. KRAFFT (2007a).

Apothekenerker in Lemgo nimmt sich ja eben dieses Programms schon zwei Jahre später an. Die chemische Arzneibereitung war nicht mehr nur ‚hoffähig' – dem Beispiel des Kaiserhofs in Prag waren auch kleinere, vor allem protestantische Höfe mit der Berufung chymiatrischer Hofärzte gefolgt, nicht zuletzt der Kasseler, an dem Moritz auch ein Laboratorium einrichten ließ –, sondern auch akademisch geworden und damit sozial aufgewertet. Der chemische Arzneien bereitende Apotheker war dem Arzt gleichgestellt; und der Lemgoer Apotheker stellte sich mit seinem Fries selbstbewusst neben ihn (der diese neue Kunst ja nicht beherrschte).

Moritz tat ein übriges, indem er in seiner Medizinalordnung von 1616 und Apothekentaxe von 1617 dieser Ausbildungsform auch die erforderliche rechtliche und wirtschaftliche Absicherung angedeihen ließ, insofern die Bereitung chymischer Arzneien darin ausdrücklich nur den Apothekern selbst sowie chymiatrisch ausgebildeten Ärzten vorbehalten wurde, welche „dieses ex fundamentis gelernet und deshalben kundig und bekannt" (§ 12) seien, die Arzneien aber nur über den Apotheker abgeben dürften.[38] Hier ist also der ursprüngliche Ort,[39] an dem die Chymiatria in die Medizinalordnungen einging. Daraufhin sah sich zwei Jahre später der Mainzer Kurfürst veranlasst, unter bestimmten Bedingungen diese von Gott gegebene Kunst und ihre Produkte wie in der angrenzenden Landgrafschaft auch in seinem Kurstaat zuzulassen.

Die Verbildlichung des Heilandsrufs durch Christus als Apotheker

Aber noch etwas anderes wurde durch diese soziale Aufwertung des Apothekers erreicht. Neben seiner biblischen Bestätigung war sie eine weitere, wesentliche Voraussetzung für die Möglichkeit einer Verbildlichung oder Visualisierung des christlichen Erlösungsgedankens in der Form der lutherischen Rechtfertigungslehre durch Christus als Apotheker – obgleich im Gegensatz zu Gott oder Christus als Arzt (oder Heiler) ‚Christus als Apotheker' nicht einmal durch Luthers Bibel vorgegeben war.[40] Den literarischen Anstoß dazu hatte höchstwahrscheinlich eine als Höhepunkt der von Luther wieder aufgenommenen *Theologia medicinalis* zu geltende, mit einer Leichenpredigt auf den am 5. Februar 1618 verstorbenen Liegnitz-Briegschen Hofarzt Flaminius Gasto verbundene, mehrfach nachgedruckte Abhandlung des schlesischen Lutheraners Valerius Herberger

38 Siehe zur Medizinalordnung Moritz' von Hessen-Kassel DÜBBER (1969), 243–279.

39 Die 'chymiatrischen' Arzneien und ihre Herstellung werden hier als hessisches Spezifikum erstmals in eine Medizinalordnung und in eine Taxe (Kapitel 17: „Von denen Artzneneyen, so auf chymische art zugerichtet werden") aufgenommen; siehe DÜBBER (1969), 271 beziehungsweise 279.

40 Vgl. im einzelnen KRAFFT (2000), KRAFFT (2001) und KRAFFT (2003a). – Die inzwischen über 160 bekannt gewordenen Bilder werden im folgenden noch nach der lediglich 133 Bilder umfassenden Liste in HEIN (1992), 15–20, identifiziert.

(1562–1627) gegeben. Sie trägt den Titel: *Jesus omnium medicorum princeps et dominus*. Nach Aufzählung der größten Ärzte bis hin zu Gasto heißt es hier:

> Aber die Warheit zu bekennen / wir haben den fürnehmesten noch nit / wenn D. Flaminius lebete / er würde es selber bekennen [...]. Wer ists denn? Der klügeste / der glückseligste / der scharffsinnigste / der thewreste vnter allen ist Jesus Christus. Der Herr mein Artzt / ist der beste. Er bekennts selber allhier durch Mosen: Jch bin der HERR dein Artzt [Exodus 15,26]. [...] Jerem. 30. Vers. 13 vnd 17. Spricht er: Es kan Dich niemand heilen / Aber jch wil dich wieder gesund machen. Matth. am 9. Cap. [12] nennet er sich ausdrücklich einen Artzt / da er sagt: Die Starcken dürffen des Artztes nicht / sondern die Krancken. [...] vnd Matth. 11 [28] sitzet er als ein allgemeiner Land Doctor / vnnd ruffet alle Krancken zu sich: Kommet her zu mir / alle / die jhr müheselig vnd beladen seyd / Ich wil euch erquicken. [...] Dieser [...] ist der fürnehmste Artzt. Sind jemals gute Aertzte gewesen / er ist jnen allen gleich / sind jemals köstliche Aertzte gewesen / er ist jnen allen sehr weit vberlegen.[41]

Das wird dann in 20 Punkten vergleichend zu den besten menschlichen Leibesärzten unter Heranziehung einschlägiger Bibelstellen ausgeführt; abschließend heißt es: „Drum kan man die Reden [von Sap. 16. V. 12] artig auff die Predigt des göttlichen Worts ziehen [...]: Es heilet sie weder Kraut noch Pflaster / sondern dein Wort / das alles heilet."

Die Verbildlichung des Heilandsrufs durch Christus als ‚himmlischen Apotheker'[42] wurde daraufhin in einem Genrebild des Nürnberger protestantischen Malers Michel Herr (1591–1661) von 1619 geschaffen (Bild 1),[43] dem man noch den Bezug zum Heilandsruf deutlich ansieht, insofern es gerade Bettler, Krüppel und Arme sind, die Christus in seiner im eigentlichen Sinne ‚öffentlichen', das heißt jedermann offenen Offizin regelrecht belagern. Für eine (un)mittelbare malerische Umsetzung des literarischen Vorbildes spricht neben den inhaltlichen Bezügen schon, dass die wichtigsten der bei Herberger zitierten Bibelstellen in derselben Reihenfolge auf die Triumphfahne des Genrebildes geschrieben sind.[44]

Dieses Sinnbildmotiv hat dann, teilweise bis in unsere Tage, eine ungeheure Nachwirkung erfahren – insbesondere in der abstrahierend konzentrierten Form eines mehr oder weniger schlichten Andachtsbildes. Die ältesten erhaltenen Beispiele stammen von 1630, wie etwa die großformatigen Bilder in den Kirchen von Plötzin[45] (Bild 2) und Werder an der Havel. Bei dieser Form des Sinnbildmotivs wird das die Himmelsapotheke aufsuchende Publikum nicht mehr mit in die Darstellungsebene des Bildes aufgenommen; es ist aus dem Bild herausge-

41 HERBERGER (1618), ediert jetzt bei STEIGER (2005), 257–321; hier 268–269 und 284–285 (Johannes Anselm Steiger hatte mich das Manuskript dankenswerterweise bereits vor dem Druck einsehen lassen).

42 Zu einem etwa gleichzeitigen anderen Entwurf Michel Herrs [noch nicht bei HEIN (1992)], der ebenfalls Nachahmung fand, siehe KRAFFT (2000), KRAFFT (2001), 206–213, und KRAFFT (2003a), 142–143.

43 HEIN (1992), Bild Nr. 110; siehe KRAFFT (2003a), 118 (Farbtafel) und 36–139 – eine Kopie im Geschworenenbuch der Nürnberger Zunft der Barbiere und Wundärzte von 1626, HEIN (1992), Bild Nr. 23; siehe KRAFFT (2003a), 119 (Farbtafel) und 140–141.

44 Siehe dazu schon KRAFFT (2005), zur näheren Begründung jetzt KRAFFT (2007a).

45 HEIN (1992), Bild Nr. 113; siehe KRAFFT (2003a), 144–147.

nommen und gleichsam in den Betrachter selbst versetzt, der sich dem Bild andächtig zuwendet. Dazu wird der Heilsakt der Erlösung von den Sünden gemäß lutherischer Rechtfertigungslehre ganz auf Christus konzentriert, der die ‚geistlichen' Arzneien – die christlichen Tugenden – zu einem individuellen Compositum mischt und dem betrachtenden Gegenüber zuwägt. Die Apotheke selbst wird nur abgekürzt angedeutet durch Apotheken-Standgefäße und einen Gewichtssatz auf einem Rezepturtisch, hinter dem Christus steht und mit einer apothekenüblichen Handwaage die sowohl heilkundlich als auch christlich-symbolisch genutzte ‚Kreuzwurz' (Madelger, Kreuzenzian, auch „Heil aller Schäden" genannt) aus einem aufgerollten Drogensack abwägt – die ‚Kreuzwurz' erhält hier die symbolische Form kleiner Kreuze als Zeichen des eigenen Leidens Christi und des dem Gläubigen zur Prüfung und Festigung seines Glaubens aufzuerlegenden ‚Kreuzes'. Die ihm für die Arzneibereitung daneben zur Verfügung stehenden Ingredienzien in den Gefäßen sind, wie ihre Signaturen ausweisen, zahlreiche christliche Tugenden, von denen das Bild von Herr nur erst die drei paulinischen, Glaube, Liebe, Hoffnung, angeführt hatte.

Von den seit Michel Herrs Genrebild auf den Bildern wörtlich zitierten Bibelversen findet sich der Heilandsruf *Matthäus* 11,28 auf fast allen und *Jesaja* 55,1 auf sämtlichen protestantischen Bildern. Letzterer („Wohlan alle die ihr dürstig seid, kommt her zum Wasser, und die ihr kein Geld habt, kommt her, Kauffet und esset, kommt her und kaufft ohne Geld und umsonst, beide, Wein und Milch") diente seit dem frühen 17. Jahrhundert als biblischer Beleg für das *sola fide*-Prinzip der lutherischen Rechtfertigungslehre; und das weist auf die eigentliche Stoßrichtung des protestantischen Andachtsbildes, das immerhin während des dreißigjährigen Glaubenskrieges entstand, als Werbe- und Propagandabild des lutherischen Protestantismus hin.[46] Dass diese Deutung nicht aus der Luft gegriffen ist, zeigt die Reaktion des römischen Katholizismus in Deutschland mit dem Entwurf eines ‚Gegenbildes', das demgegenüber die Eucharistie als das Allheilmittel propagieren und verkünden lässt und den Beginn einer letztlich bis in unsere Tage nachwirkenden Tradition darstellt.[47]

Zu den abweichenden Details der katholischen Fassung gehört, dass Christus nicht eine Seelenarznei für den Betrachter abwägt und bereitet, statt des Wägeaktes die Waage vielmehr im Gleichgewicht hängt und lediglich als Symbol der Gerechtigkeit fungiert. Dadurch geht dann die Assoziation zur Seelenwägung am Tag des Jüngsten Gerichts verloren, die im Bild von Michel Herr und in den Andachtsbildern mitklingt. Das Jüngste Gericht hat allerdings im Luthertum nicht mehr die ausschließliche Entscheidungsbedeutung für das Ewige Leben der Seele des Sterblichen. An seine Stelle tritt dessen Glaube an Christus als Gottes Sohn, der keiner weiteren Vor- und Gegenleistung zur Rechtfertigung und sofortigen Erlösung durch Christus bedarf (*sola fide*), aber natürlich gestärkt und gefestigt werden muss. Insofern diente das protestantische Sinnbildmotiv auch

46 Siehe dazu KRAFFT (2003b).

47 Siehe dazu KRAFFT (2001), 108–116.

der Bekräftigung des Gläubigen in seinem Glauben, während die rundum wohnenden Katholiken in diesem Punkte weiterhin traditionell eingestellt blieben und ihr Seelenheil durch Gute Werke, Gebet, Beichte und Ablasszahlungen erkaufen zu können dachten (die dann übrigens auch in den Signaturen auf den katholischen Bildern als Seelen-Arzneien auftreten).

Christus – der Arzt, „welchem kein Patient jemals ist gestorben"

Was schon in den Titel von Valerius Herbergers Schrift Aufnahme gefunden hatte, dass dem Arzt Jesus „keiner unter seinen Patienten ist gestorben", hatte dann auch seinen Einstieg in die Thematik gebildet:

> Das walt der Herr mein Artzt [...] Jesus Christus / welcher mir und dir (lieber Leser vnd Zuhörer) vielmal das Leben hat gerettet / welcher die meisten Patienten hat / vnd welchem kein Patient jemals ist gestorben / der sich seiner Cur hat vntergeben / ohne welchen auch kein Doctor auff Erden mit Ehren kan bestehen [...].[48]

Dementsprechend gingen dann auch Verse aus dem *Johannes-Evangelium* (6,47: „Wer an mich gleubet, der hat das ewige Leben")[49] und der *Offenbarung des Johannes* (2,10: „Sey getrew bis an den Tod / So wil ich dir die Krone des lebens geben")[50] in Bildbeispiele ein, die zur Zeit und im Sinne des Pietismus entstanden – wie beispielsweise ein Bild des ausgehenden 17. Jahrhunderts aus der lutherischen Reichsstadt Biberach im Württembergischen,[51] welches das älteste mir bekannte ikonographische Beispiel für die pietistische Wiederbelebung des lutherischen *sola scriptura*-Prinzips bildet: Es reichen nicht mehr die Signaturen, es wird auch das allein zählende Schriftzeugnis für diese Tugend erläuternd hinzu gesetzt, wie es literarisch Konrad Rosbach in seinem *Paradeißgaertlein* 1588 erstmals für die Pflanzen getan hatte.

Dieses Prinzip wird dann auf einem großformatigen Bild von 1730 aus Nürnberg mit dem Titel *Wohlbestellte Seelen-Apotheke*[52] und auf einer etwas variierenden Replik, die für die 1740 geweihte Kirche auf Schloss Wittgenstein, einem Zentrum des radikalen Pietismus, gemalt wurde,[53] auf die Spitze getrieben: Mehr als hundert mit Bibelstellen versehene Signaturen konnte ich auf ihnen entziffern, daneben Bibelverse, und unter diesen neben *Matthäus* 11,28 und *Jesaja* 55,1 an hervorragenden Stellen etwa auf einem vom Rezepturtisch

48 HERBERGER (1618), 1 [= 361 bei STEIGER (2005)].

49 Zitiert zur Signatur ‚Ewiges Leben' in Bild Nr. 89 bei HEIN (1992).

50 HEIN (1992), Bild Nr. 118; zitiert zur Signatur ‚Beständigkeit' in HEIN (1992), Bild Nr. 89 (siehe vorstehende Anmerkung).

51 HEIN (1992), Bild Nr. 89; erstmals beschrieben in KRAFFT (2001), 45–48; siehe auch KRAFFT (2003a), 173–176.

52 HEIN (1992), Bild Nr. 25; siehe dazu KRAFFT (2001), 27–31 (hier waren die Signaturen noch nicht entziffert worden).

53 HEIN (1992), Bild Nr. 119; siehe KRAFFT (2003a), 197–207 (hier wurden die Signaturen erstmals entziffert).

herabhängenden Rezeptbogen *Römer-Brief* 10,9: „So du mit deinem munde bekennest Jesum, daß er der Herr sey, und glaubest in deinem Hertzen, daß [Gott] ihn von den todten aufferweckt, so wirstu leben", und unter der Fensterbank *Sapientia Salomonis* 16,12-13: „Es heilet sie weder Kraut noch Pflaster, sondern Dein wort, Herr, welches alles heilet; denn du hast gewalt über Leben und über Todt."

Diese Ausrichtung der Thematik auf die Heilige Schrift als Gottes Wort und auf das Sinnbildmotiv sind in der lutherischen Orthodoxie und im Pietismus so geläufig, dass ein Wissen um sie auch in anderem Zusammenhang häufig einfach vorausgesetzt werden kann und auch wurde.[54] Als Beispiel kann hierfür ein Kupferstich von Caspaar Luyken (1672–1708) zum ‚Apotheker' in Christoff Weigels (1654–1725) 1698 in Regensburg erschienenem Ständebuch[55] dienen, in dem der Darstellung der Tätigkeiten in einer Leibesapotheke erst durch den hinzugesetzten Text die zusätzliche, zu erschließende Sinnebene beigegeben wird: Über dem Bild stehen nach der Überschrift *Der Apotheker* die auf den Text zum voranstehenden ‚Materialisten' Bezug nehmenden Worte: „Der Tranck von Christi Blut Stärckt u[nd] macht wolgemut", und unter dem Bild:

> Gleich wie des Apothekers Haus,
> dem Krancken Leib theilt Mitteln aus,
> So ist für Schmertzen, die uns grämen,
> für Seelen-Leid, das uns befällt,
> ein Schatz von Mitteln auffgestellt,
> in Gottes Wort, man darff nur nehmen.

Eines wird allerdings in der medizinischen und in der Erbauungsliteratur vor den Heil-Erfolg gesetzt: die reuige Bekennung der eigenen Sündhaftigkeit, wie sie schon in der Inschrift des Lemgoer Apotheken-Erkers vorausgesetzt wird. Auch das wird im Rahmen des protestantischen Sinnbildmotivs deutlich betont in der letzten nachhaltigen protestantischen Umgestaltung des Motivs, von der insgesamt noch 18 erhaltene Beispiele bisher bekannt geworden sind, das älteste von 1713, die jüngsten aus dem deutschsprachigen Raum von 1747, denen sogar (als einzige Beispiele eines Überschreitens der deutschen Sprachgrenzen) drei schwedische Bilder und ein russischer Kupferstich folgen. Allen gemeinsam ist der grundsätzliche Bildaufbau[56] (siehe Bild 3)[57]: Christus steht hinter einem die ganze Bildbreite einnehmenden abgewinkelten Rezepturtisch mit Gefäßen und einer Lade mit Kreuzwurz, in die seine Linke greift; hinter sich ein Repositorium

54 Siehe dazu KRAFFT (2001), 215–233.

55 WEIGEL (1698).

56 Zur gesamten Bildgruppe siehe KRAFFT (2001), 50–62, KRAFFT (2003a), 188–196, sowie KRAFFT (2003c).

57 HEIN (1992), Bild Nr. 128 (noch mit dem alten Standort „Newton" [sic!]). Das Bild befindet sich seit den frühen 1970er Jahren in The Country Doctor Museum, Bailey (NC), USA. Einzelheiten zum Bild waren in Europa bisher unbekannt, auch in Krafft (2003c); siehe jedoch Blumberg (1967). Ich verdanke die näheren Angaben und die Aufnahme der Managerin des Museums Anne Anderson, wofür ihr auch an dieser Stelle bestens gedankt sei.

mit Schubladen und zwei Reihen Standgefäßen, einer Bibel mit dem Lamm Gottes sowie einem Wappen- oder vielmehr Ladenschild mit dem Vers des *Lukas-Evangeliums* 15,2: „Dieser nimpt die Sünder an"; in der oben das Bild abschließenden Kartusche wird neben anderen für das Bildmotiv üblichen Bibelversen der Heilandsruf zitiert, auf dem vom Tisch wie von einem Altar herabhängenden Tuch (Antependium), plakativ dem Betrachter entgegengehalten, zu oberst der Vers *Jesaja* 55,1. Auf der dem Beschauer zugekehrten Seite des Rezepturtisches steht eine gelegentlich männliche, ursprünglich wohl aber weiblich gedachte Person, die auf eine der Waagschalen der ihr von Christus entgegengehaltenen Waage ein Spruchband legt mit dem Anfang der zweiten Strophe des Liedes *Allein zu dir, Herr Jesu Christ, mein Hoffnung steht auf Erden* von Konrad Hubert (1507–1577),[58] dessen Anfangsverse schon Valerius Herberger herangezogen hatte: „Mein Sünd' sind schwer und übergroß / und reuen mich von Herzen". Das Lied mit den Bitten an Christus war so bekannt, dass es von jedem Leser selbst ergänzt werden konnte zu: „derselben mach mich frei und los / durch deinen Tod und Schmerzen; / und zeige deinem Vater an, / daß du hast g'nug für mich getan, / so werd ich los der Sünden Last. / Erhalt mich fest in dem, was du versprochen hast." Teufelsgestalten suchen die Waagschale herabzuziehen, während das Kruzifix all die Sünden leicht aufwiegt. Die Person soll wohl die biblische Sünderin *par excellence* Maria Magdalena darstellen.

Alle auf diesen Bildern anklingenden Einzelheiten und Assoziationen werden nun durch das eindeutige Bildzitat dieser aktuellsten protestantischen Version auf das Bekrönungsstück eines Gedenksteins für den Apotheker Gottfried Haugk in Kamenz[59] übertragen (Bild 4). Er war am 24. August 1724 fast 55-jährig gestorben und auf dem St. Marien-Kirchhof beerdigt worden; die Setzung von gleich aufgebauten Gedenksteinen für insgesamt sechs Mitglieder der verschwägerten Familien Haugk und Reichel erfolgte zwischen 1729 und 1732. Der verbindende Topos aller sechs Reliefdarstellungen ist der Tod als Knochenmann in einer auf das Sterben der Person bezogenen Szene.

Wie in der pietistischen Bildgruppe steht auch auf dem Haugk-Relief Christus mit ausgebreiteten Armen hinter einem abgewinkelten Rezepturtisch und Verkaufstresen und vor einem Repositorium. Der Bezug zur Verbildlichung des Heilandsrufs wird bestätigt durch das (hier verkürzte) Zitat aus *Matthäus* 11,28 im Zwickel rechts über Christus: „Kommet her zu / mir alle die ihr mühs[elig …]". Der ihn aufsucht ist aber ein besonderer Sünder, ein vornehm gekleideter Herr mit Stock, nämlich der Apotheker Gottfried Haugk selbst, dem der Tod huckepack im Nacken sitzt. Er ist also nach seinem leiblichen Tod bei Jesus Christus gut aufgehoben und dem ewigen Leben anvertraut worden. Das Spruchband über dem Relief enthält gleichsam das Motto des gesamten Steins: „Kein Arzt mehr zu finden ist vor mich denn nur bey Jesu Christ", der nämlich statt des begrenzten irdischen das jenseitige ewige Leben verleiht.

58 Evangelisches Gesangbuch (1992), Nr. 232, Strophe 2.

59 Siehe dazu KRAFFT (2005).

Die Inschrift des Steines enthält dann eine kurze Biographie, gleichsam eine kurzgefasste Leichenpredigt in der Tradition, wie sie Martin Luther begründet hatte. Danach sollte durch den Aufweis eines gottgefälligen Lebens mit der daraus folgenden Gewissheit eines himmlischen Weiterlebens neben dem Trost für die Hinterbliebenen gezeigt werden, dass auch im Schoße der lutherischen Kirche ein seliges Sterben möglich sei.[60] Das wird auf dem Sockel des Steines noch bekräftigt mit den Versen aus Paulus' *Römer-Brief* 7,24: „Ich elender Mensch, wer will mich erlösen von dem Leiden des Todes“ und 8, 31/32: „Jst Gott für vns / Wer mag wider vns sein?“ (fortzusetzen wäre: „Welcher auch seines eigen Sons nicht hat verschonet / Sondern hat jn fur vns alle da hin gegeben / Wie solt er vns mit jm nicht alles schencken?“).

Es ist genau dieser Trost, im Leben und im Tod, der die Wiederauferstehung verspricht, den im Sinne des *sola fide*-Prinzips einerseits die protestantische Erbauungs- und Trostliteratur einschließlich der Leichenpredigten, andererseits aber auch das Andachtsbildmotiv ‚Christus als Apotheker‘ dem Gläubigen vermitteln soll. Hatte Valerius Herbergers literarische Leichenpredigt mit ihrer ausgeprägten *Theologia medicinalis* die Ikonographie des protestantischen Andachtsbildmotivs erst angeregt, so kommen die beiden seitdem getrennten Traditionen auf diesem Gedenkstein gleichsam wieder zusammen. Herberger hatte der Leichenpredigt die mehr biographischen Gedenkworte des gemeinsamen Freundes Matthäus Vechner hinzugesetzt, die nach der Begrüssung mit den Worten beginnen: „Daß *contra vim mortis*, kein *medicamen in hortis* sey / das beweiset die sehr klägliche / aber doch selige Heimfahrt des weiland / Edlen / Großachtbaren / Hochgelahrten vnd weitberühmten Herren *Doctoris Flaminij Gastonis*“; denn obwohl er durch seine Kunst viele vor dem Tode errettet hätte, „So hat er doch / gleich allen andern Menschen / nach dem vnwandelbarem Rhat Gottes / selbst auch siechen vnd sterben müssen.“[61]

Nehmen wir statt der hier anfangs zitierten sprichwörtlichen Wendung „dagegen [meist den Tod] ist kein Kraut gewachsen“ den Vers aus *Sapientia Salomonis* 16, 12 in Luthers Übersetzung („Denn es heilete sie weder Kraut noch Pflaster / Sondern dein Wort Herr / welches alles heilet“), der gerade auf den pietistischen Bildern häufig zitiert wird,[62] so werden die Parallelen zum Haugk-Gedenkstein sehr deutlich. Dessen Inschrift beginnt: „Dieser LeichenStein erinnert Dich, Leser, daß vorm Tod kein Kraut gewachsen. Denn unweit davon liegen die Gebeine [des] Herrn Gottfried Haugkens, vornehmen Bürgers und weltberühmten Apoteckers allhier [...].“ Sie endet zweckgemäß mit den Worten:

60 Vgl. hierzu LENZ (2002) und MOORE (2002).

61 HERBERGER (1618), 134–135; bei STEIGER (2005), 298–299.

62 Neben den bereits genannten Bildern Nr. 25 und 119 bei HEIN (1992) findet sich der Sapientia-Vers in diesem Sinne auf einem nach 1917 verschollenen Andachtsbild [HEIN (1992), Bild Nr. 60] noch aus der ersten Hälfte des 17. Jahrhunderts, von dem es je eine Primär- und eine Sekundärkopie aus dem frühen 20. Jahrhundert gibt [HEIN (1992), Bild Nr. 45 und 46], dazu siehe KRAFFT (2001), 23–38. Vgl. auch die oben zitierte Passage bei DIETERICH (1627).

„Nachdem er viel Segen von Gott erlanget und manche Creuz Probe ausgehalten […] starb nach einer langwirigen Kranckheit seelig […].“ Gegen den Tod ist zwar auf Erden kein Kraut gewachsen, aber Gottes Wort verheißt das ewige Leben.

Postmortale Arznei

Ein beredtes zeitgenössisches Zeugnis für diese Form des Trostes bietet auch des Berliner Predigers Daniel Schönemann (1695–1737) Trostschrift *Der Sarg Als Ein Rechter Artzt* von 1725, auf deren aufzuklappendem Titelkupfer Christus als Apotheker an einem offenen Sarg die „Universal-Medicin“ bereitet und der Sargdeckel verkündet (Bild 5): „Wer kranck ist hat hier Artzeney / Es sey die kranckheit wie sie sey“, verbildlicht durch Pflaster und Arzneien in Apotheken-Standgefäßen, die im offenen Sarg rundherum aufgestellt sind. Einige seiner gereimten Verse mögen wenigstens die Anklänge an die *Theologia medicinalis* andeuten:[63]

Wenn Kraut und Pflaster nichts in unsrer Kranckheit nützt,
    Will keine Besserung sich bey den Krancken zeigen,
So kommt der Sarg und Hilfft; Wer hier liegt, wird beschützt,
    Er kehret Ach und Weh in einen frohen Reigen.
Was Paracelso schön, Galeno gut gedeucht,
    Kan diesem Sarge doch die Wage nimmer halten,
Weil ich allein den Sarg aus GOttes Wort beleucht. […]
Des Sarges Medicin ist wohl universal,
    Der Weisen=Stein ist nichts, es wird nichts damit werden […].
Die Aerttzte flicken nur, und es wird nichts daraus, […]
Doch nimt der Sarg uns auf in das Gesunde=Hauß,
    So finden wir allda vollkommne Wunder=Curen.
Die Apothecke ist mit allem angefüllt,
    Zur Stärckung, Linderung ist alles hier zu haben,
Das nehmen wir zu uns, wenn uns ein Tuch verhüllt,
    Da wo man Mangel glaubt, sind Wunderseltne Gaben.
Zwar vormahls war es nicht also, mein Sarg, mit dir,
    Du warst vorhin [= vorher] ein Gifft und eine Marterkammer,
Nur JEsus machet dich zu einem Lust=Revier,
    Zum Ziel gehäuffter Noth, zum Schutz für allen Jammer.
Die Apotheke hat er in dir angelegt,
    Von ihm ist nur zu dir die Artzeney gekommen […].
Mein Sarg, ob deine Feinde schreyen,
    Daß du ein Feind der Aertzte bist,
Weiß ich doch deine Artzeneyen,
    Ich glaube als ein rechter Christ […].
Nun lach ich aller andern Aertzte,
    Nachdem ich dich als Artzt erkandt;

63 SCHÖNMANN (1725), 24–25, 29 und 47.

denn Christus verteilt an seine Gläubigen kostenfrei und ohne Gegengabe ‚postmortale Arzneien', wie ich sie in der Kapitelüberschrift nenne, und die helfen gegen den ‚leiblichen Tod', gegen den keine leibliche Arznei hilft, kein Kraut gewachsen ist, indem sie ihn gegen das ‚ewige Leben' eintauschen.

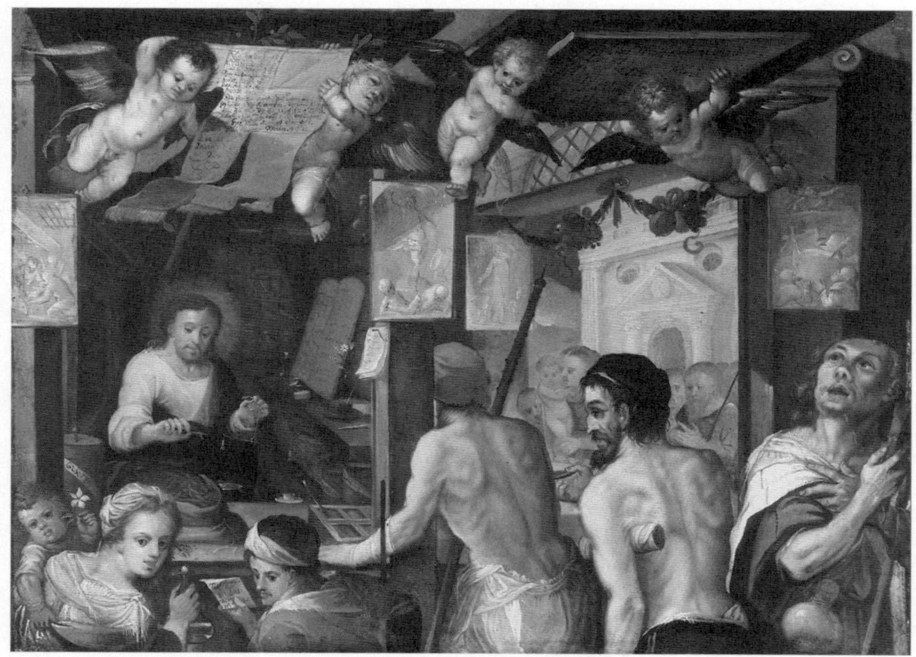

Bild 1: *Christus als Apotheker* – Genrebild (1619) von Michel Herr (Marburg, Universitätsmuseum für Kunst und Kulturgeschichte). (Foto: F. Krafft; Bildsammlung F. Krafft)

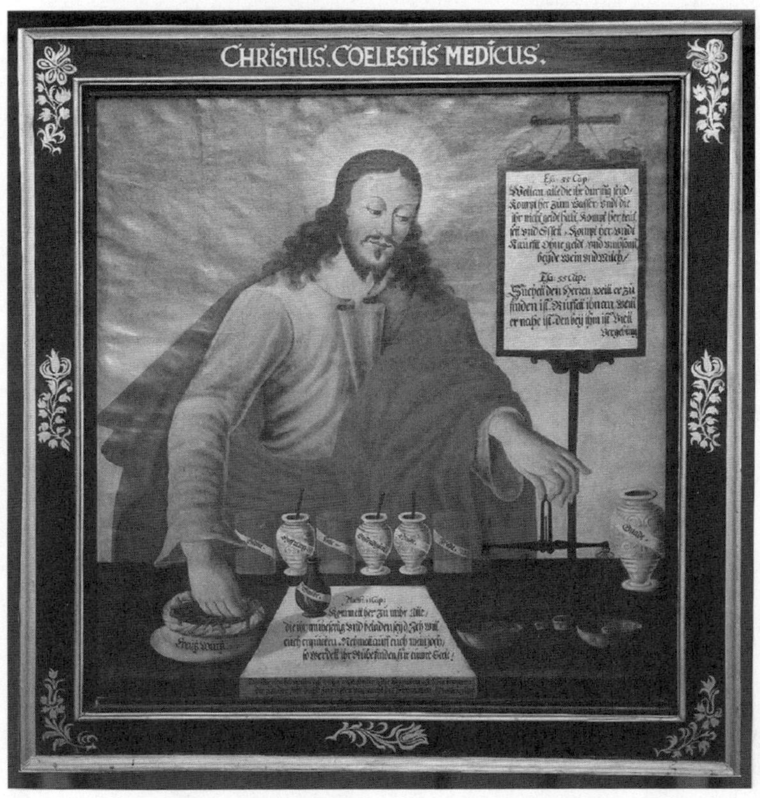

Bild 2: *Christus als Apotheker* – Lutherische Dorfkirche von Plötzin (Foto: F. Krafft; Bildsammlung F. Krafft)

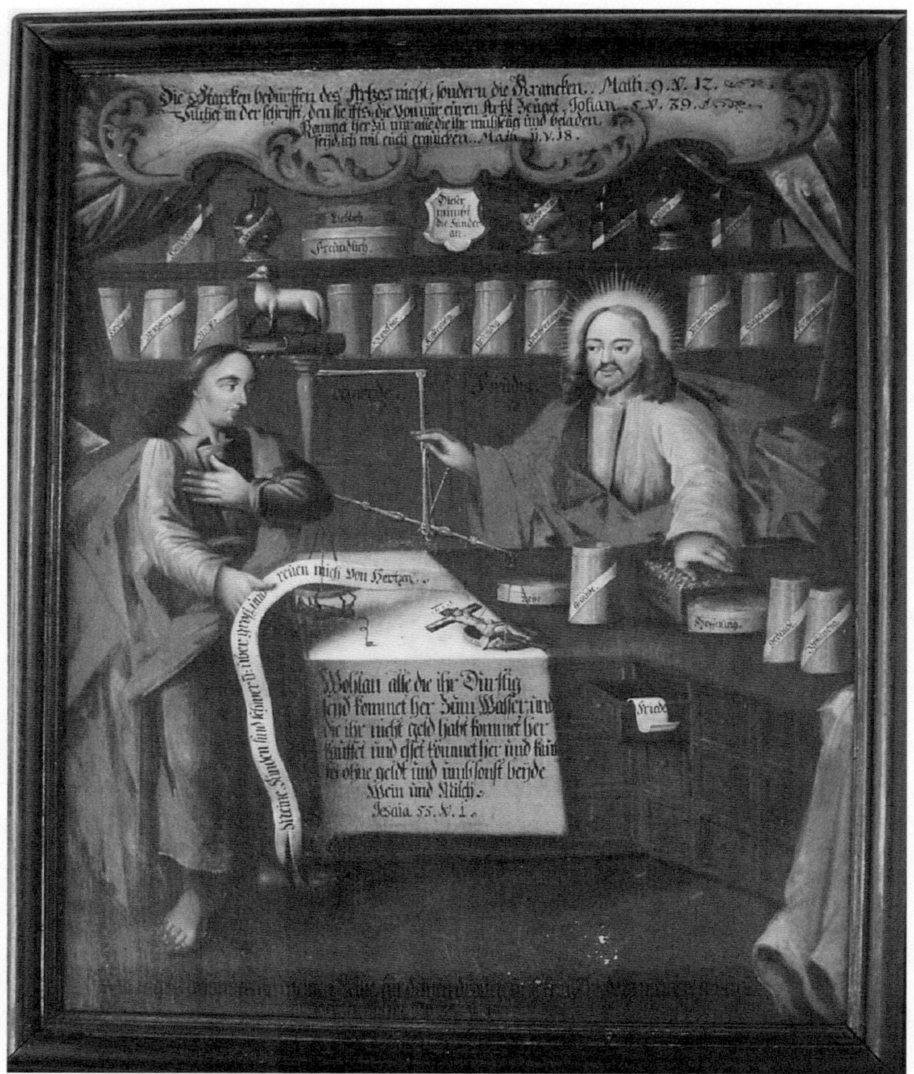

Bild 3: *Christus als Apotheker mit reumütigem Sünder* – Ölbild (1. Hälfte des 18. Jahrhunderts), 86 x 144 mm (Bailey, NC, USA, The Country Doctor Museum). (Foto: The Country Doctor Museum; Bildsammlung F. Krafft)

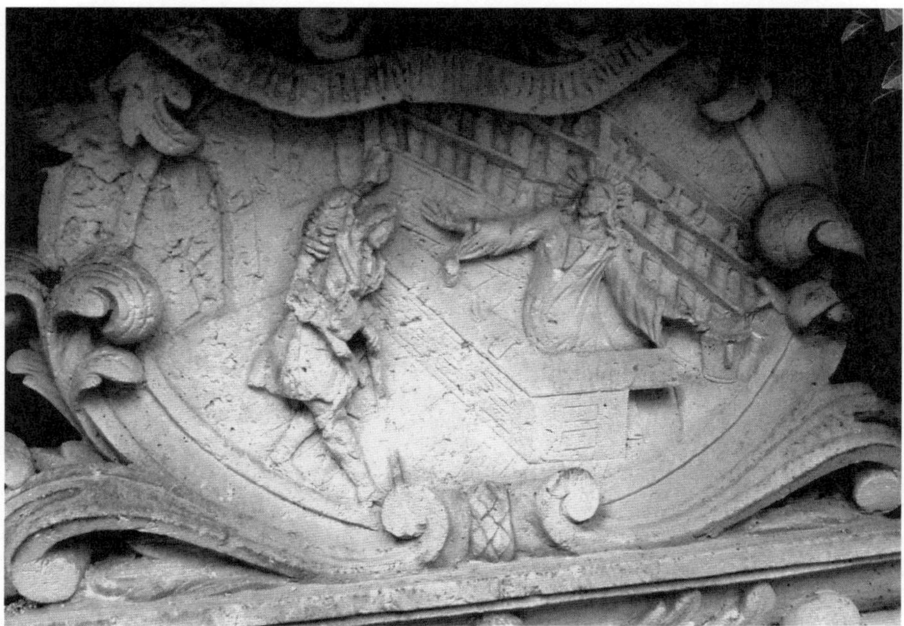

Bild 4: *Der vom Tod gepackte Apotheker Gottfried Haugk sucht Christus in der Himmlischen Apotheke auf* – Sandstein-Relief auf einem Gedenkstein (zwischen 1729 und 1732) auf dem Kirchhof St. Marien in Kamenz. (Foto: F. Krafft; Bildsammlung F. Krafft)

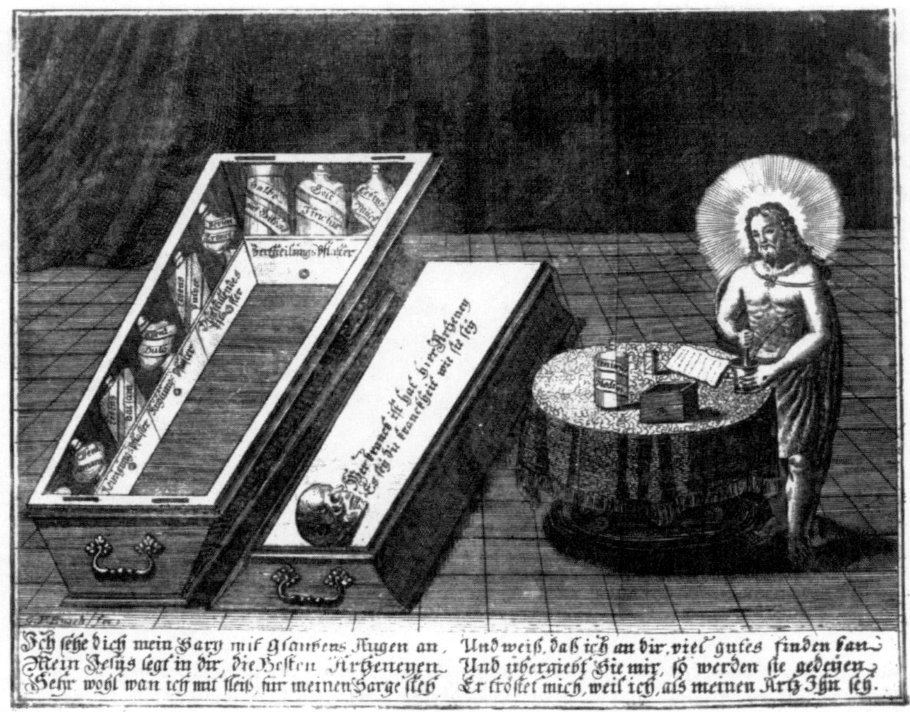
Ich sehe dich mein Sarg mit Glaubens Augen an, Und weiß, daß ich an dir, viel gutes finden kan:
Mein Jesus legt in dir, die besten Artzeneyen. Und übergiebt Sie mir, so werden sie gedeyen,
Sehr wohl wan ich mit fleiß, für meinen Sarge steh Er tröstet mich, weil ich, als meinen Artz Ihn seh.

Bild 5: *Der Sarg Als Ein Rechter Artzt* – Titelkupfer zum gleichnamigen Buch von Daniel Schönemann (Berlin 1725). (Foto: SUB Göttingen; Bildsammlung F. Krafft)

Quellen- und Literaturverzeichnis

Altmann (1972)
Altmann, Eckard: Christian Friedrich Richter. Arzt, Apotheker und Liederdichter des Halleschen Pietismus. Witten: Luther-Verlag, 1972.

Blumberg (1967)
Blumberg, Sydney N.: Christ the Apothecary of the Soul. In: Journal of the American Pharmaceutical Association NS 7 (1967), 618.

Brunschwyg (1538)
Brunschwyg, Hieronymus: Haußapotheck. Zu yeden leibs gebresten / für den gemainen man / und das arm Landuolck / Durch Hieronymum Braunschweig getrewlich zu samenn tragen unnd an tag gegeben. Augsburg: Steiner, 1538.

Dadder (1961)
Dadder, Hans: Das Apothekenwesen von Stadt und Erzstift Mainz. Mit der Mainzer Medizinalordnung und großen Apothekentaxe von 1618. Frankfurt/M.: Govi-Verlag, 1961 (Quellen und Studien zur Geschichte der Pharmazie 2).

Dehmel (1996)
Dehmel, Gisela: Die Arzneimittel in der Physikotheologie. Mit einem Geleitwort von Fritz Krafft. Münster: Lit Verlag, 1996 (Physikotheologie im historischen Kontext 5).

Dietenberger (1534)
Dietenberger, Johan: Biblia, beider Allt vnnd Newes Testamenten / fleissig / treülich vnn Christlich / nach alter / inn Christlicher Kirchen gehabter Translation / mit außlegung etlicher dunckeler ort / vnnd besserung viler verrückter wort vnd sprüch / so biß anhere inn anderen kurtz außgegangnen theutschen Bibeln gespürt vnd gesehen. Durch D. Johan Dietenberger / new verdeutscht. Gott zu ewiger ehre / vnnd wolfarth seiner heiligen Christlichen Kirchen. Mit Röm. König. Ma. Gnad vnd Freyheyt. Köln: Peter Quentel [Drucker Peter Jordan, Mainz], 1534 [Wolfenbüttel HAB Bibel-S. 2° 24].

Dietenberger (1540)
Dietenberger, Johan: Biblia, beider Allt vnnd Newes Testamenten / fleissig / treülich vnn Christlich / nach alter / in Christlicher Kirchen gehabter Translation / mit außlegung etlicher dunckeler ort / vnnd besserung vieler verrückter wordt vnd sprüch / so biß anhere in andern kurtz außgegangnen theutschen Bibeln gespürt vnd gesehen. Durch D. Johan Dietenberger / Zum andern mall Corrigieret vnn verbessert in sÿnen leben. Köln: Alopecius, 1540 [Wolfenbüttel HAB A 112 Helmst].

Dieterich (1627)
Dieterich, Conrad: Das Buch der Weißheit Salomonis also: In vnterschiedlichen Predigen erkläret und außgelegt […]. 2 Theile, Ulm: Saur, 1627, 1632 (auch Nürnberg: Endter 1641–1657 und 1667–1676; unter dem Titel: Ecclesiastes Das ist: Der Prediger Salomo […]. Ulm: Görlin 1642).

Dübber (1969)
Dübber, Irmgard: Die Geschichte des Medizinal- und Apothekenwesens in Hessen-Kassel und Hessen-Marburg von den Anfängen bis zum Dreißigjährigen Krieg. Naturwiss. Dissertation Marburg, 1969.

Francke (1701)
Francke, August Hermann: Die Fußstapffen des noch lebenden und waltenden liebreichen und getreuen Gottes, [...] durch den ausführlichen Bericht Vom Wäysen-Hause, Armen-Schulen und übrigen Armen-Verpflegung zu Glaucha an Halle [...] entdecket von August Hermann Francke. Halle: Waisenhaus, 1701.

Francke (1709)
Francke, August Hermann: Segensvolle Fußstapfen des noch lebenden und waltenden liebreichen und getreuen Gottes, zur Beschämung des Unglaubens und Stärckung des Glaubens, entdecket durch eine wahrhafte und umständliche Nachricht von dem Wäysen-Hause und übrigen Anstalten zu Glaucha vor Halle, welche im Jahr 1701. zum Druck befördert, ietzo aber zum dritten mal ediret, und bis auf gegenwärtiges Jahr fortgesetzet. Halle: Waisenhaus, 1709.

Gutmann (1975)
Gutmann, Siegfried: Alte deutsche Apotheken. Ausschnitte aus 700 Jahren deutscher Apothekengeschichte. Ausgabe 1975/10. Ettlingen: W. Spitzner Arzneimittelfabrik, 1975.

Hein (1992)
Hein, Wolfgang-Hagen: Christus als Apotheker. 2., neubearbeitete Aufl., Frankfurt a. M.: Govi-Verlag, 1992 (Monographien zur pharmazeutischen Kulturgeschichte 3).

Helm (2001)
Helm, Jürgen: Der Hallesche Pietismus und das Gesundheitswesen in Brandenburg-Preußen. In: Müller-Bahlke, Thomas (Hrsg.): Gott zur Ehr und zu des Landes Besten. Die Franckeschen Stiftungen und Preußen: Aspekte einer alten Allianz. Ausstellung in den Franckeschen Stiftungen zu Halle vom 26. Juni bis 28. Oktober 2001. Halle: Verlag der Franckeschen Stiftungen, 2001 (Kataloge der Franckeschen Stiftungen zu Halle 8), 260–272.

Helm (2004)
Helm, Jürgen: Christian Friedrich Richters Kurtzer und deutlicher Unterricht (1705) – Medizinische Programmschrift des Halleschen Pietismus. In: Toellner, Richard (Hrsg.): Die Geburt einer sanften Medizin. Die Franckeschen Stiftungen als Begegnungsstätte von Medizin und Pietismus im frühen 18. Jahrhundert. Tagungsband zum internationalen Symposion der Franckeschen Stiftungen vom 16. bis 19. April 1998. Halle: Verlag der Franckeschen Stiftungen, 2004, 25–37.

Herberger (1618)
Herberger, Valerius: Jesus omnium medicorum princeps et dominus. Sanator Fidelium aegrorum & aegrotorum, ipsorum quoque Medicinae Doctorum. JESVS Der Herr mein Artzt / der fürnemeste / klügeste vnd allerglückseligste Doctor, welchem keiner vnter seinen Patienten ist gestorben. Beschawet aus der letzten Zeil / Exod. 15, Jch bin der Herr dein Artzt. I. Zu Ehren / seiner grossen Trew / II. Zu gefallen / allen Doctoribus Medicinae, III. Zum Gedechtnis aber / des tewren H. Doctoris Flaminii Gastonis, Fürstlicher Gnaden von Lignitz vnd Brieg / so wol auch der löblichen Stadt Guraw [= Guhrau] trewen Medici. Welcher seliglich entschlaffen Anno 1618. Den 5. Februarii, vnd den 21. Hernach in grosser Versamlung begraben worden. Frawenstadt [= Fraustadt] 1618 (auch Leipzig: Thomae Schürers Erben, 1618, sowie in: V. Herberger: Trawrbinden [...] Theil 5, Leipzig: Thomae Schürers Erben, 1618 und 1622).

Hofheinz & Bröer (2003)
Hofheinz, Ralf-Dieter; Bröer, Ralf: Zwischen Gesundheitspädagogik und Kausalitätstheorie. Melanchthons „Theologie der Krankheit“. In: Frank, Günter (Hrsg.): Fragmenta Melanchthoniana, Bd. 1. Zur Geistesgeschichte des Mittelalters und der frühen Neuzeit. Heidelberg: Verlag Regionalkultur, 2003, 69–86.

Huberinus (1555)
Huberinus, Caspar: Spiegel der Haußzucht, Jesus Syrach genandt / Sambt einer kurtzen Außlegung. Für die armen Haußväter / vnd ire gesinde [...]. Nürnberg: Ulrich Neuber & Johann Vom-Berg Erben [Drucker], 1555 [zuerst Nürnberg: Hans Daubmann (Drucker), 1553; weitere Ausgaben: Nürnberg 1556, 1558, 1565, 1570, 1571, 1580, 1588, Frankfurt am Mayn: Feyerabent, 1569 (unter dem Titel: Spiegel der Geistlichen Haußzucht. Auslegung und erklerung vber das Buch Jesus Syrach ...)].

Kant (1902–1923)
Kant, Immanuel: Gesammelte Schriften, hrsg. von der Preußischen Akademie der Wissenschaften. Abt. I: Werke. 9 Bände, Berlin: Reimer, 1902–1923 [Nachdruck 1969–1972. Hier: Kritik der Urteilskraft; Kritik der reinen Vernunft. Zitiert wird nach den Seiten der Originalausgaben, die in modernen Ausgaben verzeichnet sind; A = erste, B = zweite Auflage].

Krafft (1996)
Krafft, Fritz: „Pharmako-Theologie". In: Die Pharmazie 51 (1996), 422–426; wieder abgedruckt in: Büttner, Manfred; Richter, Frank (Hrsg.): Forschungen zur Physikotheologie im Aufbruch 3. Münster: Lit Verlag, 1996 (Physikotheologie im historischen Kontext 4), 127–138.

Krafft (1999)
Krafft, Fritz: „Die Arznei kommt vom Herrn, und der Apotheker bereitet sie ...". Biblische Rechtfertigung der Apothekerkunst im Protestantismus. Apotheken-Auslucht in Lemgo und Pharmako-Theologie. Stuttgart: Wissenschaftliche Verlagsgesellschaft, 1999 (Quellen und Studien zur Geschichte der Pharmazie 76).

Krafft (2000)
Krafft, Fritz: Eine „neue" Christus-als-Apotheker-Darstellung von Michael Herr. Überlegungen zur Herkunft des Bild-Motivs. In: Geschichte der Pharmazie – DAZ Beilage 52, Nr. 1/2 (2000), 2–15.

Krafft (2001)
Krafft, Fritz: Christus als Apotheker. Ursprung, Aussage und Geschichte eines christlichen Sinnbildes. Marburg: Universitätsbibliothek, 2001 (Schriften der Universitätsbibliothek Marburg 104).

Krafft (2002)
Krafft, Fritz: Apothekenerker von Lemgo. Künstlerisches Zeugnis für ein Reformprogramm der Pharmazie. In: Pharmazeutische Zeitung 147 (2002), 2860–2865.

Krafft (2003a)
Krafft, Fritz: Christus ruft in die Himmelsapotheke. Die Verbildlichung des Heilandsrufs durch Christus als Apotheker. Begleitbuch und Katalog zur Ausstellung im Museum Altomünster (29. November 2002 bis 26. Januar 2003). Stuttgart: Wissenschaftliche Verlagsgesellschaft, 2003 (Quellen und Studien zur Geschichte der Pharmazie 81).

Krafft (2003b)
Krafft, Fritz: Die Pharmazie im Dienste der Propagierung lutherischer Rechtfertigungslehre. Zur Bildaussage eines weitverbreiteten protestantischen Sinnbildmotivs. In: Berichte zur Wissenschaftsgeschichte 26 (2003), 157–182.

Krafft (2003c)
Krafft, Fritz: Christus in der Himmelsapotheke mit reumütigem/r Sünder/in. Die pietistische Erweiterung eines protestantischen Andachtsbildmotivs. In: Friedrich, Christoph; Bernschneider-Reif, Sabine (Hrsg.): Rosarium litterarum. Beiträge zur Pharmazie- und Wissenschaftsgeschichte. Festschrift zum 65. Geburtstag von Peter Dilg. Frankfurt/M.: Govi-Verlag, 2003, 161–182.

Krafft (2005)
Krafft, Fritz: „Dieser LeichenStein erinnert Dich, Leser, dass vorm Tod kein Kraut gewachsen“. Zu der Gedenksteinsetzung für Mitglieder der Familie des Apothekers Gottfried Haugk in Kamenz. In: Zwischen Großer Röder und Kleiner Spree. Geschichte – Natur – Landschaft 3 (2005), 18–40.

Krafft (2007a)
Krafft, Fritz: Ein kurzzeitiger Aufschwung der Medizinischen Fakultät der Universität Marburg. Johannes Hartmanns Professur für Chymiatria (1609) und die Vereinigung von alter und neuer medizinisch-pharmazeutischer Denkweise. In: Dilg, Peter (Hrsg.): Pharmazie in Marburg. Historische und aktuelle Aspekte. Berlin: Verlag für Wissenschafts- und Regionalgeschichte [im Druck].

Krafft (2007b)
Krafft, Fritz: Das weitverbreitete Andachtsbild „Christus als Apotheker“. Eine aus Schlesien initiierte Visualisierung der Theologia medicinalis. In: Jahrbuch des Gerhard-Möbus-Instituts für Schlesienforschung [im Druck].

Kühlmann & Telle (1996)
Kühlmann, Wilhelm; Telle, Joachim (Hrsg.): Oswaldus Crollius, De signaturis internis rerum. Die lateinische Editio princeps (1609) und die deutsche Erstübersetzung (1623). Stuttgart: Steiner, 1996 (Heidelberger Studien zur Naturkunde der frühen Neuzeit 5).

Lenz (1992)
Lenz, Rudolf: Artikel Leichenpredigt. In: Killy, Walter (Hrsg.): Literatur Lexikon, Bd. 13 (Begriffe, Realien, Methoden, hrsg. von Volker Meid). Gütersloh, München: Bertelsmann Lexikon Verlag, 1992, 509–511.

Leo Jud (1530)
Leo Jud: Apocryphi. Biblische Bücher so wiewol bey den Alten vnder Biblischer Schrifft nit gezelt / yedoch bewerdt / nutzlich / vnd in hohem brauch. Newlich verteutscht durch Leo / genant Jud. Straßburg: Hans Knobloch, 1530 [Wolfenbüttel HAB Bibel-S. 4° 240].

Luther WA
Martin Luther: Werke. Kritische Gesamtausgabe [Weimarer Ausgabe]. Abt. I: Werke. 60 Bde., Weimar: H. Böhlaus Nachfolger, ab 1883.

Mathesius (1586)
Mathesius, Johannes: Syrach Mathesij, Das ist / Christliche, Lehrhaffte / Trostreiche vnd lustige Erklerung vnd Außlegung des schönen Haußbuchs [...].3 Theile, Leipzig: Johan. Beyer [Drucker], 1586 [auch 1588–1589 und Leipzig: Voigt, 1598].

Moore (2002)
Moore, Cornelia Niekus: Das erzählte Leben in der lutherischen Leichenpredigt. Anfang und Entwicklung im 16. Jahrhundert. In: Wolfenbütteler Barock-Nachrichten 29 (2002), 3–32.

Neuburger (1926)
Neuburger, Max: Die Lehre von der Heilkraft der Natur im Wandel der Zeit. Stuttgart: Enke, 1926.

Poeckern (1984)
Poeckern, Hans-Joachim: Die Hallischen Waisenhaus-Arzeneyen. Kommentar, Glossar und Transkription. Leipzig: Edition Leipzig, 1984.

Richter (1705)
Richter, Christian Friedrich: Kurtzer und deutlicher Unterricht Von Dem Leibe und natürlichen Leben des Menschen [...]. Halle: Waisenhaus, 1705 [Nachdrucke Leipzig: Edition Leipzig, 1984 und Zürich: SV international, Schweizer Verlagshaus, 1985].

Rohr (1740)
Rohr, Julius Bernhard von: Phyto-Theologia, oder Vernunft- und Schriftmaeßiger Versuch, wie aus dem Reich der Gewächse die Allmacht, Weisheit und Guete und Gerechtigkeit des großen Schoepfers und Erhalters aller Dinge von den Menschen erkannt und sein allerheiligster Name hiervor gepriesen werden möge. Frankfurt/M., Leipzig: Michael Blochberger, 1740.

Rosbach (1588)
Rosbach, Konrad: Paradeißgäertlein: darinnen die edelste unnd fürnembste Kraeuter nach ihrer Gestalt und Eigenschafft abcontrafeytet und mit zweyerley Wirckung, leiblich und geistlich, auß den besten Kraeuterbuechern und H. Goettlicher Schrift zusammen geordnet und beschrieben sind. Allen Haußvättern / Frawen vnd Jungfrawen / zur Leibs vnd Seelen Artzney zugebrauchen / sehr nützlich vnd auch nothwendig. Frankfurt a. M.: J. Spieß 1588; Reprint nach der Originalausgabe von 1588 [mit einem Begleitheft von Heimo Reinitzer: Anmerkungen zu Konrad Rosbachs Paradeißgaertlein]. Hannover: Edition „libri rari“ Schäfer, 1982 [2. Aufl. 1986].

Schönmann (1725)
Schönmann, Daniel: Der Sarg Als Ein Rechter Artzt, allen und jeden Zur genauen Überlegung, Gott=liebenden Gemüthern aber zur vergnügenden Erbauung In gebundener Rede fürgestellet. Berlin: Haude, 1725.

Steiger (1999)
Steiger, Johannes Anselm: Martin Luthers allegorisch-figürliche Auslegung der Heiligen Schrift. In: Zeitschrift für Kirchengeschichte 110 (1999), 331–351.

Steiger (2003)
Steiger, Johannes Anselm: Christus als Apotheker bei Martin Luther. Zugleich ein Beitrag zum Gespräch mit Fritz Krafft. In: Berichte zur Wissenschaftsgeschichte 26 (2003), 137–139.

Steiger (2005)
Steiger, Johannes Anselm: Medizinische Theologie. Christus medicus und Theologia medicinalis bei Martin Luther und im Luthertum der Barockzeit. Mit Edition dreier Quellentexte. Leiden, Boston: Brill, 2005.

Stone (1965)
Stone, Glenn C.: Christ the Apothecary of the Soul. In: The National Lutheran (April 1965), 8–9.

Toellner (1994)
Toellner, Richard: Heil und Heilung bei Martin Luther. Luthers Verhältnis zur Medizin als Anfrage an die heutige Medizin. In: Hoeppke, Hans-Jürgen; Sauer, Armin (Hrsg.): Glaubend leben. Gerhard Ruhbach zum 60. Geburtstag. Wuppertal: Brockhaus, 1994 (Monographien und Studienbücher 387), 140–152.

Toellner (2004)
Toellner, Richard (Hrsg.): Die Geburt einer sanften Medizin. Die Franckeschen Stiftungen als Begegnungsstätte von Medizin und Pietismus im frühen 18. Jahrhundert. Tagungsband zum internationalen Symposion der Franckeschen Stiftungen vom 16. bis 19. April 1998. Halle: Verlag der Franckeschen Stiftungen, 2004

Triller (1725)
Triller, Daniel Wilhelm: Poetische Betrachtungen, über verschiedene, aus der Natur- und Sittenlehre hergenommene Materien. Hamburg: Johann Christoph Kißner, 1725.

Weigel (1698)
Weigel, Christoff: Abbildung Der Gemein-Nützlichen Haupt-Stände, Von denen Regenten Und ihren So in Friedens- als Kriegs-Zeiten zugeordneten Bedienten an, biß auf alle Künstler Und Handwercker: Nach Jedes Ambts- und Beruffs-Verrichtungen, meist nach dem Leben gezeichnet und in Kupfer gebracht, auch nach Dero Ursprung, Nutzbar- und Denckwürdigkeiten kurz, doch gründlich beschrieben, und ganz neu an den Tag geleget. Regensburg, 1698 [Nachdrucke Ebenhausen: Langewiesche, 1936, Dortmund: Harenberg, 1977, Nördlingen: Uhl, 1987].

Wilson (2000)
Wilson, Renate: Pious traders in medicine. A German pharmaceutical network in eighteenth century North America. University Park, PA: Pennsylvania State University Press, 2000.

ABRAHAM WAGNER AND GEORGE DE BENNEVILLE: PHYSICIANS OF BODY AND SOUL

L. Allen Viehmeyer

Abraham Wagner and George de Benneville practiced medicine in colonial Pennsylvania. Recently, special attention has been focused on manuscripts that they authored. These bring to light much information about their medical thinking and insights into how medicine was practiced in southeastern Pennsylvania by medical providers with German training during the second half of the eighteenth century. The present paper is one of several in this volume on these manuscripts and their authors. [1]

Abraham Wagner

Religious background

Abraham Wagner (1715–1763) was born into a Protestant sect known as the Schwenkfelders. The founder of the sect was Caspar Schwenckfeld von Ossig (1489–1561), a Silesian nobleman.[2] Originally enthusiastic about Martin Luther's (1483–1546) reforms, he soon found himself in disagreement with both Rome and Wittenberg particularly in regard to communion and baptism. Due to political pressures resulting from his reform activities, Schwenckfeld went into voluntary exile in 1529 and lived the rest of his life in southwestern Germany.

Schwenckfeld interpreted communion and baptism to be spiritual, not physical, manifestations. In 1533 he proclaimed a "*Stillstand*" (hiatus) in regard to communion, advocating a suspension of the rite until all factions could agree on its essence.[3]

Schwenckfeld's followers in southwestern Germany eventually died out during the century after his death, but small pockets of the faithful continued to survive in Lower Silesia into the early nineteenth century. By the beginning of the eighteenth century only a few villages, mainly in the principalities of Liegnitz and Jauer, were inhabited by Schwenkfelders. Often brutally persecuted

1 Translations from German and Latin into English are provided by the author. Following German spelling, American scholars use the spelling "Schwenckfeld." The American Schwenkfelder community does, too, but uses for the followers of Schwenckfeld, for community matters etc. the spelling "Schwenkfelders." Other personal names, e.g. Hauptmann (Haubtmann), Hübner (Heebner), etc., have been standardized and are spelled here accordingly. – The research underlying this paper was in part supported by the national Library of Medicine, Washington, D.C.

2 For an overview of Caspar Schwenckfeld von Ossig see SCHULTZ (1977) and EBERLEIN (1999). For views on Schwenckfeld and Silesian Schwenkfelders see ERB (1986).

3 See KRIEBEL (1968). Long under congregational discussion, the "*Stillstand*" was rescinded in 1877 in the "Lower District" and about 1894 in the more conservative "Upper District" of the area in which the Schwenkfelders settled in Pennsylvania. KRIEBEL (1968), 50, 55.

in the sixteenth and early seventeenth centuries due to their heretical faith and their separatist lifestyle, the Schwenkfelders were living in relative peace with their Lutheran neighbors at the beginning of the eighteenth century. Some Lutheran clergy were tolerant of them, and they brought their children for baptism in Lutheran churches and buried their dead in Lutheran cemeteries.

Two events occurred in the first two decades of the eighteenth century that affected the lives of the Schwenkfelder faithful. Important, but of lesser significance, was the rise of Pietism, especially radical Pietism, which found enthusiastic adherents among certain Schwenkfelders.[4] The second, much more significant event was the establishment in 1719 of a Jesuit mission in Silesia with the purpose of converting all sectarians, including the Schwenkfelders, to Catholicism. The missionaries began their endeavors benignly, but they became increasingly drastic in their *modus operandi* over time because the Schwenkfelders proved to be more obstinate than had been anticipated. After twenty years of very limited success, the mission was suspended after Silesia had come under the rule of Frederick II of Prussia. During the mission years the Schwenkfelder faithful either joined the Lutheran church or emigrated. Only a very small number actually converted to Catholicism.

A medical tradition

Just four years before the Jesuit mission arrived in Harpersdorf, probably the major Schwenkfelder community at that time, Abraham Wagner was born in this Lower Silesian village. His maternal great-grandfather, George Hauptmann (1635–1722), was a Schwenkfelder practitioner of medicine, and this doubtless had a bearing on Wagner's training in medicine. In fact, Abraham Wagner seems to have been the last in a line of Silesian Schwenkfelder practitioners related either by marriage or by blood.

The first in this line of known Schwenkfelder physicians is Martin John, Jr. (1624–1707).[5] John is mentioned with some frequency in Schwenkfelder manuscripts, often as a doctor. In a contemporary dissertation from Wittenberg (*De fanaticis Silesiorum et speciatim Quirino Kuhlmanno*), John is described as a medical practitioner, specifically a botanist.[6] Chronologically, Wagner's great-grandfather, George Hauptmann (also spelled Haubtmann) is next in line. He is especially known for the harsh circumstances of the interrogation to which he was subjected by the Jesuit missionaries as they tested his faith. A contemporanean chronology of the Protestant communities in Silesia describes Hauptmann as "an *Empiricus* in medicine who helped many people with his medicines and

4 For an overview of this history, see: WEIGELT (1973); WEIGELT (1985); MESCHTER (1984); ERB (1987). For a recent American overview of Pietism with extensive references to pertinent literature see LINDBERG (2005).

5 See WEIGELT (1996).

6 "Medicinam profitebatur ac Botanices imprimis." LIEFMANN (1698), B iv: v.

became widely known."[7] He is also mentioned as a "medic[us] practicus in Lauterseifen."[8] Hauptmann's oldest son, Hans Georg (b. 1660) was "a medical doctor in Haynau. He is a Lutheran and has several children."[9]

Last in this line of Schwenkfelder physicians is Melchior Hübner (also: Heebner; 1668–1738), who practiced medicine in Hockenau just two miles from Harpersdorf before emigrating to Görlitz in Saxony, and eventually to Falkner Swamp in Pennsylvania.[10] Shortly after Hübner's death there in 1738, Wagner penned a lengthy tribute to him.[11] In this tribute Wagner describes an apprenticeship arrangement between Martin John, Jr. and Hübner, and according to which Hübner was eleven years old (1664) when he went to live with John. He remained in John's home until the latter's death in 1707. At that time Hübner took over his mentor's practice and continued to live in Hockenau until April 1726, when he and his family fled from the Jesuit mission and emigrated to Görlitz.

Birth and family

Baptized in the Lutheran Refuge Church on March 24, 1715, Abraham was the first child of Anna Jäckel (1689?–1749), née Hauptmann, and Melchior Wagner (d. 1736). Two additional children were born into the family: a daughter Susanna (1717–1742) and a son Melchior (1725–1784).[12]

Education and training

Very little is known about Wagner's childhood and formative years.[13] A handful of books and his tribute to Hübner, however, permit some speculation. The books that survive from Wagner's childhood include a Greek grammar book signed and dated 1727 when he was twelve, a comprehensive mathematics book signed and dated 1726 when he was eleven, and a fragmentary copybook in his juvenile handwriting dated throughout the year 1724 when he was nine years old.[14]

7 "[...] ein Empiricus in der Medicin, der mit seinen Artzneymitteln vielen Leuten half, und weit berühmt wurde." HENSEL (1768), 408. An extract of Hauptmann's confession of faith is given in HENSEL (1768), 681, where below with his signature Hauptmann describes himself as „ein Laborant und Medicin erfahrner in Physicis."

8 See SCHWENKFELDER MS.: Schneider, 11.

9 "D[octo]r medicinae in Haynau. Er ist lutherisch und hat viele Kinder." SCHWENKFELDER MS.: Schneider, 11.

10 MEIER (1976), chapter 3; BRECHT (1923), 220.

11 Information about Melchior Hübner comes mainly from SCHWENKFELDER MS.: Kurtze Anmerckungen.

12 For information about the Susanna Jäckel née Wagner family, see BRECHT (1923), 344; for the Melchior Wagner family, see BRECHT (1923), 1434–1440.

13 For more information about Wagner's childhood see BERKY (1954), 1–11.

14 For full titles of these books, see GRETSER (1701), HEMELING (1705), and SCHWENKFELDER MS.: Manuscript copy book.

Some assumptions about Wagner's early education might be deduced from this evidence. First, it is unlikely that Wagner ever attended a school. He was four and one-half years old when the Jesuit missionaries made Harpersdorf their headquarters. Sooner or later the missionaries probably forbade Schwenkfelder boys from attending the village school, if village authorities indeed had permitted them to do so. In 1726, when Wagner was eleven years old, a Catholic school was built in Harpersdorf by the mission. If he had been in Harpersdorf, then, as a Schwenkfelder child, he surely would have been required to attend that school, but it seems unlikely that his parents would have responded to this requirement. Second, the Greek grammar and the "self-instructing" mathematics book would seem rather advanced for an eleven and twelve-year-old attending a village school. Third, the nine-year-old's copybook is extremely persuasive evidence that Wagner was not attending a village school but tutored at home, for he copied excerpts from letters and other religious texts by Christian Hoburg (1607–1675), Martin John, Jr., and Caspar Schwenckfeld into this booklet, and his efforts were corrected by a mature hand. The second, vital piece of evidence for Wagner's tuition is the tribute that he wrote at the time of Hübner's death. In this tribute Wagner listed the books and papers in Hübner's possession, among which were writings by Christian Hoburg, Martin John, Jr., and, of course, Caspar Schwenckfeld. Surely Hübner would have been the one person who could have provided the young boy with these texts from his own library.

Several other pieces of evidence strengthen the case for Hübner's tutelage of Wagner. Wagner's lifelong vocation was medicine. Perhaps his great-grandfather Hauptmann was influential in determining this career path for the boy, but he died just as Wagner turned seven years old, so it seems unlikely that Hauptmann would have been able to provide any significant training. Perhaps his mother or his grandmother Hauptmann or both women urged the boy to follow his great-grandfather's footsteps. Whatever the case might have been, Wagner received training in and practiced medicine. Hübner, also a practitioner of medicine, surely would have had a more direct and lasting influence on the boy's pursuit of this vocation, and he could have entered easily into an apprenticeship with the boy, providing him with significant education and training him in medicine. In his tribute to Hübner, Wagner describes how Hübner had been apprenticed to John when eleven years old and had lived with his mentor until the man died. It seems that this could well have been what happened in Wagner's case.

Finally, the tribute itself suggests that more than a casual relationship existed between Wagner and Hübner. Wagner makes no reference to himself in the tribute, but it is difficult to imagine why Wagner would write such a lengthy and venerating memorial to the man, if there had not been an abiding relationship between the two, such as apprentice and mentor, for they had experienced religious persecution and forced emigration together and had a common interest in Schwenkfeldianism and the mystical as well as practicing medicine and serving others.[15]

Emigration

Within a very short time after the Jesuit mission had been established in Harpersdorf, a Schwenkfelder delegation went to the Imperial Court in Vienna where it presented multiple petitions pleading for tolerance and termination of the mission.[16] After five unfruitful years, the delegation returned empty-handed to Harpersdorf, and soon Schwenkfelder families began to flee their Silesian villages. The Hübner family was among the first to emigrate. Mission records reveal that the Hübners left Hockenau on April 26, 1726, and Görlitz records show the arrival of "Melchior Hübner, medicus, with wife and 2 children."[17] If Wagner was Hübner's apprentice, the eleven-year-old may have accompanied his master to Görlitz, but we do not have any record of his presence either in Görlitz or during the family's continued residence in Harpersdorf until 1736. While the Hübner family had been among the first Schwenkfelders to flee Silesia, the Wagner family was among the last to leave when they abandoned their Harpersdorf farm ten years later in January 1736, seeking refuge in Berthelsdorf, Saxony. The Jesuit mission records do not reveal, however, whether Abraham was with his family at that time. As early as 1726 Schwenkfelder refugees had received permission from Nikolaus Ludwig, Count Zinzendorf (1700–1760), to settle in Berthelsdorf.[18] Due to protests by Emperor Karl VI in 1731 concerning the Moravian refugees there, all refugees, Moravian and Schwenkfelder alike, were ordered on April 4, 1733, to leave Saxony. They were given a year to comply. Nevertheless, it seems not all Schwenkfelder families had left Berthelsdorf by January 1736, nine months after the deadline. But now, within a few short weeks of reaching Berthelsdorf, the Wagner family joined the other Schwenkfelder families moving from Berthelsdorf to Görlitz, also within the territory of Saxony, some fifteen miles away to the northeast. These Schwenkfelders arrived in the city on February 23, 1736.[19] They, too, had to leave Saxony within a year.

Schwenkfelder families began emigrating to Pennsylvania as early as 1733, when a first group of three families sailed there aboard the *Pennsylvania Merchant*. The largest group made the voyage in 1734. The Wagner family joined the sixth and last group of Schwenkfelder immigrants, and their ship, the "St. Andrew," landed in Philadelphia on September 26, 1737.[20]

15 BERKY (1954), 8–9.

16 GERHARD (1941), 36–38.

17 "Melchior Hübner, Arzt, mit Frau und 2 Kindern." KADELBACH [1860], 57.

18 For an overview of Count Zinzendorf and his work with extensive lists of appropriate literature see MEYER & PEUCKER (2000) and WEINLICK (2001). For a recent overview of Moravian and Schwenkfelder connections with literature see WEIGELT (2006), 64–96.

19 KADELBACH [1860], 65.

20 Details including ships' names, captains, ship lists, immigrants' names and their familial re-

Wagner in Pennsylvania

Upon arrival in Philadelphia the Wagner family split up. The two younger children and their widowed mother went to live in Mathacton with her sister Rosina, who, with husband Abraham Beyer and children, had come over in 1734 with the major Schwenkfelder migration. Abraham Wagner went to Falkner Swamp to live with Hübner, who died just nine months later. Shortly thereafter the Wagners acquired a farm about two miles from the Beyer's and moved there in December 1738. Three years later Abraham's sister Susanna married, and within a year after their mother's death in March 1749 both Abraham and Melchior married and settled on separate, near-by farms. Abraham and his wife Maria lived on this farm until her death in 1760. Abraham died three years later in 1763 at the age of forty-eight. Abraham and Maria had no children. Only his brother Melchior survived Abraham.

Like most colonists Wagner pursued several vocations. Like nearly all of the Schwenkfelder immigrants, he settled in rural Pennsylvania and engaged in farming of some sort, probably much like the environment he knew in Harpersdorf and vicinity. His spiritual life was a constant preoccupation and found expression in verse, conversations and charity.

Physician

Virtually everything known about Wagner's medical practice is preserved in his *Remediorum specimina.*[21] There are hardly any references to his practice in Schwenkfelder or any other sources. No records of specific patients are extant. The names of several persons involved in medicinal preparations or medical practice appear in Wagner's *Specimina.* Of particular interest are the names George de Benneville and Johann Adolph Meyer, fellow physicians and neighbors.[22]

De Benneville and Wagner lived just a few miles from one another while de Benneville resided in the Oley Valley between 1743 and 1757. John Adolph Meyer, another Wagner neighbor, was a physician who lived in the Moravian community in Bethlehem, Pennsylvania, from 1742 to 1750. The two men could have become acquainted, however, as early as the winter of 1736, when both were in Berthelsdorf and Herrnhut, Saxony.[23] Extant correspondence and a bequest in his will show that Wagner was an acquaintance of Heinrich Melchior

lationships are available in BRECHT (1923), 34–44: "The Migrations of the Schwenkfelders."

21 For the digitized version of the Wagner manuscript in translation, see "Eighteenth-century Colonial Formularies: The Manuscripts of George de Benneville and Abraham Wagner," College of Physicians of Philadelphia Digital Library. Recent website address: http://www.accesspadr.org/cpp/. This website publication shows the imaged German handwritten text and offers a translation into modern English.

22 MEIER (1976) devotes chapters six and seven to de Benneville and chapter four to Meyer.

23 MEIER (1976), 42.

Mühlenberg, who lived in Trappe, Pennsylvania, just five miles from Wagner.[24] The *Remediorum specimina* contains references to medicines prepared at the Francke Orphanage Foundations in Halle, Germany.[25] An emissary of the Foundations, Mühlenberg was familiar with Halle medicines and imported them for the benefit of his parishioners.[26] On one occasion Mühlenberg placed an order with Wagner.[27]

Although Melchior Wagner, ten years younger than his brother Abraham, might have been his apprentice or even his successor in the medical practice, there is no incontestable evidence that he was, although there is reference to medical instruments in the inventory of his belongings.[28]

Hymn writer

From time to time Wagner wrote religious verse, producing no less than sixty-seven hymns during his lifetime. The earliest dated hymn was written when he was seventeen. Its sophistication indicates, however, that Wagner had probably started writing verses at a much younger age. The hymns that have come down to us show that he was capable of writing on various topics in an extensive variety of poetical forms. His hymns were a personal expression of his own devotion, celebration, thanksgiving, and awe of God. Wagner's poetry constantly reveals his Pietism. Absorbed in mystical ideas since boyhood, these themes, too, are found from time to time in his hymns.

The two major sources of his hymns are an autograph manuscript, written under a pseudonym 1732–1754,[29] and the Schwenkfelder hymnal *Neu=Eingerichtetes Gesang=Buch* published in 1762.[30] Wagner's first publication was Christopher Saur's 1742 broadside of his *Kleine[s] A, B, C in der Schule Christi.*[31] Two of Wagner's hymns, *Gott Vater! Dir sey Lob und Danck* and *O*

24 A letter from Wagner to Mühlenberg from September 1, 1753, was printed in MANN, SCHMUCKER & GERMANN (1886), 690–692. For the original version of Wagner's letter to Mühlenberg, see ALAND (1987), 67–70 (letter No. 137). For an English translation see BERKY (1954), 62–66. In the codicil to his will Wagner stipulated that a book once owned by Mühlenberg should be returned to him: "7. I give and bequeath unto the Rev. Mr. H. M. Muhlenberg in Provid. Philad. a Book, called D. Pauli Antonii Collegium Antitheticum, gedruckt zu Halle 1732 in quarto, it hath been his Book before." BRECHT (1923), 1437.

25 See Crellin and Wilson in this volume.

26 See WILSON (2000) for the import of Halle medications to North America.

27 ALAND (1987), 316–317 (letter No. 177, June 22, 1757). BERKY (1954), 66–67, gives this letter in an English translation. The order is given in the footnote: "Aloes hep: Myrrhis elect: nitro puris; und pulv: Rhub – an ounce of each and one shillings worth of saffron."

28 BRECHT (1923), 1440.

29 SCHWENKFELDER MS.: Andreas Wächters Gesänge.

30 NEU=EINGERICHTETES GESANG=BUCH (1762).

31 Wagner 1755 mentions the broadside in a letter to Tersteegen, revealing the printer's name and the date of printing. Reprinted in STOUDT (1956), 152–156.

milder Heiland, Jesus Christ even found favor outside of Schwenkfelder circles, being reprinted into the early twentieth century in Brethren hymnals.[32]

Charity

Wagner's concern for his neighbor and the poor was clearly expressed in his will and codicil. He forgave all medical debts of poor people. He instructed that two-thirds of his estates go to his brother, his sole survivor, and the last third put in charge of four custodians who were to dispose of it as follows:[33]

1. Within one year £20 cash was to be distributed among poor people by four custodians having £5 each.
2. Within one year £10 cash was to be expended for the purchase of Bibles, New Testaments, Psalm books, and hymnals – Schwenkfelder, Lutheran and Reformed, in English and in German for distribution to poor adults and children.
3. As soon as possible £20 was to be contributed to the Pennsylvania Hospital.
4. All the remaining money was to be distributed by the four custodians to needy poor people within ten to twelve years.

George de Benneville

Religious background

Whereas Abraham Wagner was born into the Schwenkfelder faith, George de Benneville (1703–1793) was born into the Calvinist faith.[34] His parents were French Protestants, commonly called Huguenots, who belonged to the church founded by John Calvin (1509–1564). A reformer like the German monk Martin Luther, Calvin was a Protestant theologian living in Geneva, Switzerland. His theology differed from Luther's, especially in respect to communion and salvation. Calvin's doctrine emphasized the sovereignty of God, the supreme authority of the Scriptures, the irresistibility of grace and, especially important in de Benneville's case, the salvation of the elect by God's grace alone.

32 Thanks to Ute Evers who brought these hymns and their Brethren sources to my attention. See EVERS (2007).

33 BRECHT (1923), 1435–1437.

34 All of the information in the following about de Benneville's life in Europe is summarized from DE BENNEVILLE (1882). There is a biography of de Benneville by BELL (1953). See also JOHNSON (1969–1970). There is no independent or other source for de Benneville's childhood and formative years to corroborate what is stated in the autobiography.

The following narrative of the life of George de Benneville before his emigration to Pennsylvania is drawn almost entirely from an autobiography.[35] Written close to the end of his life and first published in English translation, it was issued a number of times in German translation in Pennsylvania after his death, attesting to his lasting popularity among many, especially separatist, Germans. Typical of Pietist autobiography, it focuses sharply on his spiritual development and is very sparse in regard to other aspects of his life. His awakening experience and two life-altering visions are paramount in telling his story.

Early years

De Benneville was born in London in 1703 into a noble Huguenot refugee family. His parents George and Marie had fled to England after the revocation of the edict of Nantes. His mother died shortly after his birth and his father died soon thereafter. Queen Anne (1665–1714) and her husband, Prince George of Denmark (1653–1708), were his godparents, but they, too had died by the time he was eleven years old.

As a twelve- to thirteen-year-old, de Benneville was put on a ship to the Mediterranean, in part to learn navigation. While the ship was docked in Algeria, de Benneville witnessed the intense compassion of two "Moors" for an injured companion, which caused him to examine his own Christianity.

Conversion and preaching

De Benneville's first conversion experience transpired after returning to England from this voyage. He related how he fell into a fit and had a vision of himself burning in hell. In another vision a little more than a year later, Christ appeared and saved him from damnation. Hearing these tales, the French Calvinist ministers attending the young de Benneville questioned his faith and could not agree that he was saved, "for they held predestination and I held the restoration of all souls."[36] As a result, de Benneville was no longer welcome at his Calvinist church.

Having received a spiritual call to preach in France, de Benneville left England, never to return. Knowing that persecution would certainly result from his preaching, he hesitated, but eventually began his pilgrimage in Normandy at the age of seventeen. After some two years of proselytizing he was arrested a second time and condemned to death. At the last minute he was reprieved and eventually released from prison.

After his near execution in France, de Benneville went to Germany in 1725 where he preached in many northern German towns as well as Holland and Flanders. After some years in this part of Europe he became extremely ill and

35 DE BENNEVILLE (1791). A reprint of this 1791 imprint is probably DE BENNEVILLE (1882). There is a German translation issued by different publishers: DE BENNEVILLE (1798), reprinted 1809, 1815, and 1824.

36 DE BENNEVILLE (1882), 16.

lapsed into a coma. Again he had visions of heaven and hell, which ended with instructions to preach the *Everlasting Gospel of Universal Love*. He began preaching, but was soon in prison again. Shortly after his release he received a call from God to preach his gospel in North America. He arrived in Philadelphia in 1741, about a year after that vision.

Medical training

Little is known about de Benneville's medical training. Bell speculates that he might have received some sort of training as a practitioner while traversing northern Germany,[37] and Meier states without documentation that de Benneville received a "doctorate from a Pietist faculty in Belgium sometime before 1739,"[38] but recent investigations discussed elsewhere in this volume are shedding additional light on his medical background.[39]

De Benneville in Pennsylvania

For de Benneville's life in North America we are on firmer ground. Anecdotes are found in several contemporary documents. These stories bring some insight into his association with various German sectarian groups, especially Schwenkfelders and the Sabbatarians at Ephrata.

Tradition holds that de Benneville first resided in Germantown with Christopher Saur, the German separatist printer.[40] Two years later in 1743 he acquired a farm in the Oley Valley, where numerous Huguenots had already settled. While residing in the Oley Valley de Benneville practiced medicine, taught school, preached the *Everlasting Gospel*, and married Esther Bertholet (1720–1796). They had seven children, of whom Daniel (1753–1827) and George, Jr. (1760–1850) became academically trained physicians. In 1757, after living in the Oley Valley for some fifteen years, the older de Benneville moved to Germantown, Pennsylvania, where he died in 1793 at ninety years of age.

Among the documents in de Benneville's legacy are a single poem of twenty-two lines to his wife Ester,[41] his will and inventory, and several religious and medical manuscripts, one of which is the *Medicina Pensylvania*.[42]

37 See BELL (1953), 4.
38 MEIER (1976), 87.
39 See Shackelford in this volume.
40 See BERKY (1954), 49.
41 See STOUDT (1956), 172.
42 For the digitized version of the bilingual de Benneville manuscript, see "Eighteenth-century Colonial Formularies: The Manuscripts of George de Benneville and Abraham Wagner," College of Physicians of Philadelphia Digital Library. Website address: http://www.accesspadr.org/cpp/. The following unpublished de Benneville manuscripts are at the Schwenkfelder Library and Heritage Center: *Tinctura Universalis. Transmutation der Metallen*, VR 42–42; *Biblical Commentaries*, VR 42–43; *Der Geist des Glaubens. Von denen Graden und Arten des Glaubens*, VR 42–44; *Von Vereinigung der Naturen. Gewisse vorgestellte Lehrsätze vom äussern und innern Menschen zu betrachten beschrieben*, VR 42–45; *Das Ewige Evangelium von Jesum Christum*, VR 42–46; *Umb Eisen zu Stahl zu*

Sabbatarian and other connections
Very little seems to have survived in regard to de Benneville's patients and his therapies as applied to individual cases. In his autobiographical *Leben und Wandel,* Heinrich Sangmeister (Br. Ezechiel; 1723–1784), a Sabbatarian at Ephrata, describes two encounters with de Benneville which refer to his medical practice. Sangmeister mentions specifically his visit to de Benneville in Oley in 1757, and de Benneville's visit to him in Virginia in 1766 while preaching at German settlements in that colony.

At the time of his visit to de Benneville's home in the Oley Valley, Sangmeister relates that upon his arrival in Oley, he [Sangmeister] had become

> [...] ill from the lingering rain, but he [de Benneville] gave me some drops, which were so effective that I was fresh and well again in the morning! [...] He [...] told me everything about how he had been guided and awakened, and finally because he was a doctor and had had many experiences, he told me some really astonishing things.[43]

After exchanging a few words with de Benneville about his gold tincture ("*Universal Goldtinctur*"[44]), Sangmeister continues:

> He said he felt impelled to offer me something he hadn't offered to anyone before; namely, if I would join him, he would teach me about medicine and everything it involved, because he felt that I had a talent for it, and that he would share his tincture with me, and should he die before I did, he would order his people orally and in writing that this bottle [of tincture] would be mine.

Another anecdote relates the misery Sangmeister endured when he contracted the "yaws." Fellow Sabbatarian and doctor Brother Samuel, "gave me a strong purge of tartar emetic [...] which I took on the following day according to [the doctor's] directions, but it stuck and didn't purge a thing."[45] Later Sangmeister asked de Benneville about this purgative and he said, "it was the worst that a person can get." Sangmeister responded that Brother Samuel had informed him,

machen durch Fermentation, de Benneville microfilm; *Fasiculus Claudit tandem* [...], VS 42–47.

43 This and the following citation are taken from SANGMEISTER (1825), 1. Theil, 57–58. "[...] so bald ich hin kam wurde ich von dem vielen Regenwetter krank, allein er gab mir einige Tropfen welche eine solche Wirckung hatten, daß ich morgends wiederum frisch und gesund war! [...] er [...] erzählte mir seine ganze Führung und Erweckung, und endlich weilen er ein Doctor und vieles erfahren hatte; so erzählte er mir wunderbare Dinge [...] er wäre getrieben um mir zu offeriren was er bisher noch niemandem gethan: daß wann ich zu ihm kommen wolte, so wolte er mich in der Medicin und in allem unterrichten, dann er fühlte daß ich eine Fähigkeit dazu hätte, und so solte ich auch an seiner Tinctur mit Theil haben, und so er vor mir sterben solte, wolte er seinen Leuten schriftlich und mündlich befehlen, daß diese Buttel mein seyn solte."

44 SANGMEISTER (1825), 1. Theil, 57.

45 This and the following two quotes are taken from SANGMEISTER (1825), 1. Theil, 13–14. "[...] gab mir eine starke Purgirung vom Tartarremetic [sic] [...] ich nahm solche nach seiner Direction des folgenden Tages, und die blieb stecken, und trieb gar nichts [...]. [...] es seyen die schlechtesten die man bekommen könne [...] Ja wohl pflegte Bruder Beneville zu sagen, die Prediger ermorden die Seelen und die Doctor[es] den Leib."

"it was the best one, and he often sold it to poor people. – Yes, indeed, as Brother Benneville liked to say, the preachers murder the soul and the doctors [murder] the body."

Schwenkfelder connection

Additional references to de Benneville as a doctor survive in a diary kept by David Schultz (1717–1797), a Schwenkfelder who lived about seventeen miles from de Benneville while the doctor had his residence in the Oley Valley. Here are excerpts from Schultz's 1750 diary entries:[46]

> At night it became better because of medicine from Benneville, but Mother is again somewhat worse. [February 24]
> [...] went to Oley to Benneville. [April 9]
> Anna Rosina [his wife] purged – but little. [April 11]
> Benneville at D.M. [David Meschter] and M.S. [Melchior Schultz] for bleeding. [April 16]

At the back of the 1768 diary a recipe for constipation attributed to de Benneville is listed among several "Remedies."

De Benneville may have been equally, if not better, known as an itinerant preacher. Both Sangmeister and Schultz include information about this activity. Sangmeister mentions de Benneville's preaching to German settlers in Sandy Hook, Virginia, during de Benneville's visit to him there in 1766. Schultz records several incidents of de Benneville preaching in the Schwenkfelder community, especially at the home of David Meschter: "George Beneville preached at Hereford – D. M. [David Meschter]" [May 27, 1756]; "Beneville is to preach" [September 12, 1756]. At the end of daily entries for August 1757, Schultz noted: "George Beneville sold his plantation this month." Nevertheless, de Benneville continued to preach in Schwenkfelder homes after moving about thirty miles away to Germantown, as evidenced by Schultz: "Beneville preached at D. M. [David Meschter]" [September 2, 1759]; "George Benneville preached at David Meschter's" [May 18, 1780].

The Universalist Church in America traces its roots back to George de Benneville. Like many other separatists, de Benneville did not wish to found a church, an external organization with rules and a hierarchy. While his gospel may have been the inspiration of the Universalist Church, Elhanan Winchester (1751–1797) and John Murray (1741–1815) were actually more instrumental in establishing the denomination.

46 Between 1743 (earliest extant) and 1790 (latest extant) David Schultz kept a diary in each annual almanac printed on the Saur press. Of the possible forty-seven only fifteen are known (1743–1744, 1750, 1752, 1756–1757, 1759, 1768–1769, 1774, 1780, 1782, 1786, 1790). All citations are taken from the two-volume edition by BERKY (1952–1953).

Good neighbors: de Benneville, the Schwenkfelders, and Wagner

There is clear evidence in David Schultz's diaries of de Benneville's connections to the Schwenkfelder community as both physician and preacher. Yet it is difficult to say when de Benneville first became acquainted with the Schwenkfelders. De Benneville mentions in this autobiography that he wandered into Germany as far as Altona and Hamburg in the north, and then to Magdeburg and the territory of Brandenburg during the sixteen years (1725–1741) he spent in that part of Europe. Perhaps he met with some Schwenkfelders in those places. On their trek to Philadelphia in 1733, the second group of Schwenkfelder emigrants passed through Magdeburg, Hamburg, and Altona. In his diary of this journey, David Schultz specifically mentions meeting the shipping agent Heinrich van der Smissen in Altona on May 8 and 9. Perhaps de Benneville encountered Schwenkfelder immigrants then. A month later in Haarlem the Schwenkfelders met Cornelius van Putten and the three Byuschanse brothers (Abraham, Isaac, and John)[47] early in June. In a 1770 letter to the Schwenkfelders in Silesia, Christopher Schultz noted that Heinrich van der Smissen's sons remained friends of "our Benneville."[48]

In 1771 the Pennsylvania Schwenkfelders had a book published in Lower Silesia, since 1742 under Prussian rule, in which they defended Caspar Schwenckfeld's theology. In the appendix of this book is a pastoral letter dated January 9, 1769, from de Benneville to the Silesian Schwenkfelders.[49]

While the possibility exists that de Benneville could have become acquainted with some Schwenkfelders in Altona or Holland during their emigration, he may well not have met them until he arrived in Germantown or even until he moved to the Oley Valley. His acquaintance with Wagner is, however, documented in a letter Wagner wrote to Gerhard Tersteegen (1697–1769). In his introductory letter[50] to the famous quietist, Wagner (1755) alludes to de Benneville, a mutual friend, who had encouraged him to write, reporting that he "had become acquainted with him [de Benneville] by the grace of God in this country [Pennsylvania]."

With so many shared interests and living in rather close proximity, it seems very possible that de Benneville and Wagner would have been friends. Besides their practice of medicine, the two men shared some religious views, especially the doctrine of the Restoration of all Things. Both men had a radical Pietist background and in their youth were persecuted for their non-conformist religious practices. Both admired and corresponded with Tersteegen,[51] whom they

47 Nothing is known about Cornelius van Putten and the three Byuschanse brothers beyond what David Schultz mentions in his diary.

48 SCHWENKFELDER MS.: Letter to Heintze.

49 *A Letter from Bristol, Pennsylvania*. See SCHULTZ (1771), 461–464.

50 SCHWENKFELDER MS.: Letter to Tersteegen.

51 For Tersteegen's medical and Christian care of people and souls see HABRICH (1997). Tersteegen's letter to Pennsylvania from May 15, 1753, probably addressed to Wagner, touches

considered to be a kindred spirit. De Benneville had visions in which he was called to preach the *Everlasting Gospel*; Wagner recorded no visions, nor has any conversion experience come down to us. Wagner was neither a preacher nor a leader of any sort. The impression Wagner leaves is one of a quiet, learned, introspective man, although he did not shy away from written and verbal discourse with fellow Schwenkfelders in regard to certain doctrinal issues.

Retrospective

The *Medicina Pensylvania* and the *Remediorum specimina*, essentially handbooks for the practicing pharmacist-physician, afford glimpses into the medical knowledge and therapies of two relatively obscure, Central European medical practitioners in eighteenth century Pennsylvania. Today, their manuscripts are primarily of interest to medical historians, for they expand knowledge about the extent to which traditional European therapies and receptures had penetrated North America.

As physicians of the body, Wagner and de Benneville sought to bring healing to many. As physicians of the soul, Wagner and de Benneville reached out in very different ways. De Benneville spent some seventy years preaching a *Gospel of Universal Love* and the salvation of all. Wagner witnessed to his deep faith by writing hymns, many of which were sung by generations of Schwenkfelders.

Many Schwenkfelders seem to have held de Benneville in high regard as a person with deep spirituality. From time to time he preached in their homes and witnessed in other ways to his faith. Schwenkfelders had great respect for Wagner, too, who left them two abiding legacies: his religious verse for many occasions and his example as generous provider of assistance in times of pecuniary or physical misfortune, not only within the Schwenkfelder community, but the world at large.

on matters of the religious scene in Pennsylvania and in Europe as well. It was published and discussed by WEIGELT (1974). For the context of the radical pietist physician's network in Europe, see HABRICH (2002).

Unpublished Sources and References

Schwenkfelder Library & Heritage Center, Pennsburg, PA (Schwenkfelder Mss.)
Schwenkfelder Ms.: Schneider
Schneider, August Friedrich Heinrich: Carl Regent's Verzeichniß aller Schwenckfelder in Langen-Neudorf, Armenruh, Lauterseiffen u. Harpersdorf [1878].

Schwenkfelder Ms.: Letter to Heintze
Schultz, Christoph: Letter [from] Pennsylvania to Carl Ehrenfried Heintze, December 15, 1770. VC 3–7.

Schwenkfelder Ms.: Andreas Wächters Gesänge
Wagner, Abraham: Andreas Wächters Gesänge und Lieder wie er sie hinter einander von Zeit zu Zeit gedichtet [1732–1754]. VN 22–61.

Schwenkfelder Ms.: Manuscript Copy Book
Wagner, Abraham: Copies [1724] of Selected Writings About Caspar Schwenckfeld and Letters to Schwenkfelders by Christian Hoburg [Manuscript Copy Book]. VS 3–5[1].

Schwenkfelder Ms.: Kurtze Anmerckungen
Wagner, Abraham: Kurtze Anmerckungen vom Leben u. Sterben des Sel. Melchior Hübners Med: Pr: von Hockenau [1738]. VS 3–5[1].

Schwenkfelder Ms.: Letter to Tersteegen
Wagner, Abraham: Letter to Gerhard Tersteegen. Skippack PA, August 27, 1755. Wagner Papers, VOC W[1].

Aland (1987)
Aland, Kurt (Ed.): Die Korrespondenz Heinrich Melchior Mühlenbergs. Aus der Anfangszeit des deutschen Luthertums in Nordamerika, Vol. 2: 1753–1762. Berlin, New York: de Gruyter, 1987.

Bell (1953)
Bell, Albert D.: The Life and Times of Dr. George de Benneville (1703–1793). Boston, MA: Department of Publication of the Universalist Church of America, 1953.

de Benneville (1791)
de Benneville, George: A True and Most Remarkable Account of Some Passages in the Life of Mr. George de Benneville, of an Ancient and Noble Protestant Family in Normandy [...]. Translated from the French of His Own Manuscript, by Elhanan Winchester. [...]. To Which is Prefixed a Preface by the Translator. [...] London: Sold by the editor at his house, and at the chapel, Glasshouse-Yard, 1791.

de Benneville (1798)
de Benneville, George: Der Merkwürdige Lebens-Lauf, die Sonderbare Bekehrung, und Entzückungen, Des Ohnlängst Bey Germantaun (in Pennsylvanien) wohnenden und verstorbenen Dr. George de Benneville. Von seiner eigenen Handschrift aus dem Französischen in die englische Sprache übersetzt und mit einer Vorrede begleitet, von E[lhanan] Winchester. Nun aber in der deutschen Sprache sorgfältig herausgegeben. Baltimore, MD: S[amuel] Saur, 1798. (Further editions of this Winchester german traduction: Libanon, PA: J[acob] Schnee, 1809; Libanon, PA: Joseph Hartman, 1815 and 1824).

de Benneville (1882)
de Benneville, George: Life and Trance of Dr. George De Benneville, of Germantown, PA. An Account of What He Saw and Heard During a Trance of Forty-Two Hours, Both in the Regions of Happiness and Misery; Together with a Short Account of His Cruel Persecutions in France for Preaching the Gospel. Translated from the French of His Own Manuscript. Schwenksville, PA: N. Bertolet Grubb, 1882.

de Benneville (2005)
de Benneville, George: Medicina Pensylvania Or The Pensylvania Physician. In: Eighteenth-century Colonial Formularies. The Manuscripts of George de Benneville and Abraham Wagner. The College of Physicians of Philadelphia Digital Library.
Recent website address (access date: June 23, 2008): http://www.accesspadr.org/cpp/.

Berky (1952–1953)
Berky, Andrew S. (Ed. and Trans.): The Journals and Papers of David Schultze. Vol. I (1726–1760), Vol. II (1761–1797). Pennsburg, PA: The Schwenkfelder Library, 1952–1953.

Berky (1954)
Berky, Andrew S.: Practitioner in Physick. A Biography of Abraham Wagner, 1717 [sic]–1763. Pennsburg, PA: The Schwenkfelder Library, 1954.

Brecht (1923)
Brecht, Samuel K. (Ed.): The Genealogical Record of the Schwenkfelder Families. Chicago: Rand McNally & Company, 1923.

Eberlein (1999)
Eberlein, Paul Gerhard: Ketzer oder Heiliger? Caspar von Schwenckfeld, der Schlesische Reformator und seine Botschaft. Metzingen: Ernst Franz, 1999 (Studien zur Schlesischen und Oberlausitzer Kirchengeschichte 6).

Evers (2007)
Evers, Ute: Das geistliche Lied der Schwenckfelder. Tutzing: Schneider, 2007 (Mainzer Studien zur Musikwissenschaft 44).

Erb (1986)
Erb, Peter C. (Ed.): Schwenckfeld and Early Schwenkfeldianism. Papers Presented at the Colloquium on Schwenckfeld and the Schwenkfelders. Pennsburg, PA: Schwenkfelder Library, 1986.

Erb (1987)
Erb, Peter C. (Ed.): Schwenkfelders in America. Papers Presented at the Colloquium on Schwenckfeld and the Schwenkfelders. Pennsburg, PA: Schwenkfelder Library, 1987.

Gerhard (1941)
Gerhard, Elmer S.: Balthasar Hoffmann (1687–1775). Scholar, Minister, Writer, Diplomat. In: Schwenckfeldiana 1, No. 2 (September 1941), 35–52.

Gretser (1701)
Gretser, Jacob: Rudimenta Linguae Graecae Ex Primo Libro Institutionum. Hannover, Wolffenbüttel: Gottfried Freytag, 1701.

Habrich (1997)
Habrich, Christa: Heilkunde im Dienst der Seelsorge bei Gerhard Tersteegen. In: Kock, Manfred (Ed.): Gerhard Tersteegen – Evangelische Mystik inmitten der Aufklärung. Köln: Rheinland-Verlag, 1997, 161–180.

Habrich (2002)
Habrich, Christa: Johann Samuel Carl (1677–1757) und die Philadelphische Ärztegemeinschaft. In: Lehmann, Hartmut; Schrader, Hans-Jürgen; Schilling, Heinz (Eds.): Jansenismus, Quietismus, Pietismus. Göttingen: Vandenhoeck & Ruprecht, 2002, 272–289.

Hemeling (1705)
Hemeling, Johann: Neu vermehrter vollkommener Rechenmeister oder selbst=lehrendes Rechen=Buch. Dillingen: Johann Caspar Bencard, 1705.

Hensel (1768)
Hensel, Johann Adam: Protestantische Kirchen=Geschichte der Gemeinen in Schlesien. Nach allen Fürstenthümern, vornehmsten Städten und Oertern dieses Landes, [...] in acht Abschnitten [...]. Leipzig, Liegnitz: David Siegert, 1768.

Johnson (1969–1970)
Johnson, David A.: George de Benneville and the Heritage of the Radical Reformation. In: Journal of the Universalist Historical Society 8 (1969–1970), 25–43.

Kadelbach [1860]
Kadelbach, Oswald: Ausführliche Geschichte Kaspar v. Schwenckfelds und der Schwenckfelder in Schlesien, der Ober-Lausitz und Amerika, nebst ihren Glaubensschriften von 1524 bis 1860, nach den vorhandenen Quellen bearbeitet. Lauban: M. Baumeister [1860].

Kriebel (1968)
Kriebel, Martha B.: Schwenkfelders and the Sacraments. Pennsburg, PA: The Board of Publication of the Schwenkfelder Church, 1968.

Liefmann (1698)
Liefmann, Gottlieb: Dissertatio Historica de Fanaticis Silesiorum et Speciatim Quirino Kuhlmanno. Wittenberg: Christian Schrödter, 1698.

Lindberg (2005)
Lindberg, Carter (Ed.): The Pietist Theologians. An Introduction to Theology in the Seventeenth and Eighteenth Centuries. Malden, MA: Blackwell, 2005.

Mann, Schmucker & Germann (1886)
Mann, Wilhelm Julius; Schmucker, B. M.; Germann, Wilhelm (Eds.): Nachrichten von den vereinigten deutschen evangelisch-lutherischen Gemeinen in Nord-America, absonderlich in Pensylvanien. Allentown, PA: Brobst, Diehl & Co., 1886.

Meier (1976)
Meier, Louis A.: Early Pennsylvania Medicine. A Representative Early American Medical History. Montgomery County, Pennsylvania 1682 to 1799. Boyertown, PA: Gilbert Print. Co., 1976.

Meyer & Peucker (2000)
Meyer, Dietrich; Peucker, Paul (Eds.): Graf ohne Grenzen. Leben und Werk von Nikolaus Ludwig Graf von Zinzendorf. Herrnhut: Comeniusbuchhandlung, 2000.

Meschter (1984)
Meschter, W. Kyrel: Twentieth Century Schwenkfelders: A Narrative History. Pennsburg, PA: The Schwenkfelder Library, 1984.

Neu=Eingerichtetes Gesang=Buch (1762)
Neu=Eingerichtetes Gesang=Buch in sich haltend eine Sammlung (mehrenteils alter) schöner lehr=reicher und erbaulicher Lieder, [...]. Nach den Haupt=Stücken der Christlichen Lehr und Glaubens eingetheilet, [...]. Germantown: Christoph Saur, 1762.

Sangmeister (1825)
Sangmeister, Heinrich: Leben und Wandel des in Gott ruhenden und seligen Br. Ezechiel Sangmeisters [...] frey und offen ans Licht gestellt [...]. Ephrata, PA: Joseph Bauman, 1825 (The English version: Sangmeister, Heinrich: Life and Conduct of the Late Brother Ezechiel Sangmeister, translated from the German Leben und Wandel. 1825, was reprinted: Ephrata, PA: Historical Society of the Cocalico Valley, 1979).

Schultz (1771)
[Schultz, Christoph:] Erläuterung für Herrn Caspar Schwenckfeld, und die Zugethanen seiner Lehre [...]. Jauer: Heinrich Christian Müller, 1771 (English translation by Elmer S. Gerhard [Ed.]: A Vindication of Caspar Schwenckfeld von Ossig [1771]. Allentown, PA: Edward Schlechter, 1942).

Schultz (1977)
Schultz, Selina Gerhard: Caspar Schwenckfeld von Ossig (1489–1561). Spiritual Interpreter of Christianity, Apostle of the Middle Way, and Pioneer in Modern Religious Thought. New edition by Peter C. Erb. Pennsburg, PA: The Board of Publication of the Schwenkfelder Church, 1977 (1st ed. Norristown, PA: The Schwenkfelder Church, 1946).

Stoudt (1956)
Stoudt, John Joseph: Pennsylvania German Poetry 1685–1830. The Pennsylvania German Folklore Society, Vol. 20. Allentown, PA: Schlechter, 1956.

Wagner (1742)
[Wagner, Abraham]: Das kleine A, B, C, in der Schule Christi, Aus denen Wercklein des gottseligen Thomae à Kempis, In Reimen verfasset, und mit H. Schrifft concordiret. [Germantown, PA]: [Christoph Saur] [1742].

Wagner (2005)
Wagner, Abraham: Remediorum Specimina aliquot ex Praxi A. W. In: Eighteenth-century Colonial Formularies. The Manuscripts of George de Benneville and Abraham Wagner. The College of Physicians of Philadelphia Digital Library.
Recent website address (access date: June 23, 2008): http://www.accesspadr.org/cpp/.

Weigelt (1973)
Weigelt, Horst: Spiritualistische Tradition im Protestantismus. Die Geschichte des Schwenckfeldertums in Schlesien. Berlin, New York: de Gruyter, 1973 (Arbeiten zur Kirchengeschichte 43).

Weigelt (1974)
Weigelt, Horst: Ein unbekannter Brief Gerhard Tersteegens. In: Monatshefte für Evangelische Kirchengeschichte 23 (1974), 50–55.

Weigelt (1985)
Weigelt, Horst: The Schwenkfelders in Silesia. Translation of Weigelt (1973) by Peter C. Erb. Pennsburg, PA: The Schwenkfelder Library, 1985.

Weigelt (1987)
Weigelt, Horst: The Emigration of the Schwenkfelders from Silesia to America. In: Erb, Peter C. (Ed.): Schwenkfelders in America. Papers Presented at the Colloquium on Schwenckfeld and the Schwenkfelders. Pennsburg, PA: The Schwenkfelder Library, 1987, 5–19.

Weigelt (1996)
Weigelt, Horst: Der Arzt und Botaniker Martin John. Eine führende Gestalt des Schlesischen Schwenckfeldertums im 17. Jahrhundert. In: Jahrbuch für Schlesische Kirchengeschichte, Neue Folge 74 (1996), 101–117.

Weigelt (2006)
Weigelt, Horst. Zinzendorf und die Schwenckfelder. In: Brecht, Martin; Peucker, Paul (Eds.): Neue Aspekte der Zinzendorf-Forschung. Göttingen: Vandenhoeck & Ruprecht, 2006 (Arbeiten zur Geschichte des Pietismus 47), 64–96.

Weinlick (2001)
Weinlick, John R.: Count Zinzendorf. The Story of His Life and Leadership in the Renewed Moravian Church. Bethlehem, Winston-Salem: Abington Press, 2001 (originally published 1956).

Wilson (2000)
Wilson, Renate: Pious Traders in Medicine. A German Pharmaceutical Network in Eighteenth-Century North America. University Park, PA: Pennsylvania State University Press, 2000.

SCHWÄGERINNEN. ADLIGE FRAUEN IN DER FRÜHPHASE DER HALLESCHEN MEDIKAMENTENEXPEDITION

Elisabeth Quast

Der folgende Beitrag stellt Ergebnisse der Erschließung einer Sammlung von Briefen[1] dar, die von Christian Friedrich Richter (1676–1711) und seinem Bruder Christian Sigismund (1673–1739) vornehmlich an Baron Carl Hildebrand von Canstein (1667–1719) in Berlin gesandt wurden. Die beiden Briefautoren waren Ärzte an den von August Hermann Francke (1663–1727) in Halle gegründeten Anstalten; ihre Namen sind mit der Gründung der Halleschen Medikamentenexpedition verknüpft. Die Briefsammlung ist bekannt wegen der in ihr enthaltenen Berichte von der Entwicklung der *Essentia dulcis*, der Halleschen Variante eines *Aurum potabile*, und der weiteren Waisenhausmedikamente.

Daneben lassen die Briefe aber auch Hintergründe zum allmählichen Aufbau des Medikamentenvertriebs, zur Werbekampagne für die *Essentia dulcis* und zur Erstellung von „Exempeln" (beispielhaften Krankengeschichten) erkennen. Überraschend ist die Beteiligung von adligen Frauen an der Organisation des Vertriebs, z. T. in der Form von Arbeitsgemeinschaften. Die Spuren, die ihre Tätigkeiten in der Briefsammlung hinterlassen haben, erlauben Rückschlüsse auf Bedingungen und Dispositionen, die dem traditionellen, eindeutig auch geschäftsorientierten Handlungsspektrum von begüterten Frauen entsprachen.[2] Von dem weltweiten Exporthandel im Kielwasser der von Halle ausgehenden pietistischen Missionen[3] lassen diese Briefe allerdings noch kaum etwas ahnen.

Die Adligen, die Essenz und die Hauswirtschaft

Der erste Fall einer Medikamenten-Expedition im buchstäblichen Sinn,[4] also der Versendung eines Medikaments aus der Produktion des Waisenhauses in Halle

1 AFSt/H C 285:15.

2 Zu Frauen (Hausfrauen, „Hauswirtinnen") und „Geschäften" im Rahmen der Hauswirtschaft im 18. Jahrhundert siehe FRÜHSORGE (1976), 137–139. HARTMANN (1983), 151–154 betont die (gleichwertige) Aufgabenteilung von Hausvater und -mutter. Über die „pietist benefactresses" im Umfeld der Halleschen Anstalten siehe WILSON (2000), 31–41. In WILSON (2001), 3, heißt es dazu: „They participated by investment, involvement in trade, or by hands-on labor […]."

3 Zu den „pious traders" in Amerika siehe WILSON (2000).

4 Wann der Beginn der Medikamentenexpedition als eines von der Apotheke zu unterscheidenden Unternehmens anzusetzen ist, wurde noch nicht abschließend geklärt. GITTNER (1948), 26, nimmt mit Bezug auf Wilhelm Fries das Jahr 1700 an, ALTMANN (1972), 87, Anm. 209, und WELSCH (1955), 65, bestimmen das Jahr 1702; ihr Beleg ist eine einzelne

im Rahmen einer Therapie, muss schon im Jahr 1701 erfolgt sein – zumindest legt dies die erste publizierte Fallgeschichte nahe.[5] Der Weg des Präparats ging ins Hessische zu einem adligen Fräulein. Ihre Krankengeschichte berichtet von einem siebenjährigen Leiden, verbunden mit Bettlägerigkeit und schweren, offenbar chronischen Entzündungen verschiedener Art. Außerdem war sie *contract*. Die Anwendung des Halleschen *Aurum potabile* bewirkte, so heißt es, ihre völlige Genesung.

Mit ihrem *Casus* leitete Christian Friedrich Richter die Sammlung von Exempeln ein, welche die *Berichte von der Essentia dulcis*[6] durch „Beweise" von deren Heilkraft stützen sollten, und unverändert übernahm er ihn auch in sein Werk *Kurtzer und deutlicher Unterricht von dem Leibe und natürlichen Leben des Menschen* von 1705.[7]

Es stellt sich die Frage, was dieses Fräulein, eine Hofdame in Berleburg in der Wetterau, dazu bewogen haben mag, ihre umfangreiche Kranken- und Heilungsgeschichte der Propaganda für Waisenhausmedikamente aus Halle zur Verfügung zu stellen. Und nicht nur dies – einige Jahre später gab sie Richter sogar die Zustimmung zur Veröffentlichung ihres Namens: Anna Gertraud v. Dalwig (ca. 1665–ca. 1737), Tochter eines alten Adelsgeschlechts aus Dillig. Sie bürgte also mit ihrer ganzen Person für die Güte und Heilkraft der Arznei. Sie war eine enge Freundin der regierenden Berleburger Gräfin und wie diese (und der gesamte kleine Grafenhof um 1700) eine bekennende Philadelphierin.[8] Mit der Ent-Anonymisierung ihrer „Exempel" hatten bereits um 1702 verschiedene Berliner adlige Patientinnen C. F. Richters begonnen: so Barbara Cordula Astmann, geborene v. Lauter (1670–1710), und Dorothea Juliana v. Löben, geborene v. Krosigk (1669–1711). Die zuletzt genannten Damen waren nicht nur geographisch viel dichter an der Quelle der Essenz als v. Dalwig. Aus den Briefen der Brüder Richter geht hervor, dass sie darüber hinaus zusammen mit weiteren Freundinnen Tätigkeiten im Bereich von Werbung und Distribution ausübten: In der

gesonderte Abrechnung aus diesem Jahr. Der Begriff selbst entstand zu einem späteren Zeitpunkt.

5 EXEMPEL (1702), [3]–[8], hier [6]. August Hermann Francke bezieht sich in den Berichten über seine Anstalten, den *Segensvollen Fußstapfen*, auf diesen Fall, FRANCKE (1994), 168–169. REITZ (1716), 277–287, fügt Franckes Bericht in die 20. Geschichte der *Historie der Wiedergebohrnen* ein. Er weist darauf hin, dass die Protagonistin „annoch in der Hütten ihres Leibes" wohne – die Historien handeln in der Regel von bereits Verstorbenen.

6 BERICHT (1701).

7 RICHTER (1705), 458–468.

8 Über diese Szene, die die kirchlichen und außerkirchlichen Frommen im protestantischen Deutschland (und darüber hinaus) aufregte, siehe SCHNEIDER (1993), 420. Über v. Dalwig siehe SCHRADER (1989), 80–85, 396 (Anm. 60), und HOFFMANN (1996), 90–91, 234 (Anm. 45, 46), mit Korrekturen an Schrader. Nach diesen beiden Autoren war sie mit radikalpietistischen Ärzten befreundet: Sie stiftete Hector de Marsays Ehe mit einer ihrer Freundinnen. Mit Gerhard Tersteegen führte sie eine Korrespondenz. Zu Tersteegen siehe HABRICH (1997). Zu Marsay siehe KNIERIEM & BURKARDT (2002), 78–95.

Residenzstadt Berlin hatte sich das kleine, aber schrittmachende Vertriebszentrum der Waisenhausmedikamente um Carl Hildebrand von Canstein gebildet.

Canstein gilt zu Recht als einer der wichtigsten Förderer von August Hermann Franckes Anstalten in Halle.[9] Vor allem die Planung und Durchführung der Wirtschaftsprojekte in der Anfangszeit einschließlich der Beschaffung von Geldspenden für deren Anschubfinanzierung sind ihm zuzuschreiben. Canstein trat als Sachwalter eines adligen Gemeinwesens auf, als Führungsfigur in einer Gruppe von reformorientierten und religiös gefestigten Adligen. Diese Formation im Berliner Establishment gehörte sicher nicht zu den großen Fraktionen der dortigen Aristokratie, grenzte sich aber andererseits nicht sektiererisch von den anderen ab. Zu dieser Gruppe zählte eine Reihe pietistischer Geistlicher in der Nachfolge Philipp Jakob Speners (1635–1705). Gemeinsam war diesen Personen ihre Bindung an Franckes Projekt zur Verbesserung aller Stände,[10] das Canstein und seine Freunde – meist, aber nicht nur lutherische Adlige – offensichtlich als ein ihnen gemäßes Programm zur Erneuerung und Reform der Gesellschaft auffassten. Der Freundeskreis bestand aus einer Reihe von Militärs und Geheimen Räten (Ministern) sowie deren Familien, Freunden und Freundinnen.

Die inneren Verhältnisse der beteiligten Häuser bis hin zu den Freundinnen/Freunden und zum Personal, vor allem die Interaktionen zwischen den Häusern sind für diese Gruppe noch kaum erforscht und bearbeitet worden, auch hinsichtlich der Frauen nicht. Ihre Leistungen, bestehend aus einer Vielzahl von Impulsen, Initiativen und Zuarbeiten sowohl philanthropischer als auch geschäftlicher Art verschwanden wohl gerade deswegen schnell aus dem Blick, weil sie überwiegend Teil des Alltagshandelns gewesen sind und daher im Abarbeiten täglich wiederkehrender Aufgaben bestanden. Diese Tätigkeiten hingen oft mit Versorgung und Erwerb zusammen. Wie bekannt, basierte die adlige Ökonomie auf dem Grundbesitz und der Revenue daraus. Aus der Perspektive der einzelnen Häuser stellen sich die „Ökonomien" als subsistenzerhaltende wirtschaftliche Einheiten von Produktion und Konsum dar. Innerhalb der häuslichen Wirtschaft lassen sich bestimmte Tätigkeiten ausdifferenzieren, für die haushaltende Frauen verantwortlich waren. Damit verbunden waren auch (zurechenbare) Einkünfte: Anke Hufschmidt hat in ihrer groß angelegten Untersuchung über adlige Frauen im Weserraum u. a. eine Reihe von Tätigkeiten im Rahmen einer gutswirtschaftlichen Haushaltsführung isoliert – sie bezeichnen gleichzeitig die allgemeinen Qualifikationen, über die Frauen verfügten, und die auch in unserem Kontext zur

9 Siehe hierzu SCHICKETANZ (2002), 2. Kapitel, besonders 37–43. Ausführlich über die Wirtschaftsprojekte Cansteins mit C. F. Richters Beteiligung schon ALTMANN (1972), Kapitel 8. Siehe auch HINRICHS (1971), 71–73.

10 Dieses Projekt ist dargelegt in Franckes *Großem Aufsatz*, den er seit 1701 immer wieder neu bearbeitete, teils unter Cansteins Mitwirkung. Er wurde in variierten Abschriften ausgewählten Personen überreicht, die seinen Plänen nützen konnten: PODCZECK (1961), 17–25.

Anwendung kommen. Neben der Verwaltung (und Vermehrung) ihres eigenen Vermögens sind zu nennen:[11]

- Führung von Haus- und Lagerbüchern, Verwaltung,
- Produktion marktfähiger Güter (Leinen, Butter, Produkte aus Viehwirtschaft usw.),
- Abrechnungen in diesen Bereichen: Rechnungsbücher, Einnahme-Ausgabebilanzen,
- Auszahlungen (z. B. von Armengeld, von Deputat an den Küster),
- Kreditgeschäfte.

Großbäuerinnen ähnlich, betrieben sie Garnspinnen, Kräuterkultur, Flachsbleichen und dgl. häufig selbst.[12] Sie waren vertraut mit haushälterischen Disziplinen wie der Vorratshaltung, der sparsamen Anwendung von Mitteln und der Organisation von Arbeitsabläufen, darunter die Einteilung, Anweisung und Aufsicht des Personals. Bei funktionierenden größeren Hauswirtschaften kann gelegentlich, hinsichtlich der Teilung der Arbeit und Kooperation, von Manufakturen gesprochen werden. Der Begriff der Manufaktur wird in diesem Beitrag noch eine Rolle spielen. Als „modernes Beispiel" in der Herausbildung der Manufaktur aus der Kombination verschiedenster handwerklicher Tätigkeiten nennt Marx eine „patriarchalische" Variante, in der alle Beschäftigten nicht nur ohne das Kommando eines Werkstattleiters arbeiten, sondern auch räumlich voneinander entfernt, in ihren Häusern oder Gärten[13] – eine Enklave ländlicher Bewirtschaftungsformen, wie sie die *Adligen Hausväter*[14] beschreiben, eingebettet in eine marktbestimmte Gesellschaft, verbunden mit ihr durch Tausch- und Handelsbeziehungen.

Ein Element der traditionellen Hauswirtschaften ist die häusliche Medizin. Sie taucht nicht in allen *Hausvätern* auf, in der Sekundärliteratur fast ausschließlich dann, wenn diese aus medizingeschichtlicher Perspektive verfasst wurde.[15] Hufschmidts sozialhistorischer Ansatz fasst medizinisches Handeln, das sie bei den Weseradligen vorfand, unter dem Begriff der Mildtätigkeit (Verteilen von Arzneimitteln an die Armen). Das Phänomen der Herstellung und Weitergabe von Arzneien durch Frauen konzentriert sich in der Forschung auf zwei Bereiche, (1) als Praxis von Fürstinnen, deren Nachlässe in hauseigenen Archiven

11 Vgl. HUFSCHMIDT (2001), 269; 193–208 (Rechercheergebnisse). Auch die städtischen Adligen besaßen Landgüter und bewirtschafteten sie. Viele der Tätigkeiten (und Qualifikationen) kamen im stadtwirtschaftlichen Bereich ebenso vor wie im landwirtschaftlichen.

12 HUFSCHMIDT (2001), 193–194.

13 MARX (1970), 357, Anm. 26. Es handelt sich um die Seidenindustrie von Lyon und Nîmes. U. a. heißt es da: „Sie beschäftigt viele Frauen und Kinder, aber ohne sie zu übermüden [...], sie lässt sie in ihren schönen Tälern und Gärten [...], um dort Seidenraupen zu züchten. [...] Alle sind sie unabhängig." „Patriarchalisch" ist hier in einem fürsorgenden Sinn gemeint.

14 Stellvertretend: FLORIN (1725), der die Arbeitsabläufe recht umfangreicher „Haus=Wesen" für „hohe" und „niedere" Stände auf größeren Gütern beschreibt.

15 Wie z. B. HARTMANN (1983).

überdauerten,[16] (2) als von Frauen ausgeübte „Volksmedizin“, die u. a. durch die Beschäftigung der Gerichte überliefert ist.[17]

Karitative Verteilung von Arzneimitteln fand bei den Berliner Adligen statt – sie soll hier nicht weiter behandelt werden. Für eine Herstellung von Arzneimitteln in ihren Haushaltungen gibt es in der Korrespondenz nur wenige Anhaltspunkte.[18] Dagegen finden sich in den Briefnachlässen der Brüder Richter und Cansteins sehr viele Hinweise auf Vertriebstätigkeiten.[19]

Im Folgenden soll vornehmlich anhand der Briefe der beiden Halleschen Waisenhausärzte an Baron Canstein das weibliche Netzwerk der frühen Medikamentenexpedition dargestellt werden. Die Analyse wird zeigen, dass die weiblichen Aktivitäten und Anstöße in dem Berliner Umfeld nicht vereinzelt, sondern arbeitsteilig und kooperativ organisiert waren.

Analyse der Briefquellen

Der Briefwechsel wurde zwischen 1701 und 1711, dem Todesjahr Christian Friedrich Richters, geführt.[20] Cansteins Schreiben an die beiden Brüder sind zwar nicht erhalten, wohl aber dessen Briefe an August Hermannn Francke, geschrieben zwischen 1697 und 1719. Die Entwicklung der Arzneiherstellung und -erprobung sowie der Aufbau des Medikamentenhandels als Betrieb oder „erwerbende Anstalt“ des Waisenhauses gehörten zu den Hauptanliegen der Direktion. Daher gab es einen permanenten Austausch zwischen Francke und dem Baron über das Projekt und, in diesem Zusammenhang, auch über die Brüder Richter. Denn nicht nur Francke, sondern – informell – auch Canstein nahm

16 BERNSCHNEIDER-REIF (2004), 163–167, stellt einige Rezeptsammlungen von Gräfinnen vor. Sie fand Berührungspunkte mit der Volksmedizin und kann die medizinische Betätigung einer Gräfin als „Laienärztin“ und Apothekerin nachweisen. Sie rekonstruiert den Weg einer Rezeptur von einer Frau „aus dem Volk“ in eine gräflichen Sammlung. Sie weist Fälle der Zusammenarbeit von Fürstin und Apotheker nach: BERNSCHNEIDER-REIF (2004), 163, 164, 165–166.

17 DANNINGER (1998) schildert die Verwerfungen, in die traditionelle Heiltätigkeit von Frauen geriet, als die neuen landesweiten Medizinalordnungen der politischen Aufklärung sie aus ihrem Gewerbe vertrieben.

18 Siehe unten Frau v. Pannewitz, Frau v. Bülow. Deren Bibliotheken sind (anders als bei Fürstinnen) kaum rekonstruierbar. Zu einschlägigen Büchern, die sie vielleicht besaßen, siehe SZASZ (1997).

19 Dies stellt mit Bezug auf C. H. v. Canstein Schicketanz fest, der ihn als Pharmavertreter einstuft: „Noch ehe die Halleschen Medikamente ab 1703 auch an anderen Orten durch Agenturen vertrieben wurden, war Canstein schon ihr erster unbezahlter Vertreter in Berlin“, SCHICKETANZ (2002), 43. Eine Druckschrift *Kurtze Nachricht von der Tinctura Polychresta* des Waisenhauses gibt als Berliner Bezugsadresse für das Präparat das Cansteinische Haus, „dem Post=Hause gegenüber“, an: AFSt/W IX/II/9.

20 Eine kritische Edition der Briefe wird von Jürgen Helm und Elisabeth Quast vorbereitet.

ihnen gegenüber Direktorenfunktionen wahr. Dies alles ist in Cansteins Briefen an Francke dokumentiert.[21]

Rechnet man die Namen der (mit den Briefschreibern interagierenden) dritten Personen, die in den Richterschen Briefen genannt werden, zusammen, dann kommt man auf etwa 140 Männer und Frauen: Patienten und Arzneikonsumenten beiderlei Geschlechts, Kommentatoren, Kritiker und Ratgeber (Ärztekollegen, auch etwa Georg Ernst Stahl), Studenten (die mittlerweile qualifiziert waren und Stellen benötigten), Informanten (aus Bereichen von Politik, Höfen, Großhandel, Chemie), Gelehrte und Projektanten (u. a. Ehrenfried Walther von Tschirnhaus). Von diesen ca. 140 Personen sind 35, also rund 25% weiblich, und von diesen 35 Frauen sind wiederum 30 adlig. Die wenigen Frauen des Hochadels sind nicht in die hier zu untersuchenden Prozesse involviert und werden, ebenso wie die wenigen bürgerlichen und Dienstfrauen, vernachlässigt. Die große Gruppe der Fräulein und Baroninnen sind Ehefrauen und weitere Angehörige von Freunden Cansteins: Personen aus der Spitze des Militärs – er war vor seiner Hinwendung zu Francke Offizier gewesen[22] –, u. a. der Generäle Natzmer und Löben, und von Hof- und Regierungsamtsträgern in Berlin: Bülow (Oberhofmeister), Pannewitz (Oberjägermeister), Schweinitz und Chwalkowski (Geheime Räte). Nach dem kulturellen Muster des Amts- oder Arbeitspaares[23] sind die Gattinnen in den Wirkungskreis und die Amtsführung der Ehemänner einbezogen. Bei dem Paar Bülow ist er Oberhofmeister des Königs, sie Oberhofmeisterin der Königin. Einige der Baroninnen stammen aus verschiedenen alten Familien Magdeburgs (Lethmate, Legat), des Saalkreises (Krosigk)[24] und Sachsens (Gersdorf). Die Biografien einiger dieser Frauen hat Ulrike Witt recherchiert. Sie hat deren Beziehungen zu dem Franckeschen Projekt minutiös rekonstruiert[25] und diese Spenderinnen und Förderinnen, deren Anteil am Werk schnell in Vergessenheit geraten war, wieder bekannt gemacht.[26] Von dreien ist überliefert, dass sie jeweils als Leiterin des Frauenzimmerstifts arbeiten sollten: die Witwen Astmann[27] und v. Geusau sowie die noch unverheiratete Bartha v. Krosigk. Frau v. Geusau übernahm das Amt für mehrere Jahre, während die beiden anderen

21 Vgl. ALTMANN (1972), Kapitel 9.

22 Siehe HINRICHS (1971), 129. Zum Verhältnis von Pietismus und preußischem Militär siehe HINRICHS (1971), Kapitel II.

23 Siehe WUNDER (1992), 137–138.

24 Zu den v. Krosigk im Halle-Saalkreis siehe DREYHAUPT (1750), Anhang genealogischer Tabellen, 208–213; 212 (die hier betroffene Generation).

25 Siehe WITT (1996), 127–135, über die Förderinnen des Frauenzimmerstifts. Über Henriette Katharina v. Gersdorf und ihre Zusammenarbeit mit Francke und Canstein, auch spätere Konflikte: WITT (1996), 157–164.

26 Zur Überlieferung weiblicher Hinterlassenschaften und zu unterbliebener Traditionsbildung in Bibliothek und Archiv der Franckeschen Stiftungen seit dem 18. Jahrhundert: KLOSTERBERG (2007).

27 Barbara Cordula Astmann, geb. von Lauter. Die von ihr selbst verfasste Lebensgeschichte ist Teil der 16. Historie in Reitz' Sammlung von Biographien „Wiedergebohrner": REITZ (1716), 230–241.

Frauen Mitarbeiter Franckes heirateten, Frau Astmann den zeitweiligen Leiter des Pädagogiums Kalckberner und Bartha v. Krosigk Canstein selbst. Bartha und Canstein hatten schon in den 1690er Jahren kooperiert: Überliefert ist eine ausdauernde Überzeugungsarbeit dieser beiden in ihren weit verzweigten Familien mit dem Ziel, dem Franckeschen Pädagogium und dem Gynäceum (der entsprechenden Schule für Mädchen aus dem Adel und „von Stand") Sprösslinge zahlungskräftiger Eltern zuzuführen.[28] Von fast allen Frauen wissen wir aus den Korrespondenzen vor allem Cansteins, dass sie gemeinsam reisten und sich wiederholt in Halle aufhielten.

Die Damen werden in den Richterbriefen insgesamt 52 Mal, besonders häufig aber zwischen Oktober 1701 und April 1703 erwähnt.[29] Anfangs geschieht dies meist in Verbindung mit einer Diagnose von Beschwerden, die zuvor wohl brieflich mitgeteilt worden waren, und mit Empfehlungen von Arzneimitteln oder einer Diät, seltener mit einer ausführlichen Verordnung (Bülow: Nr. 4, 50; Friedeborn: Nr. 39, 43).[30] Andere wenden sich wegen der Erkrankung von Kindern (Astmann: Nr. 33, 36; Pannewitz: Nr. 4) oder des Ehemanns an Canstein und die beiden Ärzte. Aber die Diagnosen und die therapeutischen Empfehlungen und Anweisungen bilden gar nicht den größten Teil der mit diesen Frauen verknüpften Briefinhalte, dies ist nur bei 12 von 32 Namensnennungen bis April 1703 der Fall. In den 20 verbleibenden Erwähnungen (bis 1703) stehen die Namen der Frauen eher für die Kennzeichnung ihres Falls: Die Nennungen verteilen sich auf allgemeine Diskussionen über Arzneimitteltherapie, etwa bei der Übertragung von Einzelfallerfahrungen auf neue Fälle (Verfahrensmuster „Behandeln wie Astmannkinder": Nr. 33) oder bei Kritik (Dr. Abel zu Astmann: Nr. 4, Stahl zur Behandlung der Astmannkinder: Nr. 43).

In zwei Erwähnungen der v. Pannewitz geht es um die Mitteilung eines Rezepts (Opiumbereitung: Nr. 62 und 64).[31] Siebenmal sind die Namen mit der Ausarbeitung abgeschlossener Kuren zu „Exempeln" verbunden: C. F. Richter bereitet Publikationen über die Waisenhausmedikamente vor (v. Friedeborn: Nr. 39, 40 und 42; Astmann: Nr. 35, 36, 40, 49). Zwei der Erwähnungen v. Krosigks betreffen Absatzfragen: Einmal die Werbung für die *Essentia dulcis* und Einwände gegen deren hohen Verkaufspreis, das andere Mal hat sie eine fehlerhafte Abrechnung Richters moniert (Nr. 30 und 36). Bei Frau v. Schweinitz geht es um den Wunsch nach „Chocelate zur Probe", über die Richter wohl im Rahmen des mit der Apotheke verbundenen Materialienhandels verfügen konnte (Nr. 50).

28 Dies gelang z. B. mit den Fräulein v. Meysebuch (Cansteins Nichte) und v. Legat, zwei Knaben v. Löben und einem namens v. Legat (alle aus Barthas Familie).

29 In diesem Zeitraum ist auch das Briefaufkommen am höchsten. Es fehlt allerdings noch eine Einschätzung darüber, wie vollständig die Sammlung ist.

30 Die Nummernangaben entsprechen der Nummerierung der Briefe in der Akte AFSt/H C 285:15.

31 Es handelt sich um die einzige in dieser Briefsammlung nachweisbare Kenntnis und Weitergabe einer Rezeptur aus dem Haushalt einer Adligen.

Frau v. Lethmate wird fast ausschließlich im Zusammenhang mit Finanztransfers nach Halle genannt (Nr. 27, 28, 29 und 81).

Ab 1704 ist die Korrespondenz erheblich ausgedünnt: Waren es von 1701 bis Ende 1703 ca. 80 Briefe, so sind es von 1704 bis 1711 nur noch ca. 76 Briefe. Die zwischen 1704 und 1711 auf Frauen bezogenen Briefstellen (23 an der Zahl) betreffen in neun Fällen Krankheitsanlässe, darunter die missglückte Schwangerschaft der Baronin Löben, die zu ihrem Tod führte (Nr. 119, 124 und 158).

Die Frauen, welche auf weiterführende Weise mit den Halleschen Waisenhausmedikamenten zu tun hatten, waren zwar meist auch Patientinnen der Brüder Richter. Aber sie nahmen anscheinend auch Medikamente ab, ohne selbst krank zu sein oder unmittelbar kranke Kinder oder Ehemänner damit zu versorgen. Es waren etwa acht bis zehn sehr aktive Frauen. Sie gaben die Arzneien weiter an Freundinnen und Freunde, zur Probe und zur Bevorratung, als Ware im Handverkauf, hatten kleine Mengen davon in Kommission, und sie warben für die Richterschen Medikamente. Da dies alles in einem überschaubaren Kreis von Bekannten stattfand, wurden sie über Güte oder Mängel der Waisenhausmedikamente schnell informiert und konnten entsprechend reagieren. Die Generalin v. Lethmate[32] besorgte den Transfer des beim Verkauf eingenommenen Geldes nach Halle. Bartha v. Krosigk erledigte verschiedene Vertriebs- und Abrechnungsaufgaben und führte eine Kunden- bzw. Patientenkorrespondenz. Einige dieser Damen schrieben in Vorbereitung der Richterschen Publikation ihre Fallgeschichte auf, sie sammelten im Freundeskreis weitere *Casus* und waren Christian Friedrich Richter behilflich, die für die *Essentia dulcis* werbenden Berichte zusammenzustellen. Auf die wichtigsten Frauen in dieser Gruppe und auf deren Tätigkeit am Beginn des Medikamentenvertriebs soll nun eingangen werden.

Prima inter pares: Bartha von Krosigk

In einem kurzen Brief der Bartha Sophia v. Krosigk (1663–1718) in Berlin an August Hermann Francke in Halle,[33] unterzeichnet mit der Formel „Ihre Freundin und Dienerin“, findet sich in schnörkelloser Sprache und ohne nähere Angabe die Bestellung von *Essentia amara*, *Magisterium solare* und *Essentia dulcis* von der stärkeren Sorte. „Ich habe zwar noch welche“, heißt es da, aber die Gelegenheit sei gut, da ein gemeinsamer Freund die Medikamente auf dem Weg von Halle nach Berlin mitbringen könne. Auf diese Weise werde das Postgeld gespart. Dann folgt die Ankündigung: „so balt es müchlich [ist,] werde ich wieder gelt schicken vor die Es[s]ens“, mit dem erläuternden Zusatz: „Den[n] es noch meist in Schulden besteht.“

32 WITT (1996), 133, 140 und 141, beschreibt sie als Förderin Franckes. Besonders unterstützte sie das Frauenzimmerstift. Siehe auch das Testament der v. Lethmate, AFSt/W X/I/36.

33 Krosigk an Francke, AFSt/H C 5, 238–239 (Berlin, 9. Mai o. J.).

Sonst steht nicht viel in dem Brief; diese Form von Bestellung ist offenbar Routine. Dass es hier nicht um den Arzneibedarf in einem akuten Krankheitsfall geht, sondern um die Erneuerung eines Vorrats, und zwar offenbar zur Belieferung eines weiteren Personenkreises, darauf weist ihre Bemerkung über die Schulden hin, verbunden mit der Ankündigung einer so bald als möglichen Geldsendung für „die Essenz". Kurzum: Wir haben es hier mit einem wirtschaftlichen Vorgang zu tun, genauer mit der Abwicklung eines Kommissionsgeschäfts zwischen v. Krosigk und dem Direktor des Waisenhauses. Und diese Art wirtschaftlicher Tätigkeit scheint eingespielte Übung zu sein: So muss sich Christian Friedrich Richter als Hersteller der Waisenhausarzneien um ein Defizit von 60 Talern kümmern, die der Dame zustehen, und deren Verbuchung auf seiner Seite offenbar nicht korrekt erfolgt ist. Er schreibt an den Baron v. Canstein:

> Die Medicamenta, so sie in beyden Schreiben verlanget, sende hiebey, nebst der Rechnung, in welche sie eingeschrieben [...] Ich erinnere mich, daß sie einmal sagten, die Frl. v. Crossigk käme 60 thl in ihrer Rechnung zu kurtz, solte sichs nach der Zeit noch nicht gefunden haben, worinnen der Irthum stehe, dürffte das Geld nur künfftig abgezogen werden, damit die gute Fräul. bey ihrer großen Mühe nicht auch großen Schaden leide.[34]

Die spätere Bartha v. Canstein war Tochter einer der alten adligen Familien des Saalkreises, des Hohenerxlebenschen Zweiges der v. Krosigk. Einige ihrer Schwestern waren mit Berliner Hof- und Regierungsamtsträgern verheiratet. Sie selbst war zwischen 1684 und 1688 Hoffräulein am Sachsen-Coburger Hof, zusammen mit ihrer Mutter, die als Hofmeisterin im Dienst der Herzogin stand. Um 1688 hat ihr die preußische Königin eine Stelle im Mindener Stift verschafft. Im Jahr 1693 kam sie in das Haus ihrer Schwester v. Löben nach Berlin zu deren Gesellschaft und Unterstützung. Aus ihren Briefen geht hervor, dass sie sich auch um die Erziehung der zahlreichen Kinder dieser Schwester kümmerte. Im Haus des Generals v. Löben lernte sie Canstein kennen.[35]

Die Aufgaben, die sie im Zusammenhang mit den Waisenhausmedikamenten wahrnahm, waren Teil eines umfangreicheren Engagements in Franckes Halleschen Einrichtungen. Sie reiste häufiger nach Halle und war mit der dortigen Entwicklung vertraut.[36] Bartha v. Krosigk war eine der wichtigen Verbindungspersonen zwischen den Franckeschen Anstalten in Halle und den Franckefreundinnen und -freunden in Berlin. Dort hat sie eine so genannte Frauenzimmerma-

34 AFSt/H C 285:15, Nr. 36 (28. Mai 1702). Die Wirtschaftstäigkeit wird auch durch eine Stelle in einem Brief Cansteins an Francke vom 24. August 1703 belegt: „ich bitte einliegendes Schreiben an die frl. Kroseck zu bestellen, weilen darin eine assignation, dem H. D. Richter wegen der medicamenten 125 th. zu zahlen. Es ist vergeßen worden. also ist an der schleunigen bestellung gelegen", SCHICKETANZ (1972), 237.

35 Ihre Personalia finden sich in der Leichenpredigt, SYMPATHIAE TESTIMONIUM (1718), 33, ergänzende Angaben in den Personalia ihrer Schwester Juliana Dorothea v. Löben in deren Leichenpredigt: MARGGRAF (1711), 56.

36 Siehe z. B. Cansteins Brief an Francke vom 20. August 1703, in dem er „in Eyl" ihren Besuch in Halle ankündigt, bei dem sie einige, beide betreffende Angelegenheiten besorgen werde. SCHICKETANZ (1972), 237.

nufaktur ins Leben gerufen zu dem Zweck, Sachspenden und Geldbeträge an das Hallesche Waisenhaus zu überweisen.[37] Nach Barthas Tod wurde diese Einrichtung von der Generalin Natzmer[38] weitergeführt. Bartha v. Krosigk speiste in Berlin täglich eine Gruppe von Armen aus dem Viertel.[39] Sie nahm August Hermann Francke die Sorge um dessen Schwester, eine verheiratete Frau Hoyer, ab, die verarmt und in offenbar desolatem Zustand nach Berlin gekommen war und sowohl materielle Unterstützung als auch ärztliche Hilfe benötigte.[40]

Aus ihrem Bekanntenkreis bekam sie Anfragen zu Medikamenten sowie „Zettel“[41] von Personen mit akuter Erkrankung, die sie an die Waisenhausärzte weiterleitete. Der Umgang der v. Krosigk mit Kranken gewann mit der schnellen Entwicklung des Halleschen Arzneiwesens 1701 eine neue Dimension: Bartha nahm die Korrespondenz mit Klienten Christian Friedrich Richters auf und leitete sie, offenbar mit Kommentar und weiteren Hinweisen versehen, an ihn bzw. seinen Bruder weiter. Eine nachfolgend zitierte Briefpassage belegt, dass sie für die *Essentia dulcis* warb und sich auch an dem Dauerstreit über deren Preis beteiligte (Canstein und Francke hielten im Gegensatz zu den Brüdern Richter den Verkaufspreis der *Essentia dulcis* für zu hoch). Richter schrieb an Canstein:

> Der Frln. von Krosigk bitte bey gehorsamer recommendation zu melden, daß dero lezteres Schreiben empfangen hätte, wäre aber an deßen Beantwortung wegen einer dazwischen kommenden unvermutheten Reise gehindert worden. Die Gräfin, deren sie gedacht habe sich noch nicht gemeldet, so sie sich aber melden wird, so solte schon wegen des pretii der essentiae dulcis concentratae remonstration gethan werden.[42]

Liest man die Briefe Nr. 30 bis Nr. 49 von Ende Juni bis Ende Dezember 1702 im Zusammenhang, dann gewinnt man einen recht guten Eindruck, wie aus den mittlerweile vorliegenden Erfahrungen mit den Waisenhausarzneien publikationsfähige „Exempel“ wurden. Es scheint, dass das Redigieren dieser Heilungs-

37 AFSt/W X/I/150, 8. Zu dieser Manufaktur siehe SCHICKETANZ (2002), 38. FRANCKE (1994), 267, führt mit Bezug auf das Jahr 1707 aus, es hätten „einige Herren-Standes, Adeliche, und andere in gutem Vermögen stehende Personen“ eine „Manufactur (wie Sie dieselbe zu nennen beliebet)“ gegründet, in der sie zugunsten des Waisenhauses teils selbst etwas arbeiteten, teils durch andere etwas arbeiten ließen.

38 SCHICKETANZ (2002), 38. Charlotte Justine v. Natzmer, Ehefrau von Cansteins Freund und pietistischem Kombattanten Dubislav Gneormar v. Natzmer, ist die Tochter der Baronin Henriette Katharina v. Gersdorf. Frau v. Natzmers Sohn aus erster Ehe, Nikolaus Ludwig Graf v. Zinzendorf, gründete später die Herrnhuter Brüdergemeine.

39 „Unsere armme werden Noch immer erqwickt und vermehrett sich die Zall es seynde Nun 17 persohnen alle tage.“ Brief an Francke, AFSt C5, 235 (Berlin, 3. April o. J.). Vgl. hierzu HUNTER (1997), 91: Sie berichtet von einer Hofdame Queen Annes (Elizabeth Gray), diese habe eine „reputation as a physician and apothecary” gehabt, und „[...] also she dayly fed and cared for more than seventy poor people in her community”.

40 Siehe Briefe Bartha v. Cansteins an Francke: AFSt/H C5, 13–16 und 234–235 (Berlin, 8. Februar bzw. 3. April, beide o. J.). Anna Elisabeth Hoyer, geb. Francke, 1656–1710/11.

41 Siehe z. B. AFSt/H C 285:15, Nr. 36 (28. Oktober 1702).

42 AFSt/H C 285:15, Nr. 30 (29. Juli 1702). Die Passage deutet darauf hin, dass es einen Briefwechsel auch zwischen Richter und Bartha gegeben haben muss, der verschollen ist.

berichte im Rahmen einer Arbeitsgemeinschaft geschah, in der auch über Formatfragen diskutiert wurde. So z. B. im Fall der Frau Astmann, die den Bericht von ihren Kindern selbst verfasste. Diesen Aufsatz will Richter in die Form eines Briefs bringen[43] und bittet um ihr Einverständnis; publiziert wurde er schließlich in der von Astmann gelieferten sachlichen Form.[44] Die ausgearbeiteten Berichte erfolgreicher Kuren werden sowohl den Haus- und Reiseapotheken beigepackt als auch von den Brüdern Richter in Broschüren veröffentlicht und in mehreren Auflagen herausgegeben. Die Exempel gelungener, durch die *Essentia dulcis* bewirkter Heilungen waren auch intern von großer Bedeutung: Der akademische Lehrer und – nolens volens – auch Supervisor der beiden Waisenhausärzte, Georg Ernst Stahl, war ein Skeptiker des *Aurum potabile*. Christian Friedrich Richter bediente sich der Briefe geheilter Patienten, um seine Argumente zu untermauern. Er schrieb an Francke:

> Ich producirte ihm unterschiedene Briefe einiger Patienten, so an die Frl. Kroßig geschrieben waren, und benahm ihm seine dubia, so gut ich konte, so schien es doch, als wenn er sich faßte, in übrigen war er sehr freundl.[45]

Bartha v. Krosigk fungierte hier also als Korrespondentin und als eine Art Sachbearbeiterin oder auch Sekretärin Richters – dessen Position sie in diesem Punkt stützt.

Auch auf einen direkten und ganz praktischen Bezug Barthas v. Krosigk zur Medizin ist noch einzugehen: Sie hat sich auf die Krankenpflege verstanden und sie anscheinend habituell ausgeübt. Sie pflegte „schwer“ Erkrankte „in ihrem Haus“, wie es heißt, gesund,[46] war also eine Heilperson und eine Krankenpflegerin. Diese Tatsache bietet eine Erklärung für relativ umfangreiche Arzneibestellungen in Halle sowohl durch sie als auch durch Canstein.[47] Wegen ihrer medizinischen Tätigkeit ist sie eine ideale Adressatin des Richterschen *Kurtzen und Deutlichen Unterrichts von dem Leibe und natürlichen Leben des Menschen*, ein Werk, das sich ausdrücklich auch an „Ungelehrte“ wendet und eine Auswahl von acht „der sichersten und besten Artzneyen“ vorstellt, die auch Laien mit Aussicht auf Heilerfolg anwenden könnten.[48] Über eine medizinische Ausbildung Barthas (im engeren Sinn) ist nichts bekannt. Vorstellbar ist, dass sie im Mindener Stift

43 AFSt/H C 285:15, Nr. 36 (28. Oktober 1702).

44 Einen weiteren Diskussionsfall beim Redigieren – zwischen Richter und Canstein – schildert Jürgen Helm im vorliegenden Band.

45 AFSt/H C 285:15, Nr. 167 (Brieffragment, von Bearbeiterhand datiert auf Oktober/November 1702). In Nr. 36 (28. Oktober 1702) beschreibt Richter dieselbe Situation unter Auslassung von Barthas Part: „Als ich zu ihm kam, producirte ich ihm unterschiedene Briefe, so die Patienten selbst geschrieben, und so wohl ihre Kranckheit, als auch die völlige Genesung mit sonderbaren expressiones enthalten.“

46 Johann Jakob Rambach in seinem Epicedium in SYMPATHIAE TESTIMONIUM (1718), 66.

47 Vgl. SCHICKETANZ (2002), 42–43 über Canstein als einen der „eifrigsten Kunden“ der Brüder Richter.

48 RICHTER (1705) im Titel. Über die Popularisierungsfunktion dieses Werks siehe HELM (2001), 263–264.

unterrichtet wurde – vom Franckeschen Fräuleinstift ist z. B. die „Apotheckerey" als Unterrichtsfach überliefert.[49] Wohl ebenso wahrscheinlich ist ein beobachtendes Lernen von der Mutter und/oder deren Kolleginnen am Hof.[50]

Es ist bemerkenswert und wohl ein seltener Fall, dass eine Frau, die nicht Professorenfrau und eben keine Universitätsverwandte war, durch eine von Professoren verfasste Leichenpredigt geehrt wurde. Dies geschah Bartha, die 1718 am Friesel starb: Ihr widmeten „die Professoren der Friedrichs=Universität" – also Francke und seine Kollegen an der theologischen Fakultät der Universität Halle – eine umfangreiche, in Berlin herausgegebene Trauerschrift. Die Personalia und die Gedächtnispredigten benennen ihre Wohltätigkeit, wie es üblich war, pauschal. In den zahlreichen Epicedien allerdings finden sich einige konkretere Hinweise.[51] Sowohl der Orientalist Johann Heinrich Michaelis als auch der Theologe Johann Jakob Rambach, damals noch Student, beide enge Mitarbeiter August Hermann Franckes, gedenken als zeitweilige Patienten Barthas ihrer Heilung „von schwerer Krankheit", die sie „nächst Gott" ihrer Sorge und Pflege zuschreiben. Bartha v. Canstein, geb. Krosigk, wurde in der Leichenfeier gewissermaßen als eine Hallesche Projektverwandte gewürdigt.

Schwägerinnen: Weitere an der Medikamentenexpedition beteiligte Frauen

Dorothea Juliana v. Löben

Mit Bartha v. Krosigks Schwestern gewann Canstein gleich mehrere philanthropische Schwägerinnen. Dorothea Juliana, Ehefrau des Generalleutnants Carl Hildebrand v. Löben, ging durch ihr Exempel einer gelungenen Kur in die Literatur ein: Sie schilderte ausführlich und sehr genau die Wirkungen der *Essentia dulcis*, die sie bei einer Geburt – insgesamt absolvierte sie deren 24 – wahrgenommen hat. Christa Habrich schreibt der Autorin eine bemerkenswerte Beobachtungsgabe und hohe laienmedizinische Qualifikation zu.[52] Frau v. Löben kommt darüber hinaus als Vermittlerin von Waisenhausmedikamenten in der Generalität in Be-

49 So WITT (1996), 138, Anm. 333.

50 HUNTER (1997), 102, schreibt zu dieser Frage: Eine Ausbildung (education) „in chemical technology and medical preparations was acquired by observation, by many while in service and appreticeship, and by aristocratic women while in their houses observing their mothers, their own apothecaries, their friends [...]. It also seems reasonable to assume that the women may have formed circles exchanging receipts and experiences [...]". Zu den einschlägigen Zuständigkeiten der Hofmeisterinnen siehe unten Anm. 58 und 60.

51 SYMPATHIAE TESTIMONIUM (1718), 57, 66. Trauergedichte widmeten ihr als erster Francke selbst, weiter Breithaupt, Anton, zwei Michaelis, Lange, Rambach, Lindhammer, Herrnschmidt.

52 „Eine Baronin von Löwen [...]": HABRICH (1982), 110; die Schreibweise entspricht der in RICHTER (1705). – Christian Sigismund Richter berichtet von der komplizierten letzten Schwangerschaft der v. Löben, „welche bereits 24 Kinder gehabt". AFSt/H C 285:15, Nr. 158 (2. Mai 1711). – Außer dem toten Kind, so heißt es in ihrer Leichenpredigt, sei ein Gallenstein „von weißer Couleur" gefunden worden: MARGGRAF (1711), 61.

tracht. Von ihr ist, wie von der Generalin Natzmer, überliefert, dass sie ihren Mann „ins Feld" begleitete.[53] Im Fall von Frau v. Natzmer belegt die Korrespondenz Cansteins,[54] dass Lieferungen von Medikamenten aus Richters Produktion für Natzmers Truppe an ihre Adresse stattfanden. Sie leitete die Sendungen dann an v. Natzmer weiter und nahm von diesem Bestellungen nach Halle entgegen. Nach diesem Muster könnte auch das Ehepaar v. Löben tätig gewesen sein.

Dorothea Juliana gehörte, wie aus Cansteins Briefen zu entnehmen ist zum (informellen) diplomatischen Corps von Franckes Anstalten: Im Zusammenspiel mit dem pietistischen Hofprediger Porst, dem Beichtvater der preußischen Königin Sophie Luise, war sie eine sehr wichtige Verbindungsperson zwischen dieser (lutherisch) frommen, wohltätigen Frau und August Hermann Francke.[55]

Christiana Antonia v. Bülow

Barthas jüngere Schwester Christiana Antonia, verheiratet mit dem Oberhofmeister und Kammerherrn Wilhelm Dieterich v. Bülow hatte ein Amt als Oberhofmeisterin der Königin. Sie war die erste Patientin, deren Beschwerden in den Briefen der Richterbrüder an Canstein ausführlich diagnostiziert und erklärt werden, vermutlich auf der Basis einer Beschreibung durch diesen.[56] Die „Schärffe", an der sie litt,[57] wurde auf „Zorn" und „Schrecken" zurückgeführt. Der Grund dieses „Zorns" und „Schreckens" mochte mit ihrer Tätigkeit am Hof[58] zusammenhängen, außerdem womöglich mit einer affektiv hofkritischen Haltung: Sie war eine fromme Frau, die gegenüber der Hofgesellschaft Vorbehalte oder gele-

53 Zumindest bereitete sie sich darauf vor. SCHICKETANZ (1972), 282: Canstein teilte Francke mit, „die fr. von loben meinet mit ihrem mann ins feldt zu gehen", weswegen deren Schwester v. Krosigk nicht abkömmlich sei, denn sie müsse deren Kinder hüten (9. 12. 1704).

54 SCHICKETANZ (1972), 525. Canstein an Francke (16. Juli 1712): „H. und fr. von Natzemer verlangen nach den Medicamenten, und wäre damit zu eylen, weilen der H. v. Natzemer Seine frau muß zu sich aus Douay nehmen, indem die armée ihren zurückmarsch darauf nicht nehmen möchte", und am 26. Juli 1712: „die Medicamente seind dem 17. dieses noch nicht bey der armée gewesen. ich sorge, da die fr. v. natzemer von douay weg, es werden selbige nicht leicht zur armée können gebracht werden".

55 Siehe z. B. SCHICKETANZ (1972), 425, besonders 399. Sophie Luise v. Mecklenburg war die 3. Ehefrau Friedrichs I. von Preußen.

56 Allerdings reiste Christian Friedrich Richter auch selbst gelegentlich nach Berlin und begutachtete dort Cansteins Klientel.

57 Zur „Schärffe" siehe STOLBERG (2002), 139–144.

58 Katrin Keller schildert den Tagesablauf von Hofdamen des Wiener Hofs. Der Arbeitsalltag ist streng reglementiert und lässt, auch wegen der Pflicht zu unbegrenzter Verfügbarkeit, wenig Ruhepausen und Rückzugsmöglichkeiten zu. Laut Keller obliegt der Oberhofmeisterin die Haushaltsführung der Königin, dies verlangt die entsprechenden Organisationsleistungen. Sie strukturiert das Besucherprogramm und die Audienzzeiten, bearbeitet Eingaben aller Art. Sie begleitet und besorgt sowohl den repräsentativen als auch „privaten" Tagesablauf der Königin. KELLER (2005), 110–118.

gentlich sogar Aversionen hatte.[59] Ihr *Casus* ging nicht ein in die Richtersche Galerie gelungener Kuren, zumindest ist sie in der Sammlung nicht identifizierbar. Es scheint, dass Frau v. Bülow als Schulbeispiel für die Einarbeitung Cansteins in hoftypische Beschwerdeprofile von Frauen zu betrachten ist – und wohl auch für Christian Friedrich Richter, der schließlich Cansteins Patientenbeobachtungen medizinisch umzusetzen hatte. Allerdings konnte v. Bülow auch selbst im Sinn einer praktischen Übung von dieser Konstellation profitieren, nicht nur als Mutter und Hausmutter, sondern auch wegen ihres Amtes: Als Oberhofmeisterin hatte sie die Zuständigkeit für das körperliche Wohlbefinden der Königin und verfügte sicherlich über eine umfangreiche Hausapotheke.[60] Auch sie ist in besonderer Weise zu dem Adressatenkreis von Richters *Unterricht* zu rechnen. Womöglich war sie die Herstellerin eines „büloischen Balsams", der in einem Vermerk über die oben erwähnte Frauenzimmermanufaktur[61] zu finden ist.

Ihre weiteren Beziehungen zu den Franckeschen Anstalten bewegten sich in dem üblichen Spektrum: Finanzielle Förderung, auch durch Stipendien an arme Begünstigte;[62] Nachfrage von Dienstpersonal, das von Francke empfohlen wurde;[63] Ankauf von großen Posten Bibeln, die Francke nach Gutdünken verschenken sollte.[64] Durch ihre amtsbedingt große Nähe zum Herrscherpaar konnte sie Informationen beschaffen, die für die Franckeschen Anstalten überlebenswichtig waren.[65]

Brigitte Maria v. Legat und Katharina v. Hackeborn

Auch die beiden ältesten Schwestern Krosigk gehörten zum Netzwerk. Sie waren nach dem bisherigen Kenntnisstand vorrangig durch Patientenbeziehungen mit den Richterbrüdern verbunden. Brigitte Maria v. Legats Tochter namens Rosimunde Juliana lebte, von ihr des Öfteren besucht, im Franckeschen Frauenzimmerstift. Sie wurde von Christian Sigismund Richter ärztlich betreut, der auch zu Bäderkuren mit ihr reiste.[66] Katharina v. Hackeborn war selbst Richtersche Patientin. Ihre Unpässlichkeiten wurden zum Anlass einer Hinzuziehung von Georg

59 Sie sei anscheinend schon „von Gott ergriefen", so Canstein am 26. 4. 1701 an Francke, und lebe, obgleich Hofmeisterin der Königin „nicht am hofe, sondern wohnet in der Stadt, [...]". SCHICKETANZ (1972), 115.

60 KELLER (2005), 118, beschreibt das Wiener königliche „Frauenzimmer", zu dem sowohl ein Raum für Erkrankte als auch eine Küche zur Bereitung von Diät- und Krankenkost gehörte. Über medizinisch gebildete englische Hofdamen und *Lady experimenters*: HUNTER (1997).

61 AFSt/W X/I/150, 8.

62 SCHICKETANZ (1972), 388 („für die arme studiosos").

63 SCHICKETANZ (1972), 72, 115.

64 SCHICKETANZ (1972), 523 (sie lieferte 1.200 Exemplare des NT).

65 Zur Bülowschen Diplomatie siehe z. B. SCHICKETANZ (1972), 342: „So baldt ich [...] durch die fr. von bülau den konig selbst haben sondiren lassen, denn an diesem letztern ist [...] das meiste gelegen, so wollen wir zusammen unsere resolution nehmen [...]". Sie sollte in diesem Fall herausfinden, ob der König beabsichtige, die Universität von Halle zu verlegen.

66 So nach Karlsbad, siehe AFST/H C 285-15, Nr. 86 (1. Juni 1704).

Ernst Stahl: Canstein hatte anscheinend den Eindruck gewonnen, die beiden Waisenhausärzte seien den Beschwerden der Dame nicht gewachsen. In dieser Situation wandte er sich, wie auch sonst in kritischen Fällen, wegen einer qualifizierten Stellungnahme an ihn.[67]

Anna Justine v. Pannewitz

Die Oberjägermeisterin Anna Justine v. Pannewitz (1664–1719) gehörte zu den Förderinnen der Franckeschen Anstalten.[68] Ihr Ehemann war ein langjähriger Freund Cansteins, überdies mit ihm verschwägert (über die Familie v. Arnim) – auch hier liegt also eine verwandtschaftsbasierte Verknüpfung vor. Er wurde einer der Berliner Patienten der Brüder Richter.

Mit Frau v. Pannewitz führte Christian Sigismund Richter einen Austausch über Opiumbereitung.[69] Anlass dazu gab wohl die Erkrankung des Herrn v. Pannewitz an einer „Species von der Gicht", wie C. S. Richter diagnostizierte.[70] Zu der Opiumbereitung der Ehefrau des Patienten meinte er, dass „man damit noch viel fürsichtiger umb gehen müßte als mit demjenigen [Opium], so auf gewöhnl. Weise, mit Essig praepariret und corrigiret wird". Sie hatte ihm außerdem eine Probe davon mitgesandt, die er analysierte und kritisch kommentierte.[71]

Johanna Ilsa v. Lethmate

Die „Generalin" Johanna Ilsa v. Lethmate, geborene v. Legat (gest. 1705), war die kinderlose Witwe eines Generalmajors. Sie erweist sich als eine Fachfrau für Finanzen:

> Der H. Prof. [Francke] hat von der Fr. General. Lettmatt kein Geld empfangen weil er das Blanqvet Ew. Gnad. wider zurück senden müßen (Brief 27).
> Von der Fr. Generalin [Lethmate] habe das übrige Geld empfangen und in die Rechnung, so hiebey zurücksende, eingetragen [...] (Brief 29).

67 Stahls Stellungnahme ist abgedruckt in MEYER-HABRICH (1981), Anhang, 48.

68 Frau v. Pannewitz arbeitete zusammen mit Canstein verschiedenen Projekten Franckes zu, z. B. der Lehre osteuropäischer Sprachen am Waisenhaus im Rahmen des Collegium Orientale. Sie schlug Lehramtskandidaten vor und sorgte für deren Bezahlung: SCHICKETANZ (1972), 152, 206 und 279, Anm. 55, und SCHICKETANZ (2002), 29.

69 AFSt/H C 285:15, Nr. 62 (6. März 1703).

70 AFSt/H C 285:15, Nr. 61 (3. März 1703).

71 Bei der Probe stellte er eine Abweichung von der Beschreibung fest: AFSt/H C 285:15, Nr. 62 (6. März 1703). Christian Sigismund Richter argwöhnte bei zwei weiteren Patienten, ihnen sei zu ihrem Nachteil Opium verabreicht worden: Adelheid Sibylle Schwartz, siehe Nr. 69 (21. April 1703), und Philipp Jakob Spener, siehe Nr. 84 (1. Juli 1704). Christian Friedrich Richter warnt im *Unterricht* vor der Anwendung von Opiaten, besonders, wenn sie „übel" zubereitet würden: RICHTER (1708), 165. 44–45, im 1. Teil des *Unterrichts,* berichtet er dagegen auch von einem kerngesunden gewohnheitsmäßigen Opiumesser.

> Die Ubersandte Rechnungen wil in Ordnung bringen, und überschicken. Zur Nachricht melde, daß das Geld von der Fr. von Lettmat noch nicht ausgezahlet worden. Es hat eben nicht zu eylen (Brief 81).[72]

Aus diesen Stellen geht hervor, dass Frau v. Lethmate die Buchhaltung und den Zahlungsverkehr des Berliner Vertriebs übernommen hatte (zumindest Teile davon). Der letzte Hinweis datiert vom April 1704. Ihr Testament zeigt, dass sie begütert war. Sie hinterließ ein Gut, das Vorwerk Schafsee bei Röblingen in der Nähe von Halle, mit dem Inventar „an Wies, Schiff und Geschirr", das als landwirtschaftlicher und wohl auch fischwirtschaftlicher Betrieb anzusehen ist und dessen Wert sie auf 10.000 rth veranschlagte. Dem Waisenhaus vermachte sie ein Kapital von 2.000 rth, von dessen Zinsen zwei Stiftsstellen finanziert werden sollten (eine davon bestimmt für ihre Nichte Rosimunde Juliana v. Legat),[73] außerdem noch einmal 200 rth (während die Armen der Stadt Halle mit 100 rth bedacht wurden). Sie hatte Francke auch einmal ein Haus aus ihrem Besitz zur Unterbringung des Stifts angeboten,[74] war also mit Finanz- und Vermögensplänen und -transfers mehrfach den Anstalten verbunden. Wie die Wege des Geldes bei der Medikamentenexpedition im einzelnen verliefen, welche Rolle genau Frau v. Lethmate dabei spielte – das „Blanquet", also eine Art Blankoscheck, gibt zu denken – ist hier nicht zu klären. Als geborene v. Legat war v. Lethmate mit den Krosigkschwestern verschwägert. Es scheint, dass als einzige Ausnahme in diesem Kreis Frau Astmann eine nichtverwandte Freundin ist.

Der religiöse Hintergrund der adligen Frauen

Mit Barbara Cordula Astmann möchte ich auf die religiösen Bindungen des Berliner Kreises zurückkommen, insbesondere zu den bekennenden Autorinnen von Richterschen Exempeln[75]. Obwohl die vorgestellten Briefzeugnisse Sachlichkeit und Nüchternheit spiegeln, ist mit den Personen eine religiöse Dramatik verknüpft. Sie sammelten sich um den pietistischen Erneuerer des lutherischen Protestantismus, Philipp Jakob Spener, und um Canstein, dessen engsten Freund und

72 Alle Briefe in AFSt/H C 285:15. Siehe auch SCHICKETANZ (1972), 178, 184, 187: Canstein nennt Frau v. Lethmate ausschließlich im Zusammenhang mit Zahlungs- und Buchungsvorgängen.

73 Siehe WITT (1996), 140, Anm. 342. In ihrem Testament bestimmte v. Lethmate als Nachfolgerin eine weitere ihrer Nichten. Die weiteren Nutznießerinnen der Stelle sollten Francke und die Verwaltung (des Stifts) frei auswählen können, AFSt/W X/I/36, fol. 2v, 3r. Eine lebenslange Rente hinterließ v. Lethmate einer Frau, die sie als „meine Türkin", welche sich habe christlich taufen lassen, bezeichnete: Fol. 3r, v.

74 WITT (1996), 133.

75 HABRICH (1982), 109–111, wählte bereits diese drei „Exempel" aus, um an ihnen das Niveau des medizinischen Wissens und Urteilsvermögens von Patientinnen aus der Bildungsschicht zu demonstrieren.

Vertrauten der Berliner Zeit.[76] Die Adligen waren von den Verwerfungen in der lutherischen Kirche nicht nur als Patronatsherren betroffen, sondern auch insofern, als die rebellischen, aufgewühlten Studenten und Magister aller Fakultäten, vor allem Theologen, in die Häuser kamen: Als Hauslehrer der Kinder, Sekretäre der Patrone, Seelenbeistände und schließlich Beichtväter nicht nur der Frauen, Prediger, Seelsorger, reisende Kandidaten oder Besucher, schließlich als Freunde.[77] Von der Mutter der „Astmannkinder" existiert eine nachgelassene Lebensbeschreibung.[78] Darin stellt sie sich als Konvertitin und in der Folge als eine Art Religionsflüchtling dar. Sie stammte, eine geborene v. Lauter, aus einer katholischen süddeutschen Adelsfamilie und trat schon als junges Mädchen zum lutherischen Protestantismus über. Zweimal war sie verheiratet, beide Male waren es lutherische Prediger aus dem engeren Kreis Speners.[79] Und auch ihr Weg von Dresden nach Berlin ist wohl im Zusammenhang mit Spener zu sehen. In Dresden war sie Hofdame der Kurfürstin Christine Eberhardine gewesen, sie schied aus deren Dienst aus zu dem Zeitpunkt, als der Kurfürst wegen des Erwerbs der polnischen Krone zum Katholizismus übertrat. Als Wahlverwandte Speners war Cordula Barbara Astmann in Berlin ein quasi natürliches Mitglied des Cansteinkreises. Zu der Bibel, die sie nach dem Tod ihres Mannes fertig stellte,[80] der sogenannten Astmann- oder Berliner Bibel, schrieb Spener ein Vorwort. Der Druck wurde durch Spenden bezuschusst, um den Preis niedrig zu halten und vor allem den Berliner Armen zu ermöglichen, die Bibel zu erwerben.[81]

Auch Dorothea Juliana v. Löben war eine bekennende Fromme. Sie hat ebenfalls einen Bericht ihres Lebens hinterlassen.[82] Darin schreibt sie, sie habe

76 Zu Philipp Jakob Spener, Senior der pietistischen Bewegung, siehe z. B. WALLMANN (2005), 66–102. Über Speners Rolle bei der Entwicklung Franckes hin zu einem Strategen und „Politiker" des Pietismus siehe STRÄTER (2007), 103, 104. Canstein setzte als Berater Franckes die Linie Speners fort.

77 So z. B. auch Magister August Hermann Francke, bevor er zum Professor ernannt wurde. Über Francke in Quedlinburg siehe DE BOOR (1968/69), 39–40. Über die Studentenbewegung der 1690er Jahre, studentische Reisetätigkeit und strategische Wohnortwechsel siehe die Studie von MORI (2004), II. Kapitel und 286–296 (Karten im Anhang). Es ist noch nicht abschließend geklärt, ob Christian Friedrich Richter zu den rebellischen Studenten in Erfurt gehörte, wie von ihr behauptet: MORI (2004), 257.

78 Sie ist in elegantem Stil verfasst und als Beschreibung des frommen gehobenen Milieus lesenswert. Der Text wurde in ihrer Leichenpredigt verwendet, ebenso von REITZ (1716) in der *Historie* von der Astmann.

79 Johann Paul Astmann (1660–1699) und Peter Kalckberner (1661–1733). Spener widmete dem Paar v. Lauter/Astmann – Kalckberner zur Hochzeit eine umfangreiche (und grundsätzliche) Schrift über die Würde des Ehestandes, in der er die Eigenschaften und die christliche Lebensführung der Braut als vorbildlich pries: SPENER (1704).

80 So REITZ (1716), 237 über ASTMANN (1699). Die 2. Auflage mit dem ausführlichen Vorwort Speners erschien 1702. Reitz erwähnt außerdem, dass sie „davon [...] in ihrem Witwenstand viele hundert Exemplaria armen Leuten verschenckt" habe.

81 So LÄCHELE (2001), 253. Er misst dieser Bibel eine „bleibende Wirkung" zu, erklärt ihre Fertigstellung indessen, anders als Reitz, zu einem Werk Speners.

82 Er wurde in ihre Leichenpredigt übernommen: MARGGRAF (1711), 40–57.

erst nach ihrem Umzug von den Löbenschen Landgütern nach Berlin aus einem Stand der „Unwissenheit“[83] herausgefunden. Durch die (pietistischen) Kirchenmänner Spener, Astmann und Schade[84] habe sie eine „gründliche Übersicht empfangen“ über das „wahre Christenthum“, in dem sie daraufhin leben wollte. Sie war diejenige, welche als erste 1703 die Rolle der Autorin ihres „Exempels“ offensiv übernahm. Im Vorwort der Publikation schildert Richter die Situation: Die Baronin v. Löben habe in den *Exempeln* aus dem Jahr 1702 die Namen der Patienten, die ihr bekannt waren, vermisst und sie dazugeschrieben. Sie habe dann beschlossen:

> Wenn mir einmal GOTT durch diese Artzney helffen sollte / wollte ich gar gerne zugeben / daß mein Exempel / zusammt dem Namen gedruckt würde [...] indem man daraus so wohl das Elend der Menschen als auch die Macht GOTTes erkennen kann / der da tödtet und lebendig macht.[85]

In Frau v. Löbens „Exempel“ geht es um Schwangerschaft und Geburt. Anders bei der hessischen Adligen Gertraud v. Dalwig, die eine schon in der Kindheit beginnende Krankheitskarriere schildert. Inzwischen war sie mit 42 Jahren „so zugerichtet und kein Theil an ihr unbeschädiget“, dass eine Wiederherstellung ihrer Gesundheit ihr „unmüglich zu seyn“ schien.[86]

Die Calvinistin v. Dalwig gehörte zu einer radikalpietistischen Strömung, die sich auf die englische Philadelphierin Jane Leade (1623–1704) bezog. Sie war eine Freundin August Hermann Franckes. Dies belegen Briefe, die sie zwischen 1700 und 1724 an ihn geschrieben hat (ihr Gesundheitszustand ist darin ein Gegenstand neben anderen).[87] Auch in der Dalwigkorrespondenz spielen Verwandtschaft und Freundschaft eine Rolle, allerdings sind rein spirituelle Beziehungen damit gemeint: Als „in Jesu theuerer wehrdester Freund und lieber Bruder“ spricht sie Francke an, und als „Meines in Jesu geliebten Freundes und Bruders verbundenes mitglied und miterbin des herrlichen Reichs Jesu Christi“ schließt v. Dalwig.[88] Die Beziehung zwischen ihr – sie galt in ihren Kreisen als eine „Priesterin“ – und den Hallensern scheint frei von direkter Interaktion. Die lutherischen Pietisten vermieden öffentlichen Kontakt mit Separatisten. Deswegen

83 Sie habe früher aus Unwissenheit „der Welt sich gleichgestellt“. Die Prediger hätten sie über die (verwerfliche) Qualität der Mitteldinge belehrt.

84 Der Name Schade ist mit dem Berliner „Beichtstuhlstreit“ verknüpft. Über Johann Caspar Schade (1666–1699), seinen radikalen Rigorismus und die dadurch ausgelösten religionspolitischen Auseinandersetzungen in Berlin siehe DRESE (2006).

85 BERICHT (1703), 32. In derselben Publikation befindet sich erstmals auch der von Frau Astmann geschriebene und gezeichnete Bericht über die Krankheit und Heilung ihrer Kinder.

86 RICHTER (1705), 464–465.

87 Im Franckenachlass Berlin sind fünf Briefe v. Dalwigs, die als „Freundin des Prof. Aug. Herm. Francke“ bezeichnet wird, erhalten. Entwürfe zu Briefen an sie von Franckes Hand sind nicht verzeichnet. Die Briefe handeln u. a. von verfolgten Glaubensgenossen (z. B. Horche) in Hessen: Stab/F 5,1/28:2 (16. April 1700). Franckes gemeinsame Wegstrecke mit radikalen Pietisten wurde schon erwähnt. Die Korrespondenz mit v. Dalwig ist ein Beleg dafür, dass er Kontakte aus dieser Phase auf anderer Ebene weiterführte.

88 Über Bruderschaften und Sozietätsvorstellungen der Philadelphier: VOGT (2001).

bedeutete der Fall Dalwig weit mehr als nur ein Patientenexempel. Es ist eine Geschichte von göttlicher Prüfung durch Krankheit, welcher sich v. Dalwig mit einem pathetischen und affirmativen Gestus unterwarf. Die Sendung von *Essentia dulcis* aus Halle galt ihr als das Wirken der „Providenz". Ihre Geschichte war ein sowohl medizinisches als auch theologisches „Exempel": Es demonstrierte die geistliche Komponente der pietistischen Krankheitsauffassung. Ein Lehrbeispiel der „pietistischen Medizin"[89], überbrückte der Text virtuell die Kluft zwischen den separatistischen und kirchlichen Fraktionen des Protestantismus. – Eine reale, physische Anwesenheit der philadelphischen Schwester im Kreis der Berliner Schwägerinnen Cansteins[90] oder gar in den Franckeschen Anstalten wäre dagegen wohl eher zum Problem geworden.

Zusammenfassung

In diesem Beitrag wurden die Damen v. Krosigk/Canstein, v. Löben, v. Bülow, v. Pannewitz, Astmann, v. Lethmate und v. Dalwig vorgestellt. Mit Ausnahme der v. Dalwig, deren Lebensmittelpunkt in Hessen lag und die in diesem Kontext lediglich in einer Fernverbindung vorkommt, unterhielten sie enge freundschaftliche Beziehungen miteinander. Wie bekannt, wurden im Adel Freundschaft und Verwandtschaft im Prinzip gleichgesetzt. Aber es ersetzte das eine nicht das andere: Es scheint, dass bei bestehenden Freundschaften zur Bestätigung und Befestigung dennoch eine Heirat gewünscht wurde, um den Freundschaftsverband durch Schwägerschaften zu erneuern und weiter zu stabilisieren.[91] So auch bei der hier untersuchten Gruppe.

Die adligen Frauen im Berliner Medikamentenvertrieb des Waisenhauses waren nahezu alle in unterschiedlichen Graden miteinander verwandt bzw. verschwägert. Es ist insofern ein verwandtschaftsbasiertes Aktionsbündnis.

89 Siehe zu diesem Komplex HELM (2003), 200–203.

90 Von Canstein ist überliefert, dass er philadelphischen Sympathisanten kritisch begegnete. Er befürchtete z. B., der künftige Ehemann seiner Nichte, der Quedlinburger v. Stammer, sei ein Leade-Anhänger: SCHICKETANZ (1972), 236, 238.

91 Siehe hierzu ein Ergebnis der Untersuchung von SPIESS (1993), 530–531, das wohl über dessen Untersuchungszeitraum (bis 1600) hinaus Gültigkeit hat. Er weist auf die Gleichsetzung von „Freund" und „Verwandter" hin, durch welche die Verwandtenpflicht zu friedlichem Umgang miteinander und zu gegenseitiger Fürsorge und Unterstützung „besonders in Krisenfällen und allen Feldern menschlichen Handelns" charakterisiert sei. In der Politik seien Verwandtschaftspflichten der gleiche Stellenwert wie den Lehns- und Dienstverpflichtungen zugebilligt worden. Bei der Erneuerung oder Neubildung von Schwägerschaft im Rahmen der Handlungsgemeinschaft von Blutsverwandten stellt Spieß eine Steigerung des Verwandtschaftsbewusstseins fest. Er weist besonders auf die „große Bedeutung der Verwandtschaft bei der Organisation der patrizischen Handelsgesellschaften" hin. Bei diesen sei „die Verbindung von Schwägern am häufigsten" gewesen.

Allein fünf Krosigkschwestern[92] gehörten dazu. Canstein und Bartha v. Krosigk verstärkten durch ihre Heirat 1707 dieses Bündnis, das damit im Kernbereich, also auch hinsichtlich Cansteins, in der zeitgenössischen Generation verschwägert war. Durch die Heirat setzten sie nicht nur der gesamten Verwandtschafts- und Interessengemeinschaft, sondern auch der Berliner Hof- und städtischen Gesellschaft, in der sie lebten, ein Zeichen. Es liegt nahe, darin einen Akt der Selbstbehauptung im Sinn dieser Gruppierung des protestantischen Reformadels (um Spener) gegenüber anderen, religiös-politisch indifferenten Fraktionen und Standespersonen in der Residenzstadt zu sehen.[93] Die weitergehende Frage nach einem adligen „Gemeinwesen" oder einem hier möglicherweise vorliegenden Adelskommunitarismus kann an dieser Stelle nicht weiter behandelt werden. Nur soviel: Es handelte sich hier um eine traditionell vermittelte Verknüpfung von adligen Häusern[94] und nicht um eine Gelegenheitskonstellation etwa von Freundinnen August Hermann Franckes.

Der Berliner Medikamentenvertrieb war also eingebettet in eine durch Verschwägerung und programmatische Bindung an den Halleschen Pietismus definierte Gemeinschaft. Sie stand durch die hochgradige Verbindlichkeit zwischen allen Personen des Netzwerks für die Güte und Erreichbarkeit der Medikamente des Waisenhauses ein, auch über Christian Friedrich Richters Tod 1711 hinaus.[95] Allerdings scheinen Canstein und seine adligen Mitstreiter das Profil der Medikamentenexpedition aus einer Perspektive zu konstruiert zu haben, die nicht identisch war mit der späteren Form: Das Konzept der Berliner Gruppe entsprach einem Personenverbandsprinzip und wirkte nicht durch das Multiplikationsverfahren, wie es dann durch die pietistischen Prediger in der inneren wie der äußeren Mission weltweit realisiert wurde. In der hier untersuchten Frühzeit sieht man sich eher an ein hausväterisches Modell erinnert, auch wenn es schon um große Einheiten wie z. B. „das Heer" gehen konnte. Hartmann erwähnt in seiner Darstellung der Anfänge eines staatlich geregelten Medizinalwesens die älteren Einheiten öffentlicher ärztlicher und pharmazeutischer Versorgung. Mit Verweis

92 Auf diese Schwestern hat schon SCHICKETANZ (1972), 896, in einem Zusatz zur Verwandtschaftstafel Cansteins hingewiesen.

93 In diese Richtung deuten gewisse Topoi in Ansprachen bei öffentlichen Anlässen. Der Berliner Prediger Porst z. B. wendete sich bei der Gedächtnisrede für Bartha v. Canstein direkt an die Trauergemeinde: „Ich muß aber noch ein Wort sagen zu den Edlen, Freyherrlichen, Gräfflichen und anderen hohen Personen dieser Stadt. Sie haben an der sel. Frey=Frau ein Exempel, dass auch Standes=Personen Christen seyn können [...]". Siehe SYMPATHIAE TESTIMONIUM (1718), 28.

94 GESTRICH (2007): „Das Haus war eine grundlegende soziale und wirtschaftliche Einheit vorindustrieller Gesellschaften", die Haushalte „komplexe soziale Einheiten". Gestrich kritisiert mit dieser Begrifflichkeit die Vorstellung des „autarken" Ganzen Hauses (nach Otto Brunner).

95 Sogar über Cansteins Tod hinaus: Dessen Hausverwalter, Hans Henrich Bartholomaei, scheint die Geschäfte weitergeführt zu haben, siehe Cansteins Testament, Punkte 4 und 5, bei SCHICKETANZ (2002), 198. Später übernahm seine Witwe (oder eine andere Verwandte namens Bartholomaei) den Berliner Medikamentenvertrieb: Siehe HELM (2001), 268.

u. a. auf die wachsenden Städte und auf die Bergbauzentren im Mittelalter spricht er von einem „Gesundheitswesen zwischen den Häusern", ein Topos, der auch den hier geschilderten Komplex charakterisieren kann.[96]

Ein weiterer deutlicher Unterschied der Konzeption scheint mir in einem spezifischen, geschäftlichen[97] Realismus dieser adligen Frauen und Männer zu liegen. Er betrifft die spezifisch pietistische Stilisierung in der Darstellung und Bewerbung der Medikamente aus dem Waisenhaus, die für C. F. Richter höchst wichtig war. Zwar waren auch alle diese Personen sehr fromm und hatten sich die sozialpolitischen Reformziele des Halleschen Pietismus zu eigen gemacht. Aber sie waren – mit Ausnahme v. Dalwigs – weit entfernt davon, die Gegenstände ihres Alltags in der Weise zu spiritualisieren, wie es die Franckeschen Theologen und Christian Friedrich Richter taten. In ihren Briefen pflegten die Baroninnen und Fräulein einen nüchternen Stil und waren genauso sachlich orientiert wie z. B. der Briefschreiber Canstein. Gegenüber dem religiös-schwärmerischen Reden über die *Essenta dulcis* scheinen sie indifferent.

Eine noch zu klärende Frage ist, ob das Zusammentreffen von bemerkenswerten Neuerungen im Jahr 1707 ein Zufall war oder ob damit die Form geschaffen wurde, in der sich die kombinierten Tätigkeiten des hier beschriebenen Vertriebssystems in den folgenden Jahren konzentrierten:

- Heirat v. Krosigk – Canstein (im Januar),
- Umzug des Berliner Waisenhausbuchladens (mit Verkauf von Waisenhausmedikamenten) in Cansteins Haus,
- Gründung der Frauenzimmermanufaktur (nach Francke: „Adligenmanufaktur").

Und weiter: Könnten die Arbeiten dieser Manufaktur sich auch auf Medikamente (Teilherstellung, Herstellung von Hausmitteln) erstreckt haben? Als ein arzneinahes Produkt dieser Einrichtung ist bisher lediglich ein Balsam („büloischer Balsam") auszumachen. Eine weiter zu untersuchende Fragestellung bleibt die verlagsmäßig organisierte Arbeit: Nach einer These von Renate Wilson arbeiteten Dienstpersonal adliger Frauen und Waisenkinder aus den an kleinen Höfen betriebenen Waisenhäusern für die pharmazeutische Produktion des Halleschen Waisenhauses (repetitive, einfache Arbeiten).[98] Sie bezieht sich dabei auf Abrechnungsunterlagen der Medikamentenexpedition aus einer späteren Epoche, etwa der Folgegeneration. Für den hier behandelten Zeitraum liegt eine vergleichbare Buchführung nicht vor.

96 HARTMANN (1983), 170. Diese Form des Gesundheitswesens habe die Bergleute, die Armen, die Soldaten und die reisenden fremden Kaufleute einbezogen.

97 Siehe wiederum FRÜHSORGE (1976) zum Begriff der Geschäfte.

98 WILSON (2001), 3. Ich danke Frau Prof. Renate Wilson für die Überlassung des Manuskripts.

Quellen- und Literaturverzeichnis

Archiv der Franckeschen Stiftungen zu Halle / Hauptarchiv (AFSt/H)
AFSt/H C 285:15: Corresp. mit denen Herrn Christian Friedrich u. Christian Sigismund Richtern als denen Medicis des Waisenhauses. 1699 seqq.
AFSt/H C5, 13–16: Bartha v. Canstein an A. H. Francke, Berlin, 8. Februar [o. J.].
AFSt/H C5, 234–235: Bartha v. Canstein an A. H. Francke, Berlin, 3. April [o. J.].
AFSt/H C 5, 238 – 239: Krosigk (= Bartha v. Krosigk) an A. H. Francke, Berlin, 9. Mai [o. J.].

Archiv der Franckeschen Stiftungen zu Halle / Wirtschafts- und Verwaltungsarchiv (AFSt/W)
AFSt/W X /I/150: [Spendenverzeichnis].
AFSt/W IX/II/9: Kurtze Nachricht von der Tinctura Polychresta.
AFSt/W X/I/36: Der Frau General=Majorin v. Lethmat geb v. Legat Testament, darin dieselbe 2000 rs. für das Weibliche Stift legirt hat / de 1713.

Francke-Nachlass der Staatsbibliothek zu Berlin – Preußischer Kulturbesitz (Stab/F)
Stab/F 5,1/28:2: Gertraud v. Dalwig an A. H. Francke, Dillig, 16. April 1700.

Altmann (1972)
Altmann, Eckhard: Christian Friedrich Richter (1676 – 1711). Arzt, Apotheker und Liederdichter des Halleschen Pietismus. Witten: Luther-Verlag, 1972 (Arbeiten zur Geschichte des Pietismus 7).

Astmann (1699)
Astmann, Johann Paul: Biblia, Das ist / Die gantze Heilige Schrifft / Altes und Neues Testaments. Teutsch / D. Martin Luthers. Mit Summarien und vollkommenen Concordantien oder Parallelen. Berlin: Witwe David Salfelds, 1699 [Die 2. Auflage mit einer ausführlichen Vorrede Philipp Jacob Speners erschien 1702].

Bericht (1701)
Bericht von der Artzney, Essentia Dulcis genannt, durch welche unter dem Seegen Gottes allerley schwere Kranckheiten [...] curiret werden. Halle: Krebs, 1701.

Bericht (1703)
Ausführlicher Bericht von der Artzney Essentia Dulcis genannt. Durch welche unter dem Seegen Gottes allerley schwere Kranckheiten [...] bißher curiret worden. Zum drittenmahl und verbessert in Druck gegeben aus der Apothecke des Wäysen-Hauses zu Glaucha an Halle. Halle: Waisenhaus, 1703.

Bernschneider-Reif (2004)
Bernschneider-Reif, Sabine: Das laienpharmazeutische Olitätenwesen im Thüringer Wald – (adelige) Frauen als Laboranten und ihre Rezeptbücher. In: Wahrig, Bettina (Hrsg.): Arzneien für das „schöne Geschlecht". Geschlechterverhältnisse in Phytotherapie und Pharmazie vom Mittelalter bis zum 19. Jahrhundert. Stuttgart: Deutscher Apotheker Verlag, 151–168.

de Boor (1968/69)
de Boor, Friedrich: Pietismus, Enthusiasmus und Separatismus an der Wende des 17./18. Jahrhunderts. Nachrichten der Luther-Akademie (Sondershausen), 1968/69, 37–41.
Danninger (1998)

Danninger, Gabriele: „... dass sie auch vor den Krankenbetten müsten das Maul halten ...“: Frauen zwischen „traditioneller Heiltätigkeit“ und „gelehrter Medizin um 1800 anhand Salzburger Quellen. Wien: Österreichischer Kunst- und Kulturverlag, 1998 (Kulturgeschichte der namenlosen Mehrheit 2).

Drese (2005)
Drese, Claudia: Der Berliner Beichtstuhlstreit oder Philipp Jakob Spener zwischen allen Stühlen? In: Pietismus und Neuzeit 31 (2005), 60–136.

Dreyhaupt (1750)
Dreyhaupt, Johann Christoph von: Pagus Neletici et Nudzici oder ausführliche diplomatisch-historische Beschreibung des zum ehemaligen Primat und Ertz-Stiffte [...] Herzogthum Magdeburg gehörigen Saal-Creyses und aller darinnen befindlichen Städte, [...]: insonderheit der Städte Halle, Wettin, Lobegün, [...]. 2. Band. Halle: Waisenhaus, 1750.

Exempel (1702)
Merckwürdige Exempel der unter dem Seegen Gottes durch die Essentiam dulcem geschehenen Curen, zum klaren Beweiß desjenigen, was von dieser Artzney in dem davon edirten Bericht angezeigt worden. Halle: Waisenhaus, 1702.

Florin (1725)
Florin, Franz Philipp: Der Kluge Landmann Oder: Recht gründlicher und zuverlässiger Unterricht, wie man das Haus=Wesen nützlich anfangen [...] möge. Erster Theil. Allen und jeden sowohl Hohen als Niedrigen / so Land=Güther besitzen / verwalten / kauffen und verkauffen, oder auch verpachten und pachten, zu sonderbahren Vortheil und Nutzen zusammen getragen. Frankfurt, Leipzig: Christoph Riegel, 1725.

Francke (1994)
Francke, August Hermann: Segensvolle Fußstapfen. Geschichte der Entstehung der Halleschen Anstalten. Gießen: Brunnen-Verlag, 1994 [1709].

Frühsorge (1976)
Frühsorge, Gotthard: Die Einheit aller Geschäfte. Tradition und Veränderung des „Hausmutter“-Bildes in der Ökonomieliteratur des 18. Jahrhunderts. Wolfenbütteler Studien zur Aufklärung 3 (1976), 137–157.

Gestrich (2007)
Gestrich, Andreas: Artikel „Haushalt“. In: Jaeger, Friedrich (Hrsg.): Enzyklopädie der Neuzeit, Bd. 5. Stuttgart, Weimar: J.B. Metzler, 2007. Sp. 224–230.

Gittner (1948)
Gittner, Herrmann: 250 Jahre Waisenhaus-Apotheke und Medikamenten-Expedition der Franckeschen Stiftungen zu Halle an der Saale. Halle (Saale): Max Niemeyer Verlag.

Habrich (1982)
Habrich, Christa: Pathographische und ätiologische Versuche medizinischer Laien im 18. Jahrhundert. In: Eckart, Wolfgang; Geyer-Kordesch, Johanna (Hrsg.): Heilberufe und Kranke im 17. und 18. Jahrhundert. Die Quellen- und Forschungssituation. Münster: Burgverlag, 1982, 99–123.

Habrich (1997)
Habrich, Christa: Heilkunde im Dienst der Seelsorge bei Gerhard Tersteegen. In: Kock, Manfred (Hrsg.): Gerhard Tersteegen – Evangelische Mystik inmitten der Aufklärung. Köln: Rheinland-Verlag GmbH, 1997, 161–180.

Hartmann (1983)
Hartmann, Fritz: Hausvater und Hausmutter als Hausarzt in der Frühen Neuzeit. Hausgewalt und Gesundheitsfürsorge. In: Historisches Seminar der Universität Hannover (Hrsg.): Staat und Gesellschaft in Mittelalter und Früher Neuzeit. Göttingen: Vandenhoeck & Ruprecht, 1983, 151–175.

Helm (2001)
Helm, Jürgen: Der Hallesche Pietismus und das Gesundheitswesen in Brandenburg-Preußen. In: Müller-Bahlke, Thomas (Hrsg.): Gott zur Ehr und zu des Landes Besten. Die Franckeschen Stiftungen und Preußen: Aspekte einer alten Allianz [Katalog zur Jahresausstellung 2001]. Halle: Verlag der Franckeschen Stiftungen, 2001, 261–273.

Helm (2003)
Helm, Jürgen: „Daß auch zugleich die Gottseligkeit dadurch gebauet wird" – Pietismus und Medizin in der ersten Hälfte des 18. Jahrhunderts. In: Berichte zur Wissenschaftsgeschichte 26, 199–211.

Hinrichs (1971)
Hinrichs, Carl: Preussentum und Pietismus. Der Pietismus in Brandenburg-Preussen als religiös-soziale Reformbewegung. Göttingen: Vandenhoeck und Ruprecht, 1971.

Hoffmann (1996)
Hoffmann, Barbara: Radikalpietismus um 1700. Der Streit um das Recht auf eine neue Gesellschaft. Frankfurt, New York: Campus Verlag, 1996.

Hufschmidt (2001)
Hufschmidt, Anke: Adlige Frauen im Weserraum zwischen 1570 und 1700. Status – Rollen – Lebenspraxis. Münster: Aschendorff, 2001.

Hunter (1997)
Hunter, Lynette: Women and Domestic Medicine: Lady Experimenters, 1570–1620. In: Hunter, Lynette; Hutton, Sarah (Hrsg.): Women, Science and Medicine 1500–1700. Mothers and Sisters of the Royal Society. Thrupp Stroud, Gloustershire, UK: Sutton Publishing, 1997, 89–107.

Keller (2005)
Keller, Katrin: Hofdamen. Amtsträgerinnen im Wiener Hofstaat des 17. Jahrhunderts. Wien, Köln, Weimar: Böhlau Verlag 2005.

Klosterberg (2007)
Klosterberg, Brigitte: Gedächtnisspeicher des Pietismus. In: Gleixner, Ulrike; Hebeisen, Erika (Hrsg.): Gendering Tradition. Erinnerungskultur und Geschlecht im Pietismus. Korb: Didymos-Verlag, 2007, 253–268.

Knieriem & Burkardt (2002)
Knieriem, Michael; Burkardt, Johannes: Gesellschaft der Kindheit Jesu-Genossen auf Schloß Hayn: Aus dem Nachlaß des von Fleischbein und Korrespondenzen von de Marsay, Prueschenk

von Lindenhofen und Tersteegen 1734 bis 1742. Ein Beitrag zur Geschichte des Radikalpietismus im Sieger- und Wittgensteiner Land. Hannover: Wehrhahn, 2002.

Kramer (1882)
Kramer, Gustav: August Hermann Francke. Ein Lebensbild, Bd. 2. Halle (S.): Waisenhaus, 1882.

Lächele (2001)
Lächele, Rainer: „Bedenck's Berlin!" Der Hallesche Pietismus und die preußische Amtskirche. In: Müller-Bahlke, Thomas (Hrsg.): Gott zur Ehr und zu des Landes Besten. Die Franckeschen Stiftungen und Preußen: Aspekte einer alten Allianz [Katalog zur Jahresausstellung 2001]. Halle (Saale): Verlag der Franckeschen Stiftungen, 2001, 251–259.

Marggraf (1711)
Marggraf, Paschasius: I. N. J. Der Köstliche Schmuck der Kinder Gottes [...]. [Leichenpredigt für Dorothea Juliana v. Löben, geb. v. Krosigk]. Berlin: Johann Wessel, 1711.

Marx (1970)
Marx, Karl: Das Kapital. Kritik der politischen Ökonomie, Bd. 1. Berlin: Dietz Verlag, 1970 (Karl Marx/Friedrich Engels Werke, Bd. 23).

Meyer-Habrich (1981)
Meyer-Habrich, Christa: Untersuchungen zur pietistischen Medizin und ihrer Ausprägung bei Johann Samuel Carl (1677–1757) und seinem Kreis. Habilitationsschrift LMU München, 1981.

Mori (2004)
Mori, Ryoko: Begeisterung und Ernüchterung in christlicher Vollkommenheit. Pietistische Selbst- und Weltwahrnehmungen im ausgehenden 17. Jahrhundert. Tübingen: Verlag der Franckeschen Stiftungen Halle im Max Niemeyer Verlag, 2004 (Hallesche Forschungen 14).

Podczeck (1962)
Podczeck, Otto (Hrsg.): August Hermann Franckes Schrift über eine Reform des Erziehungs- und Bildungswesens als Ausgangspunkt einer geistlichen und sozialen Neuordung der evangelischen Kirche des 18. Jahrhunderts: Der große Aufsatz. Mit einer quellenkundlichen Einführung. Berlin: Akademie-Verlag, 1962 (Abhandlungen der Sächsischen Akademie der Wissenschaften zu Leipzig, Philogisch-historische Klasse, Bd. 53, Teil 3).

Reitz (1716)
Reitz, Johann Henrich: Historie der Wiedergebohrnen / Oder Exempel gottseliger / so bekannt= und benannt= als unbekannter Christen / männlichen und weiblichen Geschlechts / In allerley Ständen / Wie Dieselbe erst von GOTT gezogen und bekehret / und nach vielen Kämpffen und Aengsten / durch GOttes Geist und Wort / zum Glauben und Ruh ihres Gewissens gebracht sind. Itzstein: Joh. Jacob Haug, 1716.

Richter (1705)
Richter, Christian Friedrich: Kurtzer und deutlicher Unterricht von dem Leibe und natürlichen Leben des Menschen: Woraus ein jeglicher / auch Ungelehrter erkennen kan / Was die Gesundheit ist [...]: auch welches die menschlichen Kranckheiten / deren Ursachen und Kennzeichen sind / Und wie sie [...] bey Ermangelung eines Medici, ohne Gefahr und mit gutem Success zu curiren: Nebst einem Selectu Medicamentorum, oder XIII. der sichersten und besten Artzneyen / zu einer kleinen / auff alle gewöhnliche Kranckheiten eingerichteten Haus- Reise- und Feld-Apothecken / Mit gnugsamen Bericht von deren Eigenschafften und rechtem Gebrauch. Halle: Waisenhaus, 1705.

Schicketanz (1967)
Schicketanz, Peter. Carl Hildebrand von Cansteins Beziehungen zu Philipp Jacob Spener. Witten: Luther-Verlag, 1967.

Schicketanz (1972)
Schicketanz, Peter (Hrsg.): Der Briefwechsel Carl Hildebrand von Cansteins mit August Hermann Francke. Berlin: De Gruyter, 1972.

Schicketanz (2002)
Schicketanz, Peter: Carl Hildebrand Freiherr von Canstein: Leben und Denken in Quellendarstellungen. Tübingen: Verlag der Franckeschen Stiftungen im Max Niemeyer-Verlag, 2002 (Hallesche Forschungen 8).

Schneider (1993)
Schneider, Hans: Der radikale Pietismus im 17. Jahrhundert. In: Brecht, Martin; Deppermann, Klaus, u. a. (Hrsg.): Geschichte des Pietismus, Bd. 1. Der Pietismus vom 17. bis zum frühen 18. Jahrhundert. Göttingen: Vandenhoek & Ruprecht, 1993, 391–437.

Schrader (1989)
Schrader, Hans-Jürgen: Literaturproduktion und Büchermarkt des radikalen Pietismus. Johann Heinrich Reitz' „Historie Der Wiedergebohrnen" und ihr geschichtlicher Kontext. Göttingen: Vandenhoeck und Ruprecht, 1989.

Spener [1704]
Spener, Philipp Jacob: Des Ehe=Standes Würde Bey Ehelicher Einsegnung Herrn Petri Kalckberners / Königl. Preuß. u Chur=Fürstl. Brandenburg. Inspect. der Kirchen und Schulen des andern Holtz=Creyses im Herzogthum Magdeburg und Pastoris zu Meseberg / Mit Frauen Barbara Cordula von Lauter / Seligen Herrn Johann Paul Astmanns [...] hinterlassenen Frau Wittiben / Den 15. April. 1704 in gedachtem Berlin einfältig [...] betrachtet [...].Berlin: Salfeld, [1704].

Spieß (1993)
Spieß, Karl-Heinz: Familie und Verwandtschaft im deutschen Hochadel des späten Mittelalters: 13. bis Anfang des 16. Jahrhunderts. Stuttgart: Franz Steiner, 1993.

Stolberg (2003)
Stolberg, Michael: Homo patiens. Krankheits- und Körpererfahrung in der Frühen Neuzeit. Köln: Böhlau, 2003.

Sträter (2007)
Sträter, Udo: Spener und August Hermann Francke. In: Wendebourg, Dorothea (Hrsg.): Philipp Jakob Spener – Begründer des Pietismus und protestantischer Kirchenvater. Bilanz der Forschung nach 300 Jahren. Berlin: de Gruyter, 2007, 89–104.

Sympathiae testimonium (1718)
Professoren der Friedrichs-Universität: Sympathiae testimonium, Quod quum matronae perillustri ac generosissimae omnibusque virtutibus spectatissimae, Barthae Sophiae, natae a Krosegk, Conjugilonge desideratissimae, [...] piae defunctae, perillustris ac generosissimus, dominus Carolus Hildebrandus, Liber baro a Canstein [...] Extare voluerunt Facultatis Theol. in Acad. Frideric. Professores, uti & alii illustris Nominis Cansteiniani Cultores, suo quisque loco nominati. Berlin: Gotth. Schlechtiger, 1718.

Szasz (1997)
Szasz, Ildiko: Chemie für die Dame. Fachbücher für das „Schöne Geschlecht“ vom 16. bis 19. Jahrhundert. Königstein/Taunus: Ulrike Helmer Verlag, 1997.

Vogt (2005)
„Philadelphia“ – Inhalt, Verbreitung und Einfluss eines radikal-pietistischen Schlüsselbegriffs. In: Sträter, Udo (Hrsg. in Verb. mit Lehmann, Hartmut; Müller-Bahlke, Thomas; Wallmann, Johannes): Interdisziplinäre Pietismusforschung. Beiträge zum 1. Internationalen Kongress für Pietismusforschung 2001, Bd. 2. Tübingen: Verlag der Franckeschen Stiftungen Halle im Max Niemeyer Verlag, 2005, 837–848 (Hallesche Forschungen 17).

Wallmann (2005)
Wallmann, Johannes: Der Pietismus. Göttingen: Vandenhoek & Ruprecht, 2005.

Welsch (1955)
Welsch, Heinz: Die Franckeschen Stiftungen als wirtschaftliches Grossunternehmen. Halle (Diss.), 1955.

Wilson (2000)
Wilson, Renate: Pious traders in medicine. A German pharmaceutical network in eighteenth-century North America. University Park, Pennsylvania: Pennsylvania State University Press, 2000.

Wilson (2001)
Wilson, Renate: Women in Halle Pietism: Benefactresses, worker bees, and traders. Unveröffentlichtes Ms. eines Vortrags, gehalten beim 1. Internationalen Kongress für Pietismusforschung, Halle-Saale, 2001.

Witt (1996)
Witt, Ulrike: Bekehrung, Bildung und Biographie. Frauen im Umkreis des Halleschen Pietismus. Halle: Verlag der Franckeschen Stiftungen Halle im Max Niemeyer Verlag, 1996.

Wunder (1992)
Wunder, Heide: „Er ist die Sonn’, sie ist der Mond“. Frauen in der Frühen Neuzeit. München: Beck, 1992.

Part V:
Conclusions and Observations

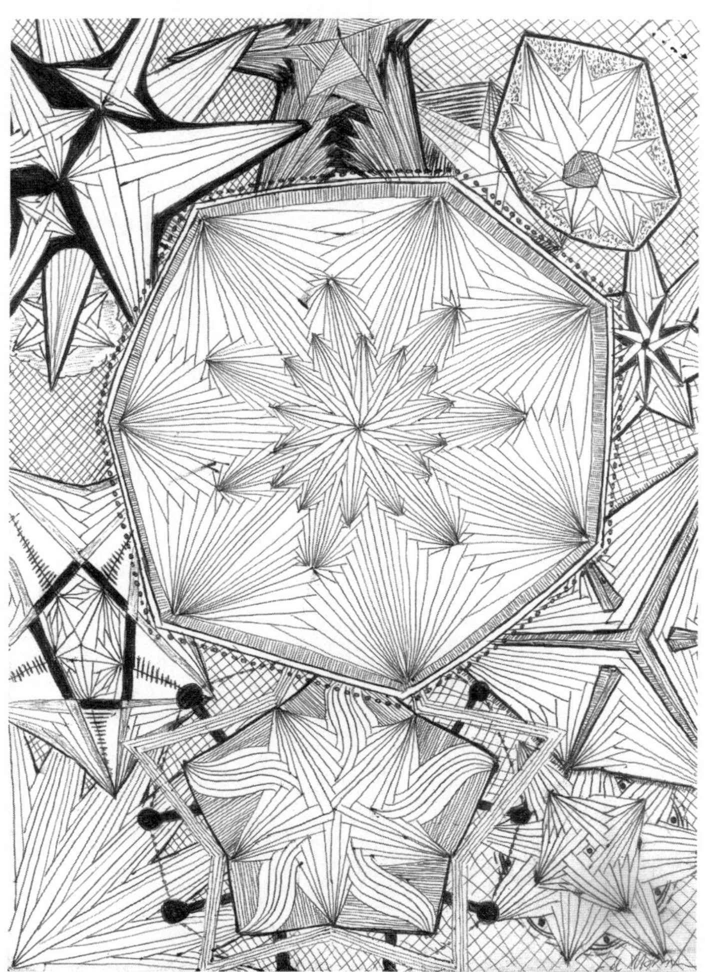

Ed Mormann, Untitled, October 2005

THE CONTEXTS OF MEDICINE IN THE SEVENTEENTH AND EIGHTEENTH CENTURY

Mary Lindemann

This volume explores a number of issues historians consider crucial to the history of medicine in the seventeenth and eighteenth centuries. It also raises a series of questions about the "doing" of that history, sometimes explicitly, sometimes implicitly. One explicitly addressed the social and religious contexts which shaped medical practice in these two centuries and in which medicine was situated. Another focused on a literal "sea change:" how German medicine migrated across the Atlantic and rooted itself in the life of the American colonies. Such contextual sets form the matrix within which historians have generally analyzed issues of theory and practice in medicine. They simultaneously lay the groundwork for a more direct discussion of the balance between theory and empiricism both in the medicine of the past and, if rather more implicitly, in how historians will approach the researching and writing of medical history early in this new century.

The use of the term "context" slides so trippingly off the tongues of historians and seems so *selbstverständlich* to us that we rarely pause to reflect on what context means or, just as importantly, to consider how we settle on certain contexts, privileging, for instance, one over another, and rejecting alternatives. I want to reflect for a while here on what we mean by context in medical history, first by evaluating how useful social and religious contextualizations are. But I also want to probe what we actually mean by such perspectives or contexts, as well as to think more rigorously about what advantages we gain from applying even broader perspectives, such as comparative, transatlantic, or transcultural ones to the history of medicine. Or is all knowledge, here knowledge about medicine, necessarily local knowledge and thus impervious to comparative analyses and unfit for building larger structural interpretations? Do we perhaps best grasp theories and practices when we limit contextualization or when we avoid rather than attempt sweeping comparisons?

To a large extent, how scholars do history (and not only medical history), depends on how they interpret that deceptively simple term: context. The real problem, the real issue, however, often lies in determining just what context and just how much context appropriately defines an investigation. We often make these decisions reflexively, without much concentrated thought. Our choices are either instinctive or determined to a larger extent by our professional training. In addition, it is not, I argue, sufficient to insist that a subject must be "contextualized" or, for that matter, to criticize a work solely as "insufficiently contextualized."

First, we need to decide where to begin and where to end our contextualizations; and that decision often resolves itself into matters of theory (or at least approach) and interpretation. It also involves matters of sources (a topic which will only be treated briefly here). Why should we adopt a certain theoretical model? When should we abandon it? To what extent can we simply be eclectic in our approach without sacrificing analytical rigor by submerging our subjects in such dense contextual soups that everything seems equally relevant? What sources work best in which contexts and with which approaches?

Second, we must remain aware of when contextualization of medical history takes us beyond that history. To raise this question in the history of medicine is, of course, perfectly legitimate, but its pursuit should also trouble medical historians who wish to preserve some sense of difference from other historians, maintain some disciplinary boundaries, and deploy an expertise that is not within everyone's grasp or training or to everyone's taste. In skillful hands, a narrow discussion within the framework of a subfield does not necessarily produce dry histories and limited conclusions.

Third, we need to figure out how debates over theory and practice in writing history intersect with concerns over contextualization. That is, do some approaches to writing history require different contexts (as well as different sources) than others? Finally, we ought to address the value of comparisons that stretch across time and place or across cultures; in particular, we need to ask ourselves what advantages a comparative or transnational perspective offers us as historians of medicine? Can certain contexts obscure as much as they illuminate?

These are large questions that are hardly unique to the history of medicine. Although they can in no way be fully answered here, I hope to address them – and especially the dual issue of contextualization and comparison – for seventeenth- and eighteenth-century medical history and its writing, based on a few examples drawn largely from the contributions to this volume.[1]

The Popularity of Medical History

Few historical disciplines have been as successfully mainstreamed or have so magnetically drawn the attention of nonspecialists (and even nonhistorians) as the history of medicine. In appealing to wide audiences, medical historians have been more effective, for instance, than historians of science, although that, too, is changing and a significant number of sophisticated general histories of science, such as recent contributions of Lisa Jardine, have bridged the gap between scholars and an educated public.[2] Especially fruitful interactions between medical history and social and cultural history have made much history of medicine es-

1 While I use essays from this volume as examples, I have not referred to all of them equally. My selection does not seek to dismiss the several excellent contributions I do not address at length.

2 Although Lisa Jardine's interests are wider in scope and although she is not a historian of science as such, her volumes on Hooke and Bacon are good examples of my point. See JARDINE (2003) and JARDINE (1974). See also her *Ingenious Pursuits: Building the Scientific Revolution,* JARDINE (1999).

sential reading not only for medical historians but for early modernists and modernists more generally. Feminist scholarship has been almost as productive in this regard. Few scholars would now limit the history of medicine to an esoteric realm. The influence of a number of mostly British and American authors has been critical and one needs only mention the name of the late Roy Porter to understand the dimensions of the achievement.

Equally characteristic of "mainstreamed medical history" is that its authors are often not trained principally in medical history, nor do they necessarily identify themselves as medical historians. Their success has, in my opinion, derived from an ability to contextualize their subjects effectively and make them immediately pertinent to several readerships. But if the task is well begun, it is hardly completed and much remains to be done. Not only will more general history benefit from the medical gaze; medical history, too, can only become stronger by varying its contextual choices and expanding its openness to Clio's other branches. Yet one must also consider the other side of the coin: what are the dangers that lurk in contextualization?

What do selected contexts tell us about seventeenth- and eighteenth-century medical theory and practice? More specifically, in what contexts have the authors in this volume – dedicated to what might seem a fairly narrow subject – embedded their stories in several contexts and stretched the boundaries of medical history? Might these boundaries have been more vigorously and productively extended?

Each set of contexts enjoys its advantages and suffers from its disadvantages and, of course, no single contextual setting is perfect. What I attempt here is an evaluation of how various subjects in medical history can be approached and how casting their discussion within other contexts produces other results, interpretations, and insights. I am not trying to define or argue for any one context as ideally suited to the study of early modern medicine, because there is no such thing. Nor do I wish us always to choose the interpretive mammoth over the punctilious mouse or vice-versa.[3]

Contexts and Medical History

Traditional histories of medicine often focused on one practitioner, producing at their worst adulatory hagiographies (although such hagiographies have pretty much vanished from the scholarly landscape). These investigations approximate, I would argue, a microhistorical approach although they rarely unearth caches of unknown archival material. Instead they explore printed sources, texts, or correspondence in depth. Yet what these studies may have lacked in breadth and immediate value for more broadly contextualized or greater structural interpreta-

3 For a discussion of the advantages of structural histories and microhistories, as well as an attempt to blend them, see EGMOND & MASON (1997).

tions, they make up for in the penetration of their gaze. The case of Friedrich Hoffmann treated in this volume by *Almut Lanz* presents an excellent example of a straightforward approach to the problem of theory and practice: between the medical theory and the pharmaceutical choices of one, extremely well-known physician. She employs her case studies to postulate the existence of a fairly direct and uncomplicated way to measure the impact of theory on practice. Plumbing Hoffmann's physiology and pathology leads us to a better grasp of his practical choices and selection of pharmaceuticals. Hoffmann's preference for six medications – his "fluids" (*flüssige Arzneien*) – corresponded, seemingly transparently, to his acceptance or articulation of his corpuscular theories (*Korpusculartheorien*). The relationship between theory and practice as laid out by Lanz is, relatively speaking, simple: "The relationship between Friedrich Hoffmann's medical theory and practice is characterized by the fact that the latter is the logical consequence of the former." This conclusion hardly floats free of context, of course. The most obvious are those of a history of medical theory and Hoffmann's own use of *ratio* and *experientia* (*Gebrauch von Ratio & Experientia*). The relationship between theory and practice thus handled allows us to eavesdrop on an internal dialogue between a theory and a practice contained within a person, constrained and affected by a personality. Obviously, of course, the broader context here is the web of academic debates about medicine that endows this single case with explanatory power.

How might individual practices and theories otherwise be treated or contextualized? While still working within the framework of medicine and "conceptual changes within medicine itself" (*Andreas-Holger Maehle*), we can readjust our focus, moving out from the theories and practices of one man to a bigger issue. In Maehle's case, that is the value of experimentation in the eighteenth century. In doing so, we must remain attentive to historical dissonances.

Maehle reminds us that the understanding of experimentation in the eighteenth century does not overlap with current perceptions. Thus, we need to set the specific conceptual meanings of eighteenth-century "experiments" within the context of their contemporary mental worlds to evaluate their purpose. In these environs, experimentation becomes less an exercise about judging efficacy than about understanding how a substance – a drug – worked and devising new ideas about when and where its application was indicated or counter-indicated. Such investigations fit well within the framework of a medical contextualization that is explicitly European in its explanatory power. The European framework Maehle picked links the "protopharmacology" of experimenters in England, France, and the Germanies and raises questions about how fully "European" theories of medicine were in these centuries. The question of whether different European types of medicine existed during the early modern period yields to discussions of trends that were more widespread and which functioned within a broadly intra-European framework. In this perspective, changes in theory or therapy are generated or determined not primarily by religious or social contexts but occur within a field of medical endeavor where medical debate and medical or natural history insights or traditions drive the discussions. Explanations rarely venture outside these discursive arenas. This essentially internalist view, which social historians have often attacked as blinkered, remains valid and valuable. One must be careful to examine if discourses that occur within fields (here, within medicine) are often only marginally influenced by broader contexts.

When we raise queries, however, about the reception of theory and responses to treatments, rather than look closely at the links between theory and practice, the emphasis on single practitioners, on medical debates, or even on how well certain practices traveled, fades in consequence. The interface between patient and practitioner, or patient and therapy, for a long time now has formed a major point of medical historical intervention. Most studies have stressed that numerous factors profoundly affect medical choices, the reception and modification of medical theories, and the acceptance of specific treatments. Those influences can be measured and comprehended in almost innumerable ways and range over the impact of climate, education, politics, social structures, cultural *habitus*, and so on. Historians have, however, frequently isolated three as especially pertinent: the patient (and his or her wishes, demands, and responses), the practitioner, and the therapies. Especially in the eighteenth century, a search for new ways of perceiving physiology and pathology that diverged from older Galenic standards characterized academic medicine. Friedrich Hoffmann, for instance, leaned toward mechanism, but other ideas, such as vitalism, competed for adherents.[4] The patient-practitioner-therapy context, however, while not insensitive to how practitioners such as Hoffmann, Franz Anton Mai, and Lorenz Heister reconceptualized physiology and pathology and crafted treatments, directs our attention more to the transmission of ideas by inquiring into "the effects of various theoretical concepts on concrete instructions on population health behavior."[5] Here *Karin Stukenbrock* enters the field of popular medical enlightenment and draws us into a conversation about the political importance of individual rights and state imperatives. Careful examination of the writings of medical practitioners, even those trimmed to the abilities of a lay or uneducated audience, however, leave us in the dark as to how such therapies were perceived, applied, adapted, or rejected. If, however, we approach the question from the perspective of the therapy itself, by isolating a therapy such as phlebotomy, we can examine "the extent to which modifications in theory had led to a change in the actual practice of bloodletting" (*Marion Maria Ruisinger*). This contextual shift toward a narrower investigation allows us to determine how some practitioners took up and applied new ideas, such as the Harveyan theory of the circulation of the blood (Ruisinger focuses on Lorenz Heister). Yet not until we explore responses – in correspondence, for example – do we comprehend how patients' expectations often shifted practice and theory.

4 See REILL (2005).

5 "Erkenntnisleitend soll dabei die Frage sein, wie sich theoretische Konzepte auf die Gesundheitsempfehlungen für die Bevölkerung auswirkten." See Stukenbrock, in this volume.

Each of these contexts allows us to penetrate the subtle interaction between how practitioners thought about practice and how they sought to practice. These and comparable sources and explorations deepen our understanding of the dynamics of what is often referred to as the medical encounter and of the responses of patients to individual therapies. By converging on one set of interactions – either dietetics or phlebotomy – we can achieve an enviable clarity of investigation that also proffers a convenient way to test reactions to one therapy or related therapies. Yet this contextual setting does not allow us to fathom the process of medical decision making per se. For that, we need to look more closely at the patient's view of, in *Michael Stolberg*'s words, "therapeutic pluralism and conflicting medical opinions."

As medical practitioners, professors, and theorists discarded or significantly modified the older Galenic humoral pathology and altered – or rather diversified – their therapies, the result proved less salutary for their "professional" standing than one might expect. The multiplicity of treatments and theories left patients uncertain about what to do and, surely as a result, probably less willing to accept medical dicta. Here, context migrates to the realm of power relationships between patients and practitioners and the situation becomes more ambiguous. Patients had increased freedom to choose, to reject, to demand, but as today they suffered agonies as they tried to reconcile divergent information and make decisions that profoundly affected their own welfare or that of family and friends. Thus, by shifting context, by moving from the interpretive framework centered on a medical marketplace and a putatively liberating medical pluralism in which people gloried in the abundance of choice, to the internal psychological implications of those possibilities, different answers emerge. Choice frightened as much as it freed. The exercise of patient power proved more unsettling or even paralyzing than empowering.

Rational planning and cool calculation rarely determine, however, the choice of a specific treatment or a certain practitioner. While it is virtually impossible to delve into minds to trace from their germination the thought processes which guide individuals in their lives, a few contexts shape choices more radically than others. And some of these factors, such as religion, are more readily accessible to historical analysis than others and, for that reason, have been extensively if not always critically surveyed. A close relationship between religion, illness, medicine, and healing has almost always pertained in human societies. Many scholars have argued that Christianity itself functions as a healing religion. It is mistaken, however, to think that the grip of Christianity and belief in the supernatural on individuals and groups in the seventeenth and eighteenth century had appreciably waned or even vanished. Quite the contrary. Indeed, it has been argued many times that the eighteenth century witnessed a strong revival of the religious element in medicine and healing, not the least in the forms of evangelical pietism (itself a complex phenomenon with varied representatives and positions) and

Methodism. John Wesley's *Primitive Physic*[6] and the series of writings that flowed out of Halle indicate the numerous and often impressive dimensions of this revival and reorientation[7] and speak volumes about the enhanced impact of religion in medicine that we ignore at our peril.[8] For the Schwenkfelder Abraham Wagner practicing in the New World, medicine remained linked to spiritual care (*John K. Crellin*) and at least in that relationship, little differentiated the western from the eastern side of the Atlantic basin.

Because so much work has already been done on the relationship of medicine, healing, and religion, we almost reflexively accept that religion was and remained a crucial referent for medicine and medical choice throughout the seventeenth and eighteenth centuries. Yet, what happens when we engage this concept differently, as *Fritz Krafft* does, in moving beyond the "end of life"? What impact does this journey have in suggesting, and then analyzing, the truly expansive reach of spiritual medicine? In the pietist framework, Christ was himself a "medicine," and this christological postmortal medicine healed physical suffering through death and resurrection into everlasting life. Critical here, of course, is the perception that "first [God's] 'power' and His will endow medicines with their healing effects."[9] This reorientation, however, merely serves as a beginning. In this model, in the context of a medicine that includes pre- and post-death, illness becomes its own "cure." To grasp these connections, we must bring into the discussion death and the dead and employ them as central factors in the writing of medical history. This continuum – this spectrum of healing stretching through death – explains, at least in part, the prevalence of the habit of using body parts – dead bodies – as medicines, siphoning from the realm of the other world its curative powers, as *Robert Jütte* astutely observes. The eighteenth-century endeavor to anchor medicine in another context altogether and to base it on reason and experience (*Vernunft* and *Erfahrung*) meant that the much older empirical medicine (*Erfahrungsmedizin*) as well as the analogical thinking (*Analogiedenken*) that justified the employment of body parts as therapeutic elements, no longer satisfied intellectual demands, as academic physicians such as Hoffmann came to insist on a theory-based medicine.

Jütte's context is, however, extensive in yet other ways. While he remains primarily concerned with elucidating a unique "turning point" in medicine, he situates his investigation within a much longer chronology. The temporal boundaries he has selected pose questions of progress and change over time but also remind us how crucial standpoint is. If eighteenth-century medicine (or at least academic medicine) had turned against a medicine that used human tissues

6 WESLEY (1759).

7 For a good guide to these complexities, see HELM (2006).

8 NUMBERS & AMUNDSEN (1986), MARLAND & PELLING (1996), and POLLOCK (1992) are only a few examples of works which treat this nexus; and on Halle, see WILSON (1996) and WILSON (2000).

9 "Erst Gottes 'Krafft' und Absicht verleihen demnach den 'Arzneien' ihre heilende Wirkung." See Krafft, in this volume.

and organs as part of a rational medicine, what happens if we project a century or two ahead, if we view the transformation he charts through a time telescope? By bookending his article with two contemporary events – a theft of body parts in 1995 and current debates on transplantation, placenta therapy, and growth hormones harvested from corpses – Jütte focuses on a number of what first may appear ahistorical questions. On riper reflection, however, we perceive how this orientation permits him to embed a series of time-specific occurrences in the eighteenth century in a far more comprehensive historical, social, and, for that matter, ethical matrix.

Atlantic Crossings

If situating questions about theory and practice in vastly expanded or unusual chronological frames generates fresh visions and realizations, what happens when we convey them to other geographical and cultural locations, moving them across the oceans? What advantages do geographically comparative perspectives promise for medical history? Early modern historians have been more adventuresome in traversing national boundaries (which often did not exist or, at the very least, were far less solid than lines on a map made them seem) than modernists. Despite considerable existing work on several aspects of the Atlantic world, medical history is still undeveloped in this context. Indeed, we are not yet even sure what questions we should be asking. But to start: how did theories and practices transfer across distance and to what extent did the unfamiliar conditions of the New World – Pennsylvania in the eighteenth century, for example – alter either or both? In terms of the chemiatric medicine handled here, Paracelsian theories apparently voyaged pretty much wholesale from the old world to the new, judging at least from the evidence of the de Benneville manuscript. Its author, however, gauged his presentation to the less familiar environment of a frontier that preferred its information to be set out quickly and directly, plain-spoken one might suggest. Thus, as *Jole Shackelford* points out, in the *Medicina Pennsylvania* George de Benneville sought to eliminate unessential theory or condense it into a table as much as possible. One cannot discount personal inclinations as to how material was marshaled. Perhaps de Benneville was less adroit in handling complex ideas than his European preceptors were, or that he had less patience for theoretical hair-splitting. Nonetheless the environment itself surely influenced how he couched his theories and, one suspects, also the very theoretical content itself. One might also argue that the hold of Paracelsian theory and therapeutics far into the eighteenth century might have been more tenacious and stronger in areas relatively remote from the European centers of medical debate and publication. Clearly, as *Renate Wilson* points out, de Benneville's and Wagner's "dispensatories cum receptures" demonstrate how practitioners sought to mold or adapt European medicines and therapies to best meet the needs of their clients in the multilingual medical market of eighteenth-century North America.

So what changed after crossing the Atlantic and why and how does this shape-shifting reveal the larger dynamics of the relationship between theory and practice not only in the specific place of Pennsylvania but across the globe? In other words, does an examination of one colonial experience open up novel ways for us to comprehend other colonial or frontier experiences? Is there a general frontier experience in medicine? Is the frontier itself a determinant structure? The results of comparative work illustrate that one should not overstate the isolation, benightedness, or primitiveness of newly-settled areas. The word "frontier" reflects something else entirely, suggesting openness and innovation or adaptation as much as backwardness and isolation. The de Benneville and Wagner manuscripts reveal sophistication and a conveyance of the therapies of the Old World – from the Germanies – into the New, albeit with modifications that reflected those circumstances. One was the multilingual character of the target population but others were social, economic, and geographical in nature.

While we learn little here about how folk medicine or indigenous customs may have inserted themselves into theory and practice, we gain at least some sense that the oceanic translocation affected how medicine was practiced. If we observe a lesser theoretical sophistication in the New World approach, we still note a considered adjustment of remedies and practices. Thus, here as elsewhere in Atlantic history studies, we cannot be satisfied with a simple "they carried their ideas with them" approach. Yet we also must be wary of postulating greater changes than those that actually occurred. What makes these two physician-authors similar is their membership in dissident religious communities, as lapsed Huguenots or persistent Schwenkfelders. If their special brands of radical Protestantism altered theories and therapies in some way, little evidence demonstrates how differently a Schwenkfelder physician would think and act from a lapsed Huguenot one; rather, both, seemingly in equal measure, reflected German medical and pharmaceutical practice and the shared corpus of early modern medical traditions. Thus, translocation apparently mattered little, and added little, to their theories. As to their practice, except as reflected in their manuscripts and some local correspondence (as reported by *L. Allen Viehmeyer* in this volume), we know next to nothing. Thus, we can only surmise that the sociogeographical context may have made a difference in how medicine was practiced on the ground, but as yet, no firm evidence substantiates what seems a perfectly plausible supposition.

Thoughts in Lieu of a Conclusion

My purpose in writing this piece was not to set myself up as a critic or proponent of any one particular approach to the history of medicine. Nor do I want to privilege or push one context over another. Rather, I would like to act as a mediator between approaches and contexts. It is banal to say, but nonetheless true, that each context discussed here – from the narrowest to the broadest, from the ones focused most closely on medical theory to those most expansive in their catchment area – offers advantages and disadvantages to the medical historian. Certainly, some contexts as explored here are more evolved, and perhaps also more sophisticated, than others. The investigation of case studies, for instance, or the examination of the impact of religion on medical theory and practice, have long and venerable pedigrees. Less common are approaches that reach across oceanic expanses. For the first group, we have well-developed methodologies and equally well-developed historiographical frameworks in which to slot individual studies. The latter context – the comparative or Atlantic – remains a brave new world, uncrowded and thus exciting and promising, but also uncertain and unproven. Yet one of the glories of all history is its ecumenicalism; to survive and to flourish, it must allow, indeed must encourage, historians to follow a wide range of perspectives. As these jostle and wrangle with one another, they also cross-fertilize and enrich by challenging us to ask new questions, to direct our thoughts into new channels, and to try out new methods.

References

Egmond & Mason (1997)
Egmond, Florike; Mason, Peter: The Mammoth and the Mouse; Microhistory and Morphology. Baltimore: Johns Hopkins University Press, 1997.

Helm (2006)
Helm, Jürgen: Krankheit, Bekehrung und Reform. Medizin und Krankenfürsorge im Halleschen Pietismus. Tübingen: Verlag der Franckeschen Stiftungen im Niemeyer Verlag, 2006 (Hallesche Forschungen 21).

Jardine (2003)
Jardine, Lisa: The Curious Life of Robert Hooke. The Man Who Measured London. London: Harper Collins, 2003 .

Jardine (1999)
Jardine, Lisa: Ingenious Pursuits. Building the Scientific Revolution. London: Little, Brown and Co., 1999.

Jardine (1974)
Jardine, Lisa: Francis Bacon. Discovery and the Art of Discourse. London: Cambridge University Press, 1974.

Marland & Pelling (1996)
Marland, Hilary; Pelling, Margaret (Eds.): The Task of Healing. Medicine, Religion and Gender in England and the Netherlands, 1450–1800. Rotterdam: Erasmus Publications, 1996.

Numbers & Amundsen (1986)
Numbers, Ronald; Amundsen, Darrel W. (Eds.): Caring and Curing. Health and Medicine in the Western Religious Tradition. New York: Macmillan, 1986.

Pollock (1992)
Pollock, Linda: With Faith and Physic. The Life of a Tudor Gentlewoman, Lady Grace Mildmay, 1552–1620. New York: St. Martin's Press, 1992.

Reill (2005)
Reill, Peter: Vitalizing Nature in the Enlightenment. Berkeley, Los Angeles: University of California Press, 2005.

Wesley (1759)
Wesley, John: Primitive Physic. Bristol: John Graham, 1759.

Wilson (1996)
Wilson, Renate: Pietist Universal Reform and Care of the Sick and the Poor. The Medical Institutions of the Francke Foundation and Their Social Contexts. In: Finzsch, Norbert; Jütte, Robert (Eds.): Institutions of Confinement. Hospitals, Asylums, and Prisons in Western Europe and America, 1500–1900. New York: Cambridge University Press, 1996, 113–54.

Wilson (2000)
Wilson, Renate: Pious Traders in Medicine. A German Pharmaceutical Network in Eighteenth-Century North America. University Park, PA: Penn State University Press, 2000.

SUMMARIES – ZUSAMMENFASSUNGEN

Part I: Theory and Therapy

Jole Shackelford

PARACELSIAN UROSCOPY AND GERMAN CHEMIATRIC MEDICINE IN THE MEDICINA PENSYLVANIA OF GEORGE DE BENNEVILLE

PARACELSISTISCHE HARNSCHAU UND DEUTSCHE CHEMIATRISCHE MEDIZIN IN DER MEDICINA PENSYLVANIA DES GEORGE DE BENNEVILLE

Recent study of a German-English medical manual left in manuscript by the immigrant physician George de Benneville has revealed a wide-ranging and sometimes perplexing pharmaceutical therapeutics. Jole Shackelford shows that roughly 40 pages of the approximately 170 page *Medicina Pensylvania* offer a therapeutics that is unambiguously grounded in the theory and practice associated with the late sixteenth and early seventeenth-century followers of the eccentric and radical German physician Theophrastus Paracelsus. Paracelsus' ideas about the medical use of uroscopy to reveal metabolic failures in the human body were elaborated into an astrological-chemical pathology and diagnostic semiotics by Johann Hayne, whose book was one of multiple sources for the *Medicina Pensylvania*. The integration of chemiatric theory and therapeutic practice that is implicit in Hayne's book and de Benneville's dispensatory plus pharmaceutical manual reveals a persistence of Paracelsian medical practice into eighteenth century North America that has not been adequately explored.

Die medizin- und pharmaziehistorische Untersuchung eines deutsch-englischen Manuskriptes aus dem Nachlass des 1730 nach Amerika eingewanderten Arztes George de Benneville erlaubt einen Einblick in dessen Therapievorstellungen, der zu überraschenden Ergebnissen führt. Jole Shackelford zeigt, dass etwa 40 Seiten des rund 170 Doppel-Folios umfassenden Arzneibuchs diagnostische und therapeutische Vorstellungen enthalten, die eindeutig in der Theorie und medizinischen Praxis der Paracelsisten des späten 16. und frühen 17. Jahrhunderts verankert sind. Die Vorstellungen des Paracelsus über die Harnschau zur Diagnose von inneren Erkrankungen wurden an der Wende zum 17. Jahrhundert von Johann Hayne in einem Traktat zur astrologisch-chemischen Pathologie dargestellt. Dieser Traktat war die Quelle der entsprechenden Abschnitte der *Medicina Pensylvania*. Die offensichtliche enge Verbindung von chemiatrischer Theorie und therapeutischer Praxis in dem Hayneschen Traktat und in einem Teil des sonst eher traditionellen Arzneibuchs von de Benneville zeigt das Fortleben paracelsistischer medizinischer Praktiken bis ins 18. Jahrhundert, das in der Medizingeschichte noch nicht angemessen gewürdigt worden ist.

Marion Maria Ruisinger

THE CIRCULATION OF THE BLOOD AND VENESECTION: ON THE RELATION BETWEEN MEDICAL THEORY AND PRACTICE IN THE EARLY EIGHTEENTH CENTURY

BLUTKREISLAUF UND ADERLASS: EIN BEITRAG ZUM VERHÄLTNIS VON MEDIZINISCHER THEORIE UND ÄRZTLICHER PRAXIS IM FRÜHEN 18. JAHRHUNDERT

In early modern medicine, venesection was embedded in the physiology of Galen. When this model was replaced by the model of the circulation of the blood proposed by William Harvey in 1628, venesection was reinterpreted in ways that departed from the original notions of organ specificity, the *revulsio* and *derivatio*. Marion Maria Ruisinger addresses the question of the extent to which this theoretical departure affected the actual practice of bloodletting. From a provider perspective, she examines the vernacular German surgical literature addressing the barber surgeon of the early eighteenth century. The patient perspective is recreated by an examination of the *consilia* rendered by Lorenz Heister. She concludes that at the time, venesection was still largely practiced according to pre-Harveyan methods, and that this continuity of Galenist practice was often due to the insistence of the patient. For the men and women who received venesection, the choice of the 'right' vein meant a conscious attempt to influence a specific part of the body. This patient autonomy in treatment was threatened by the newer models of circulation. Additionally, regular preventive venesection established a client-provider hierarchy between the healthy client and the barber surgeon which permeated their relationship.

Der Aderlass wurde zu Beginn der Frühen Neuzeit auf Basis der Physiologie Galens gedeutet. Mit der Ablösung dieses traditionellen Modells durch das 1628 veröffentlichte Kreislaufmodell William Harveys vollzog sich eine Neuinterpretation des Aderlasses, die mit der traditionellen Vorstellung der Organspezifität, der *revulsio* und der *derivatio,* brach. Marion Maria Ruisingers Studie beantwortet die Frage, inwieweit sich diese neue Aderlass-Theorie auf die zeitgenössische Aderlass-Praxis auswirkte. Für die Rekonstruktion der Perspektive der Handwerkschirurgen wird die deutschsprachige chirurgische Fachliteratur des frühen 18. Jahrhunderts herangezogen, zur Rekonstruktion der Patientenperspektive dient die Konsiliarkorrespondenz Lorenz Heisters. Es zeigt sich, dass der Aderlass zu diesem Zeitpunkt noch weitgehend nach der vor Harvey etablierten Methode durchgeführt wurde. Der maßgebliche Faktor für dieses Festhalten an einer galenistisch fundierten Praxis ist auf der Klientenseite zu suchen. Für die Frauen und Männer, die sich zur Ader ließen, hätte der Bruch mit der Vorstellung, durch die Wahl der ‚richtigen' Vene gezielt auf das Innere des eigenen Körpers Einfluss nehmen zu können, einen erheblichen Autonomieverlust bedeutet. Zudem etablierte sich durch die habituell durchgeführten präventiven Aderlässe ein Hierarchiegefälle zwischen dem gesunden Kunden und dem Wundarzt, das auch im

Behandlungsfall zum Tragen kam und das dem Chirurgen lediglich die Rolle des Befehlsempfängers zuwies.

Andreas-Holger Maehle

EXPERIENCE, EXPERIMENT AND THEORY: JUSTIFICATIONS AND CRITICISMS OF PHARMACOTHERAPEUTIC PRACTICES IN THE EIGHTEENTH CENTURY

ERFAHRUNG, EXPERIMENT UND THEORIE: RECHTFERTIGUNGEN UND KRITIK VON PHARMAKOTHERAPEUTISCHEN PRAKTIKEN IM 18. JAHRHUNDERT

According to traditional historiography, a chasm existed between the new medical theories and the therapeutic practices of the eighteenth century. In his contribution, Andreas Holger Maehle qualifies this assessment by demonstrating contemporary interactions between experimental investigations of drugs or new remedies and theoretical considerations of their mode of action and appropriate therapeutic use. Such interactions are illustrated through case studies of three medicines that were central to therapeutics during the period of the Enlightenment: opium, Peruvian bark, and lithontriptics (so-called stone-dissolving substances). It is shown how experimental studies (*in vitro*, on animals, and on patients) provided supporting evidence for various pharmacological theories and influenced therapeutic recommendations. Moreover, Maehle shows that there was a lively and critical discourse on matters of pharmacotherapy in eighteenth-century Europe.

Der traditionellen Historiographie zufolge bestand im 18. Jahrhundert eine Kluft zwischen den neueren medizinischen Theorien der Zeit und der therapeutischen Praxis. Andreas-Holger Maehle relativiert diese Einschätzung, indem er den bereits damals hergestellten Zusammenhang zwischen experimentellen Untersuchungen von Drogen oder neuen Heilmitteln einerseits und theoretischen Überlegungen zu deren Wirkungsweise sowie angemessenem therapeutischen Gebrauch andererseits aufzeigt. Diese Wechselwirkungen werden anhand von Fallstudien zu drei Arzneimitteln demonstriert, die eine zentrale Rolle in der medizinischen Therapie des Zeitalters der Aufklärung spielten: Opium, Chinarinde und die Lithontriptica (die so genannten stein-auflösenden Medikamente). Es wird dargestellt, wie experimentelle Studien (*in vitro*, an Tieren und an Patienten) verschiedene pharmakologische Theorien unterstützten und therapeutische Empfehlungen beeinflussten. Der Beitrag zeigt zudem, dass im Europa des 18. Jahrhunderts ein lebhafter und kritischer Diskurs über Fragen der Arzneimittelbehandlung stattfand.

Karin Stukenbrock

ADVICE TO THE PUBLIC: ON THE RELATIONSHIP BETWEEN MEDICAL THEORY AND DIETETIC PRACTICE

„WER SEINE GESUNDHEIT LIEBT, DER FLIEHE DIE MEDICOS UND ARTZNEYEN“ – ZUM VERHÄLTNIS VON MEDIZINISCHER THEORIE UND DIÄTETISCHER PRAXIS

The medical literature of the eighteenth century saw an increasing preoccupation with the preservation of health. Karin Stukenbrock investigates this phenomenon against the background of the changes in the medical theories of the period. She raises the question whether and to what extent these changes found their way into the dietetic and public health advice physicians directed to a populace considered in need of health education and guidance. She examines selected writings by Friedrich Hoffmann, in particular his *Kurzgefaßte Diätetic* of 1744, and a later author, Franz Anton Mai and his *Medicinische Fastenpredigten* of 1793-1794. Stukenbrock finds that despite considerable changes in medical theory, dietetic advice to the public hardly changed over the course of the century. A healthy life continued to be predicated on moderation in all situations and on appropriate diet, exercise and other measures based on one's individual constitution.

Ein wichtiger Teil der medizinischen Literatur des 18. Jahrhunderts beschäftigte sich mit der Gesunderhaltung des Menschen. Vor dem Hintergrund des Konzeptwandels in der medizinischen Theorie dieser Zeit geht Karin Stukenbrock der Frage nach, inwiefern sich dieser Wandel auf die von Ärzten an das Publikum gerichteten diätetisch-praktischen Anweisungen auswirkte. Ihr Untersuchungsgegenstand sind ausgewählte Schriften von Friedrich Hoffmann, vor allem dessen *Kurzgefaßte Diätetic* von 1744, sowie Franz Anton Mais *Medicinische Fastenpredigten* aus den Jahren 1793 und 1794. Stukenbrock kommt zu dem Ergebnis, dass sich die dem Publikum gegebenen Ratschläge trotz der im Lauf des 18. Jahrhunderts gewandelten theoretischen Vorannahmen nicht verändert haben. Als wesentliche Garanten für ein gesundes Leben wurden nach wie vor das Maßhalten in allen Lebenslagen sowie eine ausgewogene und der individuellen Konstitution angepasste Lebensführung angesehen.

Part II: Therapeutic Uncertainties

Michael Stolberg

THERAPEUTIC PLURALISM AND CONFLICTING MEDICAL OPINIONS IN THE EIGHTEENTH CENTURY: THE PATIENT'S VIEW

THERAPEUTISCHER PLURALISMUS UND WIDERSPRECHENDE MEDIZINISCHE ANSICHTEN IM 18. JAHRHUNDERT: DIE PATIENTENPERSPEKTIVE

Michael Stolberg examines patient experience with contradictory medical diagnoses and advice. Conflicting therapeutic instructions tended to disorient and rob ill and often desperate patients of confidence in their healers. Based on letters and similar documents by the patients themselves and family members, Stolberg concludes that frequent dissent among physicians and others at the bedside did not necessarily reflect the notorious pluralism of medical theories that pervaded the eighteenth century. Diagnostic and therapeutic pluralism was not so much due to the prevailing diagnostic uncertainty among physicians as to the continuing patient dominance in the eighteenth century medical market. To secure professional renown and its economic rewards, physicians had to convince their patients that they had fully considered his or her individual constitution and circumstances and that their advice was based on their own extraordinary professional experience and medical intuition. In addition to at least temporary improvement in the patient's condition, success came to those whose diagnostic judgments and therapeutic advice were distinct and distinguishable from that of their colleagues.

Gegenstand des Beitrags von Michael Stolberg ist die Bedeutung widersprüchlicher ärztlicher Diagnosen und Ratschläge aus der Sicht von Kranken und Angehörigen. Auf die verzweifelten Patienten wirkten die divergierenden Empfehlungen verunsichernd und desorientierend. Stolberg zeigt anhand von Patientenbriefen und anderen Selbstzeugnissen, dass die für die Patienten alltägliche Erfahrung von ärztlichem Dissens am Krankenbett nicht primär dem ausgeprägten Pluralismus der Theorien in der Medizin des 18. Jahrhunderts entsprang. Neben der Unsicherheit der verfügbaren diagnostischen Methoden waren es insbesondere die patientendominierten Bedingungen des zeitgenössischen medizinischen Markts und die Erwartungen der Kranken selbst, die dem diagnostischen und therapeutischen Pluralismus am Krankenbett Vorschub leisteten. Auf beruflichen und ökonomischen Erfolg konnten vor allem jene Ärzte hoffen, die ihre Patienten davon überzeugten, dass ihre Diagnose und Therapie die individuelle Verfasstheit des Patienten umfassend berücksichtigten und auf einer ganz besonderen, herausragenden Erfahrung und Intuition beruhten. Beides konnte letztlich nur dadurch gelingen, dass sich ihr Urteil und vor allem ihr Behandlungsplan von dem anderer Ärzte deutlich unterschieden und sich der Gesundheitszustand des Patienten unter der eingeschlagenen Behandlung zumindest vorübergehend besserte.

Jürgen Helm

THE HALLE ORPHANAGE MEDICATIONS: A CASE STUDY IN THE DEVELOPMENT AND DISSEMINATION OF THERAPEUTIC PRACTICES IN THE EIGHTEENTH CENTURY

DIE MEDIKAMENTE DES HALLESCHEN WAISENHAUSES. EIN BEISPIEL FÜR DIE ETABLIERUNG UND VERBREITUNG THERAPEUTISCHER PRAKTIKEN IM 18. JAHRHUNDERT

During the first decades of the eighteenth century, the so-called Halle Orphanage medications gained access to the medical markets of the Germanies and Northern Europe. In his contribution to this volume, Jürgen Helm analyses a large collection of letters by the physicians responsible for the development and trials of these medications and of a set of informational and advertising broadsheets. His sources suggest three major prerequisites for the success of these medications: (1) The explicit incorporation of Georg Ernst Stahl's theories into the printed materials provided a plausible underpinning for the assumed effectiveness of the medications. (2) While the publication of carefully selected case histories was an accepted practice in eighteenth century medical marketing, the printing and missionary activities of the Halle Orphanage endowed these marketing strategies with a special message and reach that went well beyond the customary advertising campaigns of the period. (3) Focus on the individual patient and patient outcomes during the first part of the eighteenth century, coupled with a multitude of positive patient testimonials, made it possible to overcome, at least in the public mind, contradictory reports of lacking effectiveness.

Die Medikamente des Halleschen Waisenhauses etablierten sich im Verlauf des 18. Jahrhunderts auf deutschsprachigen und anderen europäischen Gesundheitsmärkten. Jürgen Helms Beitrag stellt anhand einer Analyse von Briefen der in den Franckeschen Anstalten verantwortlichen Ärzte und von gedruckten Informations- und Werbeschriften drei wichtige Voraussetzungen des Erfolgs der Arzneien dar: (1) Mit der gezielten Übernahme von Georg Ernst Stahls Theorie in die gedruckten Texte zu den Medikamenten lieferte man eine plausible Erklärung für deren Wirkungsprinzip. (2) Zwischen der im 18. Jahrhundert durchaus üblichen Sammlung von Fallberichten zum besseren Verständnis von Arzneimittelwirkungen und den missionarischen und verlegerischen Aktivitäten der Franckeschen Anstalten kam es zu einer Synergie, deren Resultat eine für die damalige Zeit erstaunliche Werbekampagne war. (3) Der individualisierende Ansatz der Medizin in der ersten Hälfte des 18. Jahrhunderts und die umfangreiche Sammlung von Heilungsberichten ermöglichten es, Berichte über erfolglose Therapieversuche mit den Medikamenten zu entkräften.

Part III: Materia Medica and Their Uses

Robert Jütte

MENSCHLICHE GEWEBE UND ORGANE ALS BESTANDTEIL EINER RATIONALEN MEDIZIN IM 18. JAHRHUNDERT

HUMAN TISSUES AND ORGANS AS PART OF A RATIONAL MEDICINE OF THE EIGHTEENTH CENTURY

Human body parts and tissues played an important role in therapeutics until the late eighteenth century and sometimes even beyond that date. Using bones, skulls, blood, fat, skin and other parts taken from corpses of people who had been executed or died a violent death was not linked to a magical background but was considered as rational medicine. This meant that such substances were administered both by learned physicians and barber-surgeons. These rather expensive substances were provided by executioners and were also sold in pharmacies. They are listed in the official *materia medica* until the late eighteenth and early nineteenth century. In his paper, Robert Jütte describes the whole range of therapeutic use of human body parts, showing that this practice was indeed based on rational considerations.

Menschliche Organe und Gewebe spielten bis ins späte 18. Jahrhundert und zum Teil auch noch darüber hinaus in der Medizin eine Rolle. Die Verwendung von Knochen, Schädeln, Blut, Fett und Haut von Hingerichteten oder von Personen, die eines gewaltsamen Todes gestorben waren, hatte nichts mit Magie zu tun. Im Unterschied zu heute wurden diese Therapien als rationale Medizin verstanden und von Wundärzten und gelehrten Ärzten gleichermaßen angewendet. Scharfrichter lieferten die teuren Ausgangssubstanzen, die auch in Apotheken erhältlich waren. Bis ins frühe 19. Jahrhundert wurden diese Arzneistoffe auch in Pharmakopöen erwähnt. In Robert Jüttes Beitrag wird das ganze Spektrum des therapeutischen Gebrauchs menschlicher Körperteile aufgezeigt und der Nachweis geführt, dass es sich dabei um eine „rationale“ Therapie handelt.

Almut Lanz

FRIEDRICH HOFFMANN: CONCORDANCE BETWEEN MEDICAL THEORY AND PRACTICE

FRIEDRICH HOFFMANN: ÜBEREINSTIMMUNG VON MEDIZINISCHER THEORIE UND PRAXIS

Almut Lanz demonstrates the effects of Friedrich Hoffmann's medical theory on his therapeutic practice. Hoffmann's medical evolution is examined with a view to the emergence of some of the characteristics that distinguished his thinking throughout his life. Lanz shows that his preference for logic, anatomy, chemistry and medical practice can be discerned even in his early medical studies. Hoffmann's theory of physiology, pathology und therapy is explained by reference to his early *Fundamenta Medicinae* (1695), while his medical practice is illustrated by examples from the first three volumes of his *Medicina consultatoria*, published in 1721–1723. Lanz argues that this practice logically follows his medical theory, in accordance with the concepts of reason and experience, developed in his large oeuvre.

Im Beitrag von Almut Lanz wird die Auswirkung der medizinischen Theorie Friedrich Hoffmanns auf dessen therapeutische Praxis dargestellt. Zunächst wird auf den beruflichen Werdegang Hoffmanns eingegangen, da bereits dessen Ausbildung durch besondere Interessenschwerpunkte gekennzeichnet ist, die er lebenslang beibehielt: Logik, Anatomie, Chemie und ärztliche Praxis. Unter Bezugnahme auf Hoffmanns Frühwerk *Fundamenta Medicinae* (1695) wird auf Hoffmanns medizinische Theorie, nämlich die in diesem Werk dargelegten Grundzüge der Physiologie, Pathologie und Therapeutik, eingegangen. Hoffmanns therapeutische Praxis wird an Beispielen aus den ersten drei Bänden seiner *Medicina consultatoria* (1721–1723) vorgestellt und hinsichtlich des theoretischen Bezugs überprüft. Lanz weist nach, dass Hoffmanns ärztliche Praxis eine logische Konsequenz seiner medizinischen Theorie darstellt, entsprechend dem Gebrauch von Vernunft und Erfahrung, wie er ihn in seinem umfangreichen Werk entwickelt hat.

John K. Crellin

MENTORS AND FORMULAE: CONTINUITY AND CHANGE IN EIGHTEENTH-CENTURY THERAPEUTICS

MENTOREN UND REZEPTE: KONTINUITÄT UND WANDEL IN DER THERAPIE DES 18. JAHRHUNDERTS

In his current paper and elsewhere, John Crellin suggests that in his mid-eighteenth century Pennsylvania practice, Abraham Wagner, an immigrant practitioner to North America and the author of the *Remediorum specimina*, was influenced not only by the theory of Georg Ernst Stahl and of other medical authorities, but by his Silesian mentors. Crellin intends to prompt further discussion of eighteenth-century therapy by focusing in particular on how Wagner was both influenced by and monitored the practices of his three Schwenkfelder mentors, whose names – Martin John, Jr., George Hauptmann, and Melchior Hübner or Heebner – have not reached the annals of medical history. In so far as Wagner was judicious in what he wanted to pass on in his manuscript, his apprenticeship in place of a formal academic medical education is of particular interest in terms of the nature and formulation of many of his prescriptions. Crellin suggests this was a significant factor in Wagner's validation of medicines alongside theory and clinical experience. Brief mention is also made of practitioner-patient relationships as affecting treatment outcomes.

John Crellin untersucht in seinem Beitrag die medizinische Praxis Abraham Wagners, des aus Schlesien nach Nordamerika eingewanderten Autors der *Remediorum specimina.* Wagner war nicht nur von den Theorien Georg Ernst Stahls und anderer medizinischer Autoritäten beeinflusst, sondern auch von den Praktiken seiner Lehrer und Vorgänger Martin John, Jr., George Hauptmann und Melchior Hübner, die in der Medizingeschichte nur wenig bekannt sind. Crellin zufolge weisen die von Wagner in sein Manuskript aufgenommenen Rezepturen auf die Entwicklung einer auf Theorie und klinischer Erfahrung basierenden Medizin hin. In seinem Beitrag geht Crellin auch kurz auf die Arzt-Patient-Beziehung und ihren Einfluss auf den Therapieerfolg ein.

Renate Wilson

THE TRANSMISSION OF MEDICAL AND PHARMACEUTICAL KNOWLEDGE TO COLONIAL NORTH AMERICA

DIE ÜBERMITTLUNG MEDIZINISCHEN UND PHARMAZEUTISCHEN WISSENS IN DIE NORDAMERIKANISCHEN KOLONIEN

Renate Wilson places the two medical manuscripts attributed to George de Benneville and Abraham Wagner into a common linguistic and social context. Several reasons for the neglect of these manuscripts in the history of mainstream North American medicine are suggested. One is the contest for linguistic dominance and medical tradition in the scientific discourse of the late colonial period and in the New Republic. The other deals with the place of sectarian or dissident medical practitioners vs. the standard bearers of the Enlightenment, in particular its Scottish version. Both linguistic barriers and the presumed adherence to Stahlian medical theory by German-language practitioners seem to have played a part in causing and perpetuating this neglect. Wilson emphasizes that the language used in these manuscripts – the *Medicina Pensylvania* and the *Remediorum specimina* discussed elsewhere in this volume – is not so much lay vernacular as the established German medical *Fachprosa* of the early modern period. The bilingual de Benneville text as well as the Wagner compendium additionally addressed and reflected cooperation with Anglophone, German, and Dutch copractitioners in North America. Despite their affinity to spiritualist Christianity, both authors worked within the parameters of early modern medical and pharmaceutical practice and there is little to indicate a specifically spiritualist or religious provenance for their remedies and courses of treatment. Seen in conjunction, these medical compendia and receptures present themselves to the reader not so much as part of a dissident medical tradition but reflect the web of manifold and interacting European transmissions of therapeutic knowledge into North America.

Renate Wilson setzt zwei im Pennsylvanien der Kolonialzeit entstandene Arzneibücher, die den deutschsprachigen Ärzten George de Benneville und Abraham Wagner zugeschrieben werden, in den sozial- und medizingeschichtlichen Rahmen der nordamerikanischen therapeutischen Praxis des 18. Jahrhunderts. Die Vernachlässigung dieser Manuskripte in der medizingeschichtlichen Literatur erklärt sich für Wilson zum einen aus dem Konflikt um sprachliche Vorherrschaft und die ‚richtige' medizinische Tradition im wissenschaftlichen Diskurs der jungen Republik des ausgehenden Jahrhunderts, zum anderen aus dem nachgeordneten Stellenwert, der dissidenten ärztlichen Praktikern im Gegensatz zu den Protagonisten der Aufklärung, insbesondere in ihrer schottischen Prägung, zugemessen wird. Sie schreibt diese Ablehnung sowohl sprachlichen Barrieren zu, als auch dem – tatsächlichen oder unterstellten – Einfluss von Georg Ernst Stahl auf deutschsprachige Ärzte in Nordamerika. Wilson zeichnet die Sprache dieser Manuskripte im Kontext der deutschsprachigen frühneuzeitlichen medizinischen Fachprosa nach. De Bennevilles zweisprachiger Text wie auch das Rezeptbuch von Abraham Wagner wenden sich darüber hinaus an englischsprachige, deutsche und niederländische medizinische Praktiker in Nordamerika und spiegeln die bestehende Kooperation zwischen diesen Gruppen wider. Hinsichtlich der Frage der Verknüpfung von Religion und Medizin stellt Wilson fest, dass beide Autoren trotz ihrer Affinität zu einem spirituellen Christentum im Rahmen der zeitüblichen medizinischen und pharmazeutischen Praxis arbeiteten. Es gibt nur wenige Hinweise auf einen spezifischen spirituellen oder religiösen Kontext für ihre Heilmittel und Behandlungsmethoden. Zusammengenommen stellen sich diese beiden medizinischen Kompendien und Rezeptsammlungen dem Leser nicht so sehr als Teil einer unorthodoxen medizinischen Tradition dar, sondern als ein Beispiel für das vielfältige und interagierende Netzwerk europäischen therapeutischen Wissens in Nordamerika.

Part IV: Religion and Society in Eighteenth Century Medicine

Fritz Krafft

MEDICINA THEOLOGICA AS AN OUTCOME OF THE THEOLOGIA MEDICINALIS IN EARLY MODERN PROTESTANTISM

„ … DENN BIST DU NICHT BEY IHR MIT DEINER KRAFFT ZUGEGEN, SO HILFT KEIN DIPTAM NICHT, UND KEINE PANACEE.“ – MEDICINA THEOLOGICA ALS KONSEQUENZ DER THEOLOGIA MEDICINALIS IM PROTESTANTISMUS

For a non-teleological understanding of Christian medicine before the Enlightenment, Krafft proposes that the medicine of the body (as a *donum Dei*) always was connected with 'spiritual' medicine because medical use could only be successful with the help of God (obtained by saying a prayer). Also, treatment with a physical medicine only made sense if it was connected with a treatment of the soul (applying Christ's medicines of the soul). In this paper, Krafft describes the history of *Theologia medicinalis* within Protestantism from Martin Luther and Orthodoxy to Pietism, on the basis of an exegesis of the book Jesus Sirach in the literature of the oeconomia; a second section deals with the origin and history of the symbolic image of Christ as apothecary up to the special images of Pietism, which culminated in a commemorative stone and in a book of comfort *Der Sarg als ein rechter Artzt* (The coffin as a right physician) by Daniel Schoenemann (1725). Both express the firm conviction that the life of a believer in Christ is not taken away by bodily death but is changed and turned into everlasting life by His 'postmortal medicine.'

Für ein nicht-teleologisches Verständnis medizinischer Aktivitäten in der Zeit vor der Aufklärung ist es nicht nur in Bezug auf den Pietismus erforderlich, zu berücksichtigen, dass die Leibesmedizin (als verehrenswerte Gottesgabe, *donum Dei*) stets mit einer ‚geistlichen' Medizin verbunden wurde – nicht nur, weil erst durch das Mitwirken Gottes (erwirkt durch das Gebet) die Anwendung eines Medikaments erfolgreich sein könne, sondern auch, weil eine Behandlung mittels ‚leiblicher Arznei' sinnvollerweise mit einer solchen mittels ‚geistlicher' (Seelen-)Arznei zu verknüpfen sei (wenn letztere auch häufig vernachlässigt wurde). Kraffts Beitrag stellt die Geschichte der *Theologia medicinalis* innerhalb des Protestantismus von Martin Luther und der lutherischen Orthodoxie bis zum Pietismus anhand der Jesus Sirach-Exegese in der Hausväterliteratur dar; in einem zweiten Durchgang werden Entstehen und Geschichte des Sinnbildmotivs ‚Christus als Apotheker' der Seelenarzneien bis hin zu den speziellen Ausformungen durch den Pietismus dargestellt. Sie gipfelt in einem um 1735 gesetzten Gedenkstein und in dem Trostbuch *Der Sarg als ein rechter Artzt* von Daniel Schönemann (1725) als Ausdruck der Glaubensüberzeugung, dass durch den leiblichen Tod des Gläubigen nicht das Leben genommen, sondern mit Hilfe von Christi ‚postmortaler Medizin' gewandelt wird zum ewigen Leben.

L. Allen Viehmeyer

ABRAHAM WAGNER AND GEORGE DE BENNEVILLE: PHYSICIANS OF BODY AND SOUL

ABRAHAM WAGNER UND GEORGE DE BENNEVILLE: ÄRZTE VON KÖRPER UND SEELE

Allen Viehmeyer provides biographical detail and some general background on the lives of Abraham Wagner and George de Benneville. Both men were medical practitioners in Philadelphia County (today Montgomery and Berks Counties) in eighteenth century Pennsylvania. The legacy of each man includes a medical manuscript of historical importance. The issue of their early education and medical training is addressed. Wagner learned his skills as an apprentice to Melchior Hübner (Heebner). How de Benneville acquired his medical skills remains unknown. Some historical background on their emigration and acquaintance is presented as well. Both men came to Pennsylvania seeking religious freedom, having been persecuted in Europe for their sectarian views. De Benneville was a Huguenot and Wagner was a Schwenkfelder. Both were ardent and active in the pursuit of their faith and shared some religious beliefs view. In general there seems to have a special, enduring bond between de Benneville and the Schwenkfelders. In addition to their medical practice, de Benneville preached far and wide in the Piedmont and as far as Virginia. Wagner is also known for his hymns.

In Allen Viehmeyers Beitrag werden Leben und Wirken von Abraham Wagner und George de Benneville dargestellt. Beide arbeiteten als Ärzte in Philadelphia County (heute Montgomery und Berks Counties) in Pennsylvania und hinterließen medizinische Handschriften, die für die Kolonialgeschichte der amerikanischen Medizin bemerkenswert sind. Wagner erwarb seine medizinischen Fachkenntnisse als Lehrling eines älteren Arztes, Melchior Hübner. Die Frage, wie de Benneville sich sein medizinisches Wissen angeeignet hatte, kann nicht eindeutig beantwortet werden. Beide Männer waren in Europa wegen ihrer sektiererischen religiösen Ansichten verfolgt worden und kamen nach Pennsylvania, um Glaubensfreiheit zu erlangen. De Benneville war Hugenotte, Wagner ein Mitglied der Schwenckfelder-Sekte. Eine persönliche und dauerhafte Verbindung zwischen de Benneville und den Schwenckfeldern in Pennsylvania kann angenommen werden. Zusätzlich zur medizinischen Praxis war de Benneville als Prediger unter den Christen der deutschen Siedlungen von Pennsylvania bis Virginia tätig, während Wagner sich als Dichter von Kirchenliedern hervortat.

Elisabeth Quast

PIETIST NOBLEWOMEN AND THEIR NETWORKS: FEMALE COLLABORATION IN TESTING AND PROMOTING THE HALLE ORPHANAGE MEDICATIONS

SCHWÄGERINNEN. ADLIGE FRAUEN IN DER FRÜHZEIT DER HALLESCHEN MEDIKAMENTENEXPEDITION

In her contribution to this volume, Elisabeth Quast examines the active participation of Pietist women in the circle around Carl Hildebrand, Baron Canstein, in the original sales and distribution of the Halle Orphanage medications during the first phase of their development. Canstein was a close collaborator of August Hermann Francke, and his female collaborators were drawn from the Prussian nobility at the Court in Berlin. Quast uses as her sources a previously unpublished collection of letters to Canstein by the major developers of these medications, the brothers Christian Friedrich and Christian Sigismund Richter, both physicians at the Halle Orphanage. The letters date to the period 1701 to 1711 and reveal this circle of women as both users and disseminators of a famous set of medical products. They self-medicated with the *Essentia dulcis* and other Orphanage medications and can be shown to have actively participated in the writing of treatment reports published by the Richter brothers between 1701 to 1705 in several tracts, among them *Exempel sonderbarer Curen* and *Berichte von der Essentia dulcis*. Their contribution to the early trade in these medications included promotion, dissemination, and sales to others in their large networks of family and friends in the Prussian nobility. Their close ties to the Pietist movement in Halle and Berlin made them desirable promoters and permitted the establishment of a durable trading network at this level. According to Quast, the effective and efficient organization of their collaboration reflects traditional administrative and financial activities among women heading large aristocratic households – the oeconomia of the nobility – during the early modern period. This is reinforced by the establishment of a so-called *Frauenzimmermanufaktur* – a women's manufacture – in Berlin in 1707, which may well have offered a template for this collaborative effort promoting a socially acceptable and profitable cause.

Elisabeth Quast untersucht in ihrem Beitrag die Beteiligung von adligen Frauen um Baron Carl Hildebrand von Canstein am Vertrieb der Richterschen Medikamente in der ersten Phase der so genannten Medikamentenexpedition, des ca. 1701 beginnenden Versandhandels des Waisenhauses. Die Quellenlage, insbesondere eine Sammlung von Briefen der beiden Waisenhausärzte Christian Friedrich Richter und Christian Sigismund Richter, die diese zwischen 1701 und 1711 an Canstein in Berlin richteten, erlaubt eine Rekonstruktion der Tätigkeit dieser Frauen: Als aktive und qualifizierte Patientinnen und Kundinnen waren sie bei der Erprobung der *Essentia dulcis* und der weiteren Medikamente des Waisenhauses einbezogen. Ihre Mitwirkung ist nachweisbar bei der Ausarbeitung von Krankengeschichten für die Richterschen *Exempel sonderbarer Curen* und die *Berichte von der Essentia dulcis*, die zwischen 1701 und 1705 erschienen. Sie übernahmen Aufgaben der Absatzförderung, etwa Werbung, Vertreterinnentätigkeit und Verkaufstätigkeit. Die traditionelle verwandtschaftsbasierte Verpflichtungsstruktur des Adels und die nachhaltige, religiös-politisch motivierte Bindung an das pietistische Projekt garantierten eine beachtliche Tragfähigkeit und Verlässlichkeit der hier aufgebauten Beziehungen. Die Zu- und Mitarbeit der adligen Frauen beim Aufbau des Medikamentenvertriebs war planvoll organisiert. Die einzelnen Tätigkeiten können dem zeitgemäßen Handlungsspektrum von Frauen, die großen Haushalten vorstehen und in Geschäften geübt sind, zugeordnet werden. Die Tatsache, dass diese Berliner Frauengruppe 1707 eine so genannte Frauenzimmermanufaktur gegründet hat, bietet ein ökonomisch stringentes Deutungsmuster an. Quast schlägt vor, die Arbeitsorganisation einer Manufaktur als Muster für die spezifische Kombination der weiblichen Zu- und Mitarbeit an der Medikamentenexpedition zu sehen.

Part V: Conclusions and Observations

Mary Lindemann

THE CONTEXTS OF MEDICINE IN THE SEVENTEENTH AND EIGHTEENTH CENTURY

KONTEXTE DER MEDIZIN IM 17. UND 18. JAHRHUNDERT

In her concluding remarks, Mary Lindemann reflects on some of the issues involved in the "doing" of medical history. Choosing her topics from the issues raised in this volume, she first considers several reasons for the popularity of medical history and its ability to attract wide scholarly interest beyond medical history as customarily defined. Turning to an evaluation of the contexts in which researchers place that history, she explores issues of practice, personalities, and geographical scope suggested by the papers in this volume. A major question is the degree to which both established and less explored contexts tell us about seventeenth- and eighteenth-century medical theory and practice. The investigation of case studies or the examination of the impact of religion on medical theory and practice have long and venerable pedigrees, well-developed methodologies, and equally well-developed historiographical frameworks. While the comparative or Atlantic framework remains a brave new world, relatively uncrowded and thus exciting and promising, it is still uncertain and unproven in terms of its fit into more established historical approaches. Her conclusion is that each particular disciplinary or subdisciplinary approach can cross-fertilize and enrich this history by forcing the community of scholars to ask new questions, work comparatively, and try out new methods.

In ihren abschließenden Bemerkungen geht Mary Lindemann auf einige wichtige Aspekte moderner Medizingeschichtsschreibung ein. Medizinhistorische Themen üben auch auf Wissenschaftler außerhalb der eigentlichen Medizingeschichte eine erhebliche Anziehungskraft aus. Wie Lindemann anhand von Beiträgen des vorliegenden Bandes aufzeigt, betreffen die von Medizinhistorikern erforschten Zusammenhänge in aller Regel spezifische Praktiken, bestimmte Persönlichkeiten oder auch geographische Aspekte. In welchem Ausmaß kann die Untersuchung solcher mehr oder weniger erforschter Kontexte zu unserem Wissen über die medizinische Theorie und Praxis im 17. und 18. Jahrhundert beitragen? Arbeiten über Fallstudien oder zum Einfluss von Religion auf medizinisches Denken und Handeln können auf zahlreiche Vorläufer, auf eine etablierte Methodologie und einen ebenso etablierten historiographischen Rahmen zurückgreifen. Demgegenüber stellt die bislang nur in geringem Umfang erfolgte Erforschung des transatlantischen Kontextes der Medizin des 18. Jahrhunderts eine Perspektive dar, die zwar viel versprechend ist, bei der aber noch nicht mit Sicherheit gesagt werden kann, wie sie sich in die etablierten historiographischen Ansätze einfügen lässt. Lindemann folgert aus ihren Überlegungen, dass sich die jeweils spezifischen Zugänge gegenseitig befruchten und unser Wissen bereichern können, wenn die Medizingeschichte bereit ist, neue Fragen zu stellen, nach gemeinsamen Antworten zu suchen und dabei neue Methoden zu entwickeln.

LIST OF AUTHORS

John K. Crellin, MD, PhD, formerly John Clinch Professor of Medical History at Memorial University of Newfoundland, Canada, holds British qualifications in medicine, in pharmacy, and in the history of science. He now teaches complementary and alternative medicine with a sustained interest in the history of therapy.

Jürgen Helm, MD, teaches history and ethics of medicine and is managing director of the Ethics Committee (Institutional Review Board) at the Martin Luther University Halle-Wittenberg. Major publications include sixteenth century anatomy and Pietism and medicine in the eighteenth century.

Robert Jütte, PhD, is a historian of early modern public health and the social history of medicine. He is professor and head of the Institute for the History of Medicine of the Robert Bosch Foundation. He teaches general history at the University of Stuttgart.

Fritz Krafft, PhD, is Professor Emeritus of the History of Pharmacy and Science and a former director of the Institute for History of Pharmacy at the Philipps University of Marburg. He is a specialist in the history of physicotheology.

Almut Lanz, ScD, is a retired pharmacist and historian of pharmacy at the Technical University of Braunschweig. Her major publications deal with early modern pharmaceutical theory and practice.

Mary Lindemann, PhD, Professor of History at the University of Miami, Florida. She has published extensively on early modern European and German history and is known for her studies on eighteenth-century German and European medicine.

Andreas-Holger Maehle, MD, PhD, is Professor of the History of Medicine and Medical Ethics at Durham University. He has published widely on the history of animal experimentation, medical ethics, and pharmacology.

Elisabeth Quast, MA, is a social scientist. Her main fields of research are German social policy and social history in the eighteenth century. She is currently preparing an annotated edition of the correspondence between the brothers Richter, physicians in Halle, and the Baron Canstein in Berlin.

Marion Maria Ruisinger, MD, teaches at the Institute for History and Ethics of Medicine at the Friedrich Alexander University Erlangen-Nürnberg. She has published extensively on the history of surgery and of patient-physician-relationships.

Jole Shackelford, PhD, teaches history of medicine at the University of Minnesota. His publications include theoretical and practical aspects of Paracelsian medicine and medicine at the early modern Danish court, and a study of the Danish physician Ole Worm and the German physician Ambrosius Rhodius.

Michael Stolberg, MD, PhD, is Professor and Director of the Institute for the History of Medicine at the University of Würzburg. He has published extensively on the social and cultural history of early modern medicine, patient history, and the history of the body.

Karin Stukenbrock, PhD, teaches history and ethics of medicine at the Otto von Guericke University Magdeburg. She has published on the social history of medicine, on early modern anatomy, and on blood related diseases in the twentieth century.

L. Allen Viehmeyer, PhD, is Professor Emeritus of Foreign Languages (German) at Youngstown State University, Youngstown, Ohio, specializing in colonial German-American culture. Currently he is Associate Director of Research at the Schwenkfelder Library & Heritage Center, Pennsburg, Pennsylvania.

Renate Wilson, PhD, is Adjunct Professor in Health Policy and Management at the Bloomberg School of Public Health and the Institute for the History of Science, Medicine and Technology, Johns Hopkins University. She has published extensively on the transatlantic networks of the Francke Foundations. Her current research centers on the eighteenth century global trade in drugs.

Index